Avoiding and Treating Dental Complications

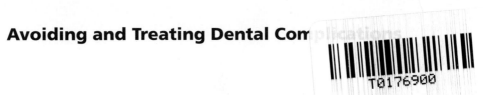

Avoiding and Treating Dental Complications

Best Practices in Dentistry

EDITED BY

Deborah A. Termeie D.D.S.

Clinical Lecturer
Department of Periodontics, School of Dentistry
University of California, Los Angeles
Los Angeles, California

WILEY Blackwell

Library of Congress Cataloging-in-Publication Data

Names: Termeie, Deborah, editor.
Title: Avoiding and treating dental complications: best practices in dentistry edited by Deborah A. Termeie.
Description: Ames, Iowa : John Wiley & Sons Inc., 2016. | Includes bibliographical references and index.
Identifiers: LCCN 2016002818 | ISBN 9781118988022 (pbk.) | ISBN 9781118988039 (Adobe PDF) |
    ISBN 9781118988046 (ePub)
Subjects: | MESH: Tooth Diseases–surgery | Intraoperative Complications–prevention & control |
    Dentistry–methods | Practice Guideline
Classification: LCC RK521 | NLM WU 166 | DDC 617.6/43–dc23
LC record available at http://lccn.loc.gov/2016002818

Set in 8.5/12pt Meridien by SPi Global, Pondicherry, India
Printed and bound in Singapore by Markono Print Media Pte Ltd

1   2016

Contents

List of contributors

Shahrokh C. Bagheri, D.M.D., M.D., F.A.C.S., F.I.C.D.
Chief, Department of Surgery, Division of Oral and
Maxillofacial Surgery, Northside Hospital, Atlanta, GA, USA
Private Practice, Georgia Oral and Facial Reconstructive
Surgery, Atlanta, GA, USA
Adjunct Assistant Professor of Oral and Maxillofacial
Surgery, School of Medicine, University of Miami, Miami,
FL, USA
Adjunct Assistant Professor of Oral and Maxillofacial Surgery,
Department of Surgery, School of Medicine, Emory University,
Atlanta, GA, USA
Adjunct Associate Professor of Oral and Maxillofacial Surgery,
Augusta University, Augusta, GA, USA
and
Diplomate, American Board of Oral and Maxillofacial Surgery,
Chicago, IL, USA

Daniel J. Boehne, D.D.S.
Lecturer
Section of Endodontics, Clinical Dental Sciences
UCLA School of Dentistry
Los Angeles, CA, USA

Behnam Bohluli, D.M.D.
Associate Professor
Oral and Maxillofacial Surgery
Azad University of Medical Sciences
Tehran, Iran

Paulo M. Camargo, D.D.S., M.S., M.B.A., F.A.C.D.
Professor
Tarrson Family Endowed Chair in Periodontics
Associate Dean of Clinical Dental Sciences
Section of Periodontics, Clinical Dental Sciences
UCLA School of Dentistry
Los Angeles, CA, USA

Thomas S. Giugliano, D.D.S., F.I.C.O.I.
Assistant Clinical Professor
Department of Prosthodontics
New York University College of Dentistry
New York, USA

Philip R. Melnick, D.M.D., F.A.C.D.
Lecturer, Section of Periodontics, Clinical Dental Sciences
UCLA School of Dentistry
Los Angeles, CA, USA

Roger A. Meyer, D.D.S., M.S., M.D., F.A.C.S., F.A.C.D.
Chief, Department of Surgery, Division of Oral and
Maxillofacial Surgery, Northside Hospital, Atlanta, GA, USA
Adjunct Assistant Professor, Oral and Maxillofacial Surgery,
Medical College of Georgia, Georgia Regents University,
Augusta, GA, USA
Diplomate, American Board of Oral and Maxillofacial Surgery,
Chicago, IL, USA
Director, Maxillofacial Consultations Ltd, Greensboro, GA, USA
Private Practice, Georgia Oral and Facial Reconstructive
Surgery, Marietta, GA, USA

Daniel W. Nelson, D.D.S.
Assistant Clinical Professor
UCSF School of Dentistry, Division of Periodontology
San Francisco, CA, USA

Elizabeth A. Palmer, M.S., D.M.D.
Clinical Assistant Professor
Department of Pediatric Dentistry, University of Washington
School of Dentistry
Seattle, WA, USA

Rebecca L. Slayton, D.D.S., Ph.D.
Law/Lewis Professor and Chair
Department of Pediatric Dentistry, University of Washington
School of Dentistry
Seattle, WA, USA

Richard G. Stevenson III, D.D.S., F.A.G.D., F.A.C.D., A.B.O.D.
Professor of Clinical Dentistry
Chair, Section of Restorative Dentistry
UCLA School of Dentistry
Los Angeles, CA, USA

Deborah A. Termeie, D.D.S.
Lecturer
Section of Periodontics, Clinical Dental Sciences
UCLA School of Dentistry, Los Angeles, CA, USA

James W. Tom, D.D.S., M.S.
Associate Clinical Professor, Dentist Anesthesiologist
Division of Endodontics, General Practice Dentistry
Herman Ostrow School of Dentistry of USC
and
Division of Public Health and Pediatric Dentistry
Herman Ostrow School of Dentistry of USC
Los Angeles, CA, USA

Hung V. Vu, M.S., Ph.D., D.D.S.
Lecturer, Section of Orthodontics,
UCLA School of Dentistry
Los Angeles, CA, USA
Orthodontist
US Department of Veterans Affairs Greater Los Angeles
Healthcare System
Los Angeles, CA, USA
Private Practice, Vu Orthodontics
Fountain Valley, CA, USA

and
Professor Emeritus
Department of Mechanical & Aerospace Engineering
California State University Long Beach
Long Beach, CA, USA

Shane N. White, B.Dent.Sc., M.S., M.A., Ph.D.
Professor
Section of Endodontics, Clinical Dental Sciences
UCLA School of Dentistry
Los Angeles, CA, USA

Acknowledgments

I would like to acknowledge my mentor, Philip R. Melnick, D.D.S., for his guidance and advice and thank the following reviewers: Dr. Thomas Hilton, Dr. Richard Trushkowsky, Dr. Jack Caton, Dr. Dennis Tarnow, Dr. Fredrick Barnett, Dr. Lenny Naftalin, Dr. Christine Quinn, Dr. Natalie Tung, Dr. Everlyn Chung, Dr. Christopher Marchack, Dr. Kumar Shah, Dr. Richard Kao, Dr. Gary Armitage, Dr. Patrice Wunsch, Dr. Kevin Donly, Dr. Man Wai Ng, Dr. Nicole Cheng, Dr. Anurag Bhargava, Dr. Anirudha Agnihotry and Dr. Patrick Turley. Lastly, I would like to also thank my loving husband, David, and my children, Gabriella and Elliot. Without their love and support, this book would not have been possible.

My appreciation is given to Wiley and the editorial staff whose knowledge and dedicated care to every word and idea made this book possible.

CHAPTER 1

Best practices: Restorative complications

Richard G. Stevenson III

Section of Restorative Dentistry, UCLA School of Dentistry, Los Angeles, CA, USA

Rubber dam challenges

Metal clamps damage tooth structure or porcelain surfaces of crowns
Prevention and management

The use of light cured provisional material can reduce the potential of metal rubber dam clamps to cause iatrogenic damage (Liebenberg, 1995). Prior to clamp placement, a small amount of composite based material may be added to the metal prongs of the clamp. Alternatively instead of metal clamps, the use of plastic rubber dam clamps is less likely to damage tooth structure or existing restorations (Madison, Jordan, and Krell, 1986).

Placing a matrix band on the same tooth as a rubber dam clamp
Prevention and management

One of the methods to solve this complication is to open the clamp with rubber dam forceps and then place the matrix under the prongs and then release the clamp on the band, securing it during the procedure. Another method is to use a sectional matrix secured with a wedge and compound, thus avoiding the clamp entirely.

Poor adaption of rubber dam to partially erupted teeth or a short clinical crown lacking a supragingival undercut is a common challenge leading to clamp instability
Prevention and management

Ford, Ford, and Rhodes (2004) advocate the use of the split dam technique along with a caulking agent to achieve an adequate seal. Morgan and Marshall (1990) recommend that a glass ionomer cement, like Fuji Plus, may be mixed according to the manufacturer's directions and loaded into a composite syringe. The material is syringed along the gingival margins of the tooth to be prepared to approximate normal tooth contours. A plastic instrument may be used to shape the material to create adequate facial and lingual undercuts. The material provides a circumferential surface against which the rubber dam may seal. After the procedure is completed, the glass ionomer/composite material may be removed with a large spoon excavator or curette.

Wakabayashi *et al.* (1986) recommend that a small amount of self-curing resin mixture be placed at the gingival margin on the reciprocal surfaces of the tooth and cured well, after which a standard clamp is set apical to the resin spots, as this will facilitate supragingival retention of a rubber dam clamp.

Class V cavity preparation and restoration complications

Lacerating gingival tissue and compromising periodontium due to poor gingival tissue management and isolation
Prevention and management

Isolation of class V cervical lesions for soft tissue displacement, moisture containment, and infection control can utilize several methods, including rubber dam isolation, placing retraction cord in the sulcus, minor gingival surgery using a radio-surgical laser, scalpel gingivectomy prior to rubber dam retainer placement, cotton roll/saliva ejector isolation, and the use of clear matrix systems for anatomical contour.

Rubber dams help prevent operative-site exposure to blood and crevicular and intraoral fluids. In order to isolate a class V lesion, the hole in the rubber dam for the tooth to be restored is positioned approximately 3 mm facial to the normal hole position, slightly larger in size, and with slightly more distance between the adjacent holes. After the dam is placed, a 212-type clamp is engaged on the lingual side of the tooth and rotated into position in the facial, while stretching the dam apically to reveal the lesion. The beak of the 212-type clamp should be positioned at approximately 1 mm apical to the anticipated preparation gingival margin of the cavity preparation. This usually requires stabilization of the retainer with thermoplastic impression compound. In apically extensive lesions, the beaks of the 212-type clamp may be modified by bending the lingal beak coronally (not apically) and rotating the 212-type clamp facially during placement, securing with one hand while the compound is added to the bow of one side until it is hard. The decision to bend the facial beak apically will lead to a more restricted access to the lesion and thus should be avoided. The teeth must be dry for the heated compound to be secure. After one side is placed, the compound is placed on the other side of the bow. A safe alternative way to use heated compound is to take the Monoject syringe and trim back the tip so you have a wider lumen. Then take green stick compound, break it up into smaller pieces, and place it into the Monoject syringe. Immerse the syringe in hot water. The compound melts and you can then inject the compound into the desired area. It is much easier and safer than messing with a flame chairside and is much easier to direct into the desired location, especially if you are using one hand, which you often are in this situation since you are using the other hand to maintain the position of the 212-type clamp. When the restoration had been completed, rubber dam forceps easily break the compound loose upon retainer removal.

A recent technique to isolate the gingival margin of class V lesions employs a paste (Expasyl, *Kerr*, or Traxodent, *Premier*) that provides reasonable gingival retraction and hemostasis. These pastes consist of an organic, clay material (kaolin), mixed with aluminum chloride as a hemostatic agent. It is thick and firm yet viscous enough to be placed into the gingival sulcus. The paste is injected directly into the sulcus from a preloaded syringe at a recommended rate of 2 mm/s, using even pressure. If necessary, this can be followed by gently tamping on the paste with a plastic instrument or cotton pellet to ensure the paste is fully established or secured into the sulcus. Once the material has been applied and absorbs moisture and hemostasis is achieved, the material should be isolated from additional moisture and saliva. The paste is left in the sulcus for 1–2 min if the tissue is thin or 3–4 min if the soft tissue is thicker. The paste should then be removed by gently rinsing, followed with drying the site, prior to restoration placement. If necessary, the process can be repeated without traumatizing the tissue. Gingival retraction will last for 4 min after the paste has been rinsed and removed from the site.

Contouring class V restorations in the gingival area

When the lesion extends subgingivally, care must be taken not to damage the cementum with rotary instruments. If the restoration is not appropriately contoured and polished, it may lead to gingival inflammation due to food/plaque traps, secondary decay, and early failure of the restoration.

Prevention and management

A technique for better contouring and polishing uses a standard mylar matrix, which has been previously cut to fit the tooth to facilitate the insertion of composite resin into the cavity. Cutting the matrix is not always required. The matrix is inserted into one side of the cavity and fixed in place with a wooden wedge. It is then carefully inserted into the gingival sulcus, involving the entire cervical wall of the cavity (Figure 1.1).

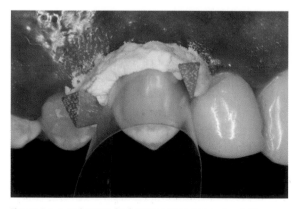

Figure 1.1 A technique for better contouring and polishing uses a standard mylar matrix.

The unattached side of the matrix is positioned by inserting another wedge into the opposite side of the cavity. A photocured gingival barrier (OpalDam, OpalDam Green, Top Dam/FGM, Joinville, Santa Catarina, Brazil) is injected around the mylar matrix to stabilize it. This procedure is not difficult to perform but has to be done with precision in order to form a large enough occlusal/incisal opening between the matrix and the tooth to allow the insertion of restorative material. This procedure also allows the necessary volume of restorative material to be inserted without any excess and adequate separation between the gingiva and tooth, forming an angle that provides an aperture, wide enough for the composite resin syringe tip insertion. Some authors recommend contouring of the gingival aspect of the matrix by stretching the middle gingival portion over the handle of an explorer to gain a shape consistent with the emergence angle on the cementoenamel junction of the tooth prior to securing the matrix against the tooth. Another option is the use of a metal matrix; however, due to the light barrier created by the metal, light curing must be completed in two or more steps, first curing the accessible portion, then removing the metal, and curing the deeper portion with the light applied directly to the exposed restorative material. Some authors think that it works better than the mylar matrix in terms of maintaining shape and stability. This option can be especially useful in situations with intrinsic anatomical difficulties, as in molar furcations. The plastic mylar matrix has a lower risk of damage to soft tissue during insertion into the gingival sulcus and better light transmission for curing and visualization of the preparation cavity (Perez, 2010).

Complications involving liners and bases

Inappropriate use and selection of liners and bases in different clinical situations
Prevention and management
The following recommendations will be based on three different cavity depths and three different restorative materials/techniques (amalgam, composite and indirect restorations) in terms of pulpal proximity:

1 Shallow preparations when the remaining dentin thickness (RDT) is greater than 2 mm
2 Moderately deep preparations when the RDT is 0.5–2 mm
3 Deep preparations when the RDT is less than or equal to 0.5 mm (Table 1.1)

Amalgam
For shallow amalgam tooth preparations (RDT > 2 mm), the use of a dentin-bonding agent may be applied as a sealing agent to the internal walls of preparation, avoiding the cavosurface margin before insertion of the restoration. The use of a self-etching adhesive system will not require a separate etching step.

For moderately deep preparations (RDT = 0.5–2 mm), a liner of glass ionomer may be placed for pulpal protection, followed by the sealing step described earlier. It is well understood that amalgam restorations are great thermal conductors, and placing a thick base has shown to predictably reduce the temperature changes at the base of the cavity (Harper *et al.*, 1980).

For deep preparations (RDT < 0.5 mm), a subbase may be placed on the deepest region in which infected dentin was excavated with a calcium hydroxide material (Dycal, LD Caulk) followed by a liner of glass ionomer on the deepest region in which infected dentin was excavated with a calcium hydroxide material (i.e., it is well understood that removal near the pulpal aspects of the preparation is not necessary to preserve pulpal health, as long as the tooth is asymptomatic or only mildly (reversibly) symptomatic, and a well-sealed restoration is placed (Maltz *et al.*, 2012b).

Glass ionomer restoratives
Since glass ionomer cements are poor conductors of temperature, no material is required to be placed except for deep preparations (RDT < 0.5 mm), in which case, a liner as described earlier should be placed (Roberson *et al.*, 2006).

Composite resin
- For shallow preparations (RDT > 2 mm), dentin-bonding agents are the only necessary material to be placed.
- For deep preparations (RDT < 0.5 mm), a liner should be placed as with amalgam and glass ionomer restorations.
- For moderately deep preparations (RDT > 0.5–2.0 mm), since glass ionomer liners have shown to improve the performance of composite resins (Arora *et al.*, 2012), a thin liner of resin-modified glass ionomer (RMGI) may be used on the deeper dentin surfaces.

> CAUTION: Do not use zinc oxide eugenol as a liner underneath dental composites as it interferes with dental composite polymerization (Roberson *et al.*, 2006).

Table 1.1 Recommended and selection of liners and bases in different clinical situations.

Restorative material	Amalgam	Composite resin	Indirect restorations
0.5–1 mm	 DBA Amalgam GIC liner MTA/Ca(OH)$_2$ Pulpal protection: MTA/Ca(OH)$_2$ (deepest portion) Liner: GIC DBA as a sealer	 DBA Composite GIC liner Pulpal protection: MTA/Ca(OH)$_2$ (deepest portion) Liner: GIC DBA as adhesive	 Indirect restoration GIC liner MTA/Ca(OH)$_2$ Pulpal protection: MTA/Ca(OH)$_2$ (deepest portion) Liner: GIC
1–2 mm	 DBA Amalgam GIC liner Pulpal protection: optional Liner: GIC DBA as a sealer *Optional base layer	 DBA Composite GIC liner Pulpal protection: optional Liner: GIC DBA as adhesive	 Indirect restoration GIC liner Pulpal protection: optional Liner: GIC
2 mm— more	 Amalgam DBA (as sealer) DBA as a sealer *Optional base layer	 Composite DBA (as adhesive) DBA as adhesive	 Indirect restoration Nothing; consider blockout for undercuts

Distance from pulp (RDT)

Ceramic and cast gold restorations

- For moderately deep preparations (RDT = 0.5–2 mm), a base is recommended under the restoration in order to create flat walls and uniform restorative material thickness. Wax patterns are more accurately fabricated if they are smooth and uniform.
- For deep preparations (RDT < 0.5 mm), to protect the pulp, a liner is placed and then a base is applied (Roberson *et al.*, 2006). Placing bases under ceramic and cast gold restorations also will aid in preserving tooth structure by blocking out undercuts in dentin, which would otherwise require overlying tooth structure removal.

Managing the integrity of calcium hydroxide liners
Prevention and management

Since calcium hydroxide liners are highly soluble, they are lost during acid etching and are subject to dissolution over time. The best way to seal calcium hydroxide liners is with the use of RMGI. The RMGIs should line the cavity preparation, covering the calcium hydroxide material, thereby securing it to improve pulpal protection and minimize bacterial microleakage (Rada, 2013).

Bacterial contamination
Prevention and management

Apart from selecting the right material for the procedure, performing it in a clean environment with the use of a rubber dam is one of the most important factors for success (Maltz *et al.*, 2012b).

Techniques to improve marginal quality include:

1 Utilizing resin-modified glass ionomer cements in a sandwich technique (Dietrich *et al.*, 1999).
2 Beveling of enamel margins prior to etching to improve adhesion by exposing the ends rather than the sides of the enamel rods to improve adhesion and reduce leakage.
3 Incremental filling with composite resin to reduce polymerization stresses.
4 The use of water-cooled tungsten carbide finishing burs as dry polishing disk techniques increases leakage (Taylor and Lynch, 1993).
5 In a study by Schwartz, there was significantly less leakage detected in glass ionomer/composite sandwich restorations (Schwartz, Anderson, and Pelleu, 1990).

In all cases, a sterile procedure is the most ideal environment to work in, and it also positively affects the outcome of most procedures (Stockton, 1999). Therefore, clinicians should practice rubber dam isolation whenever possible.

Deep caries

Comparison of the three major caries removal modalities:

1 Direct complete excavation
2 Stepwise excavation
3 Partial caries removal

Prevention and management

Performing stepwise excavation for extremely deep caries lesions is associated with fewer exposed pulps, sustained vitality, and a lack of apical radiolucency compared with performing direct complete excavation. Stepwise excavation may be a preferable management technique for these deep caries lesions (Bjørndal *et al.*, 2010).

However, it is not necessary to remove all carious dentin before the restoration is placed, because over time, sealing of carious dentin results in lower levels of infection than traditional dentin caries removal. Also, the stepwise technique incurs a second intervention, with resultant trauma to the pulp and increased time and expense for the patient (Maltz *et al.*, 2012b). The retention of carious dentin does not interfere with pulp vitality (Maltz and Alves, 2013). In another study conducted by Maltz *et al.*, partial carious dentin removal showed a statistically significant improvement with regard to the maintenance of pulp vitality as compared with stepwise excavation after a 3-year follow-up period (Maltz *et al.*, 2012a).

Sealing of carious dentin arrests the lesion progression irrespective of the dentin protection used (Corralo and Maltz, 2013). It is important to note that all of these techniques require that the DEJ and the first 2 mm from the external cavosurface margin in a pulpal direction be caries-free. Ideal caries removal end points generate a peripheral seal zone that can support long-term biomimetic restorations (Alleman and Mange, 2012). In all cases, it is critical to obtain a completely caries-free zone at dentino-enamel junction and 0.5–1.0 of remaining dentin thickness.

Pulp exposure
Prevention and management

The size of the exposure, the quality of the isolation, the age of the patient, and the presence of caries at the periphery of the preparation have a significant influence on the success of direct pulp caps. Pulp exposures, which elicit hemorrhage, must be controlled prior to attempting a direct pulp-capping procedure.

The degree of bleeding on pulpal exposure is related to the success rate of direct pulp-capping procedures (Matsuo et al., 1996). Numerous agents are used for hemostasis with pulp exposures: a 0.9% saline solution, ferric sulfate, 2.5% NaOCl, $Ca(OH)_2$ solution, and 2% chlorhexidine digluconate (Silva et al., 2006a). An alternative to 2.5% NaOCl is 5.25% NaOCl (Silva et al., 2006a). Usually bleeding is controlled within 10 min of application; however, when it cannot be stopped, within this time frame, endodontics is likely.

The two most widely used materials for pulp capping are mineral trioxide aggregate (MTA) and calcium hydroxide. Calcium hydroxide is widely used and has been found to perform better than single-bottle adhesive system (Silva et al., 2006b) and self-etch (SE) adhesives (Accorinte et al., 2007). MTA has been found to be better than a single-bottle adhesive system calcium hydroxide in the following ways:

- Pulp healing with MTA is faster than that of calcium hydroxide (Accorinte et al., 2008; Chacko and Kurikose, 2006).
- Dentin bridge formation with MTA is more homogenous and continuous with the original dentin when compared to the pulps capped with calcium hydroxide (Chacko and Kurikose, 2006).
- Calcium hydroxide shows tunnel defects and irregularity in the calcified bridge formed beneath it when used as a capping material (Parirokh et al., 2011).
- A large randomized clinical trial (Hilton et al., 2013) provided confirmatory evidence for superior performance with MTA as a direct pulp-capping agent as compared with calcium hydroxide when evaluated in a practice-based research network for up to 2 years. The probability of failure at 24 months in this trial was 31.5% for calcium hydroxide vs. 19.7% for MTA.
- Resin-modified calcium silicate-filled liner (TheraCal, Bisco), a recently introduced material, displays higher calcium-releasing ability and lower solubility than either ProRoot MTA or Dycal. TheraCal had a cure depth of 1.7 mm. The solubility of TheraCal ($\Delta - 1.58\%$) was low and significantly less than that of Dycal ($\Delta - 4.58\%$) and of ProRoot MTA ($\Delta - 18.34\%$). The amount of water absorbed by TheraCal ($\Delta + 10.42\%$) was significantly higher than Dycal ($\Delta + 4.87\%$) and significantly lower than ProRoot MTA ($\Delta + 13.96\%$) (Gandolfi, Siboni, and Prati, 2012).
- Resin composite and resin-modified glass ionomer materials can optimize healing following pulp capping, because they appear to reduce the number of defects in comparison with $Ca(OH)_2$ alone (Murray and Garcia-Godoy, 2006). After placement of $Ca(OH)_2$ over the exposed pulp, it is important to secure the material with a liner of RMGI prior to continuing with the direct restoration.

Composite complications

There are two basic techniques for the placement of composite restorations: bulk fill and incremental insertion.

With the bulk-fill technique, the entire amount of composite resin is placed into the preparation at one time and then trans-enamel polymerization is used to cure the composite. The composite material then shrinks toward the light source. This creates internal stresses in the composite material leading to increased polymerization stresses, which may challenge the bond to dentin leading to microleakage. This can also lead to significant temperature and biting sensitivity (Marangos, 2006).

Potential advantages of bulk filling are:

1 Fewer voids may be present in the mass of material, since all of it is placed at one time.
2 The technique is faster and easier than placing numerous increments when curing times are identical.

Potential disadvantages of bulk filling are:

1 Creating adequate proximal contact areas may be challenging unless adequate matrices are used.
2 Effects due to shrinkage stress may be more pronounced when bulk filled than when placed in increments, since the entire mass polymerizes at one time rather than in small increments.
3 Polymerization of resin in deep preparation locations may be inadequate.

Prevention and management

Incremental placement of posterior composites has been advocated for a long time as a means to partially mitigate polymerization contraction. Many methodologies have been suggested, including using no liner, the use of a low modulus flowable composite, or self-curing glass ionomer cement. Since there are many viscosities of composites available with various degrees of polymerization contraction, the adaptive quality of the composite or its flow as well as inherent volumetric properties will affect the final marginal adaptation and leakage patterns with these placement techniques. Currently, incremental placement is the most researched and supported filling and curing method. Current bulk-fill resins show potential improvements in some properties, but the following challenges still exist for most materials:

- Volumetric shrinkage and stress are not less than other conventional restorative resins.
- Light cure may not reach the bottom extensive (over deep 5 mm) restorations.
- Fast curing lights do not deeply cure bulk-fill resins.
- Some flowable resins cannot be used on occlusal surfaces.
- Making tight proximal contacts can be difficult.
- Preventing voids in crucial locations is unpredictable. At this time, bulk filling as a concept may have promising potential and may perform well in certain situations, but material improvements are necessary to overcome the described challenges (Christensen, 2012).

Polymerization shrinkage
Prevention and management

Incorporating commercially available fiber systems within the composite restorations has shown to reduce the polymerization shrinkage. The fiber materials are available as transparent fiber meshes which can be placed into the cavity and composite material is allowed to flow around the mesh. It is shown that marginal microleakage significantly decreases when composites are applied by the incremental technique with the incorporation of fiber meshwork (Ozel and Soyman, 2009).

As described in the previous section, incremental placement of composite resins remains the most predictable method to decrease the effects of polymerization shrinkage stresses on the tooth.

Open contacts
Prevention and management

Tofflemire matrices will not predictably establish anatomically correct physiologic contacts when used with composite resins. Due to low resistance to deformation, these matrices result in a poor contour and point contacts (Strydom, 2006). Some clinicians re-prepare such proximal surfaces, adding more composite, and a plaque and food retentive area may develop.

Light curing complications

Common complications

1 Premature failure of resin restorations is a commonly encountered problem. The median longevity for posterior resin-based restorations placed in dental offices is only about 6 years (Sunnegårdh-Grönberg et al., 2009) with the primary reasons for replacement being secondary caries and bulk fracture of the resin (Heintze and Rousson, 2012; Sunnegårdh-Grönberg et al., 2009).

2 Undercured resins are a significant cause of restoration failure due to fracture, secondary caries, or excessive wear of the restoration (Ferracane, Berge, and Condon, 1998; Hammouda, 2010; Shortall et al., 2013).

3 When composites resins are not optimally cured and thus do not reach a sufficient degree of monomer conversion, they are more likely to leach toxic substances (Chen et al., 2001).

4 Light curing delivers energy that causes a temperature increase in the tooth and surrounding oral tissues (Oberholzer et al., 2012; Shortall et al., 2013). Arbitrarily, increasing exposure times in an effort to prevent undercuring may damage the pulp and surrounding tissues.

Improper positioning of the curing light may contribute to these failures. Appropriate light curing of the entire restoration is a basic requirement when placing composite resins (Price, 2014).

Etiology

Contemporary light cure units (LCUs) deliver a wide range of spectral emissions and irradiance levels (Leprince et al., 2010; Rueggeberg, 2013). These differences are often not detectable by the eye (El-Mowafy et al., 2005), neither accurately by a dental radiometer,

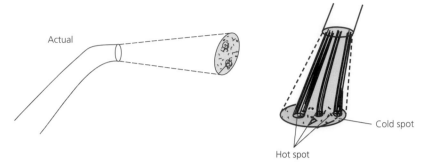

Figure 1.2 Transverse section of a fiber-optic tip of a light curing unit and light passing across it demonstrating hot and cold spot.

but they can affect the polymerization of the composite resins (Figure 1.2).

Nonuniform irradiance

Nonuniform light beam show areas of variation across the tip end of the LCU delivering more irradiance in some areas and delivering less irradiance in others. If the light is held steady, this may result in some of regions of the resin receiving an inadequate amount of energy when light curing.

Preventive measure

1 Light exposure time will have to be increased at the risk of overexposing some of the oral tissues, unless carefully managed (Rueggeberg, 2013).
2 The spectral emission from the LCU and the spectral requirements of the composite resin should be matched both to ensure optimal polymerization (Jandt and Mills, 2013; Price, Fahey, and Felix, 2010) and to minimize intrapulpal temperature increases (Leprince *et al.*, 2010).
3 Polywave light-emitting diode units (with two or more spectral peaks) have been introduced that use two or more different colors of LED, meaning that their spectral output ranges from blue (460 nm) to violet (410 nm) wavelengths of light. These lights can polymerize composite resin containing both conventional and alternative photoinitiators.

Management

The light tip should be moved around by a few millimeters when light curing (Rueggeberg, 2013). This movement should compensate for the nonuniform irradiance and spectral distributions from the LCU.

Differing irradiance

With some LCUs, the irradiance may be high close to the tip but declines rapidly as the distance from the tip end increases (Price and Ferracane, 2012). Most class II resin restorations fail at the gingival portion of the proximal box (Mjör, 2005). This is the region that is the most difficult to reach with the LCU and is furthest away from the light source (Price and Ferracane, 2012). Consequently, the resin here will receive the least amount of light and will be undercured (Shortall *et al.*, 2013). Increasing the distance decreases the dentin shear bond strength (Xu, Sandras, and Burgess, 2006) (Figure 1.3).

Prevention and management

Increasing curing time will compensate for the decreased dentin shear bond strength. It is important to learn how to use the LCU to maximize the energy delivered to the composite. Place the central axis of the tip of the light directly over the restoration surface; the emitting end should be parallel to the surface being exposed.

When using an LCU with an inhomogeneous light output, move the light tip around and increase the exposure time. This should also be done where undercuts are present that prevent straight-line access to the composite. Additionally, in this situation, use supplementary buccolingual curing (but beware of overheating). Another consideration is the distance from light tip to composite increment. If more than 2–3 mm away, then use thinner increments of composite, for example, 1 mm to insure a complete cure.

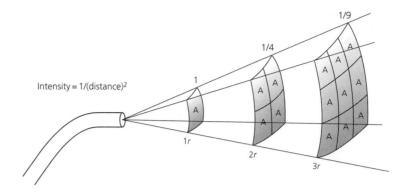

Intensity = 1/(distance)^2

Figure 1.3 The relation between the intensity and distance of the curing light.

Post complications

Maximizing post and buildup retention without compromising tooth resistance form
Prevention and management
Post length
Length is an important factor that affects the retention of the posts in the root.

The determination of the appropriate post length and the remaining root canal filling after preparation has been studied extensively. Some studies recommended that the post should be longer than the crown length, halfway between the root apex and the crest of the alveolar bone. Other studies suggest that posts with three quarters the length of the root are less likely to debond (Leary, Aquilino, and Svare, 1987). Kessler and Peters' findings showed no perforations with a size 2 or 3 Gates Glidden bur in mandibular molars and that the danger of creating thin or perforated walls was much greater toward the bifurcation.

Increasing the post length is associated with a significant enhancement in post retention (Macedo, Faria e Silva, and Marcondes Martins, 2010) while keeping in mind maintaining of 4–5 mm of the gutta-percha seal. However, in cases of curved root canals where the desired length may not be achievable, greater length into the root canals is not necessary to enhance the retention of bonded fiber posts (Braga *et al.*, 2006).

A safe and well-recognized rule to follow is to make the post at least equal to crown length however, never removing the remaining 5 mm of endodontic filling material (Figure 1.4).

Post diameter is too large
Maintaining the remaining tooth structure is an important objective while restoring endodontically treated teeth. However, an increase in post diameter may result in more reduction of root dentin. At the same time, some studies did not find any significant increase in the post retention by using a large post diameter (Hunter, Feiglin, and Williams, 1989).

Prevention and management
Studies have shown that post diameter should not be more than one third of the root diameter at any locations and at the post tip the diameter of post should be 1 mm or less (Standlee, Caputo, and Hanson, 1978). Another study suggests that the posts should be surrounded by 1 mm of sound dentin.

Complications related to post design
Post design can be classified according to two categories: shape and surface configuration.
1 According to shape, there are parallel-sided and tapered posts.
2 According to surface configuration, there are threaded, serrated, cross-hatched, and smooth surface posts.

One clinical study found that parallel-sided, serrated posts have more retention than tapered and smooth posts. Standlee and Caputo in their study reported that endodontic posts with transverse serrations or cross-hatching were retained better than posts with longitudinal threads (Standlee and Caputo, 1993). However, another study indicated that threaded posts are the most retentive (Cohen *et al.*, 1999), as threaded posts engage into the root

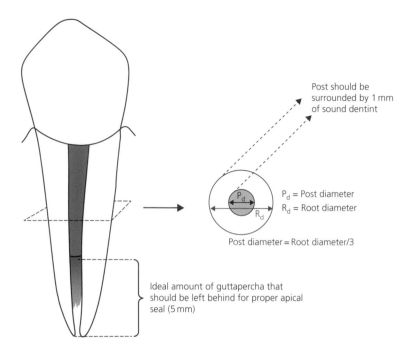

Post should be
surrounded by 1 mm
of sound dentint

P_d = Post diameter
R_d = Root diameter

Post diameter = Root diameter/3

Ideal amount of guttapercha that
should be left behind for proper apical
seal (5 mm)

Figure 1.4 Ideal post length and post
diameter for a post and core restoration.

dentin compared to smooth surface posts that depend mainly on the cement for retention.

Even though tapered posts result in less tooth reduction, they create a wedging effect and stresses on the remaining root structure.

Asmussen, Peutzfeldt, and Sahafi (2005) and Cooney, Caputo, and Trabert (1986) and another study done by Yang *et al.* (2001) reported that parallel-sided dowels distributed stress widely in the dentin leading to more stable restorations in contrast to tapered posts, which showed the greatest stress concentration and displacement under horizontal forces. However, the threads in these actively fitting posts may produce a higher stress during placement resulting in root fracture (Cooney, Caputo, and Trabert, 1986). For these reasons, most studies suggest smooth surface posts and the enhancement of cements to reach the required post retention (Hagge, Wong, and Lindemuth, 2002).

Posts leading to root fracture
Prevention and management
Several points should be evaluated and considered to reduce the possibility of root fracture. A low modulus material (less stiff, more flexible) allows greater bending under load. When strain exceeds the yield point, the material is irreversibly deformed even after the load has

been removed. The placement of endodontic posts creates an unnatural restored structure, because it fills the root canal with a material that has stiffness unlike that of the pulp and it is not possible to recreate the original stress distribution within the tooth (Ona *et al.*, 2013). Nevertheless, it is necessary to have materials whose mechanical properties closely resemble the properties of dentin (E = 18 GPa) (Bateman, Ricketts, and Saunders, 2003). According to Galhano *et al.* (2005a), posts reinforced with fibers have an modulus of elasticity of approximately 20 GPa, while cast metal alloy posts and prefabricated metal posts have an E of about 200 GPa and ceramic posts about 150 GPa (Galhano *et al.*, 2005b). Thus, posts reinforced with fibers have mechanical properties similar to dentin, which show a flexural modulus of about 18 GPa. Posts must also have adequate modulus to avoid distortion under load (Kinney, Marshall, and Marshall, 2003).

Akkayan and Gülmez evaluated the resistance to fracture of endodontically treated teeth restored with different post systems and concluded that teeth restored with posts that have properties closer to those of the dental structure, such as the glass fiber posts, showed favorable fractures; however, those restored with titanium and zirconia posts demonstrated catastrophic fractures (Akkayan and Gülmez, 2002).

Discoloration of the tooth with metal posts
Prevention and management
Discoloration can occur because of the metal post and it can be solved with the use of zirconia dowels (Meyenberg, Lüthy, and Schärer, 1995) and (Hochman and Zalkind, 1999), a tooth-colored ceramic. This avoids the discoloration of tooth structure that can occur with metal dowels, and the zirconia dowels produce optical properties comparable to all-ceramic crowns (Michalakis *et al.*, 2004; Toksavul, Turkun, and Toman, 2004), though retrieval of these posts can be difficult as they possess a hard surface and are very brittle.

Mechanical retention of the post
The zirconia dowel has a smooth surface configuration with no grooves, serrations, or roughness to enhance mechanical retention. As a result, the zirconia dowel does not bond well to composite resins and may not provide the best support for these dowels. They also have poor resin-bonding capabilities to dentin after dynamic loading and cycling due to the rigidity of the dowel (Dietschi, Romelli, and Goretti, 1998). Debonding and loss of retention are the most likely causes of failure associated with using fiber-reinforced posts (Segerström, Astbäck, and Ekstrand, 2006).

The relatively smooth surface of fiber-reinforced posts limits the mechanical bonding of resin cements into the post surfaces. Micro-abrasive surface treatments have been studied thoroughly to assess their effects on the bond strength between fiber posts and resin cements. The effects of these treatments depend on the hardness, size, and shape of the particles (Oshida *et al.*, 1993).

Prevention and management
Aluminum oxide (alumina) has angular surfaces that have the ability to create a rough surface on posts, allowing luting cements to interlock micromechanically with post surfaces. However, the volume lost from the fiber post surface might affect the mechanical properties of these posts (Goracci and Ferrari, 2011). It has been shown that micro-mechanical retention is improved greatly with the use of airborne alumina particles (Prithviraj *et al.*, 2010). Air abrasion should be used but with caution to avoid removing excess material from the post surface.

Pin complications

Dentinal failures and lateral cracks due to pin installation
Prevention and management
Lateral cracks in dentin may be caused if a dull drill is employed during channel preparation. Every time a drill is used, a small notch may be made on the drill shank, indicating the number of times it is used.

Limiting the use of presently available drills to the preparation of five channels will provide substantial assurance against cracking, although the force exerted on the drill may also be a factor (Standlee and Caputo, 1993; Standlee, Caputo, and Hanson, 1978). Using a stepwise approach may offer significant advantages in pin placement. The first step involves locating or creating a flat surface in dentin and then with stepwise approach may offer significant advantages in pin placement. The first step involves locating or creating a flat surface in the buildup or restorative material (0.5 mm minimum) and the pulp chamber. The initial drill should be smaller than the final pin drill. One technique recommended by the author is to use a drill with a 2 mm depth limiting shoulder and a diameter of 0.017 smaller than the final pin drill. A self-shearing pin (Max 021, diameter 0.023.02 Coltene–Whaledent) is then placed with a slow-speed latch-type attachment. This approach creates a straight pin channel and secure pin, and the Max 021 system uses a pin with a depth-limiting shelf to prevent pin overextension and a rounded retentively designed head to prevent untoward stresses in the final restoration or buildup material.

Periodontal problems from pin perforations into periodontal tissues
Prevention and management
Small perforations into the periodontal ligament may be repaired by the removal of the protruding pin portion. This is achieved by creating a gingival flap sufficient to gain access and cutting away the excess pin with a fine diamond bur used in an air turbine handpiece and cooled with water. The tooth surface is then polished with abrasive strips and topical fluoride applied before the gingival flap is sutured back into position (Figure 1.5).

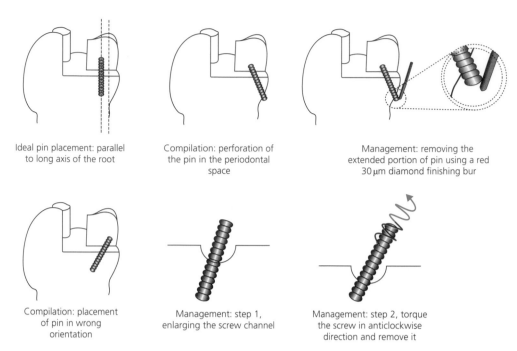

Ideal pin placement: parallel to long axis of the root

Compilation: perforation of the pin in the periodontal space

Management: removing the extended portion of pin using a red 30 μm diamond finishing bur

Compilation: placement of pin in wrong orientation

Management: step 1, enlarging the screw channel

Management: step 2, torque the screw in anticlockwise direction and remove it

Figure 1.5 Approaches in treating pin perforation.

Proximal contact complications

The placement of direct composite restorations that involve posterior proximal surfaces is common in most dental patients. Unlike dental amalgam, which can be a very forgiving material technically and can be condensed against a matrix band to create a proximal contact, proper placement of composite restorative materials presents a unique set of challenges for the restorative dentist.

The adhesion process itself is well understood by most clinicians as far as isolation and execution; however, there are some steps in the placement process that cause difficulty and may ultimately lead to a compromised proximal contact. The following areas of concern will be addressed: management of the soft tissue in the interproximal region, creation of proximal contour and contact, and finishing and polishing of the restoration.

Improper proximal contact and contour

A major challenge for the dentist is to recreate a physiologic proximal contact with the adjacent tooth and, at the same time, restore proper interproximal anatomic form given the limitations of conventional matrix systems. It is widely accepted that proximal contacts are very important features in a properly functioning dentition. A lack of proximal contacts contributes to food impaction, secondary caries, tooth movement, and periodontal complications (Lacy, 1987).

Prevention and management

The thickness of the matrix band and the ability to compress the periodontal ligaments of the tooth being restored and the one adjacent to it can sometimes make the restoration of proximal tooth contact arduous at best. When separation is required for restorative procedures, such as placement of a class II resin composite restoration, special separation rings (G-Ring, Garrison Dental; V-Rings, Triodent; Palodent BiTine rings, Dentsply) are routinely more predictable than wooden wedges (Loomans et al., 2007).

In three-surface class II MOD resin composite restorations, tighter proximal contacts were obtained when separation rings and sectional matrix bands were applied simultaneously for both proximal surfaces (Saber et al., 2011).

The use of a sectional matrix band helps achieve a tight proximal contact, and the centripetal restorative technique can help to obtain contour and anatomy, minimizing the use of rotary instruments during the finishing procedures (Santos, 2015). The centripetal

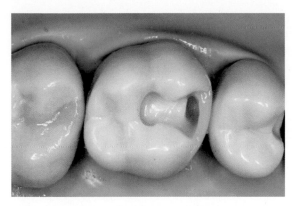

Figure 1.6 Figure showing centripetal (wall) technique.

composite filling technique is a variation of the incremental buildup technique with composite for class II restorations. In the centripetal technique, the first layer of composite is placed at the site of missing proximal wall, against the band, and light cured. The matrix assembly is then removed, affording the operator greater access. Subsequent increments are then placed as if filling an occlusal restoration (Figure 1.6).

Anatomically, the posterior proximal surface is convex occlusally and concave gingivally. The proximal contact is elliptical in the buccolingual direction and located approximately 1 mm apical to the height of the marginal ridge. As the surface of the tooth progresses gingivally from the contact area toward the cementoenamel junction, a concavity exists that houses the interdental papilla. Conventional matrix systems are made of thin, flat metallic strips that are placed circumferentially around the tooth to be restored and affixed with some sort of retaining device. While contact with the adjacent tooth can be made with a circumferential matrix band, it is practically impossible to recreate the natural convex/concave anatomy of the posterior proximal surface because of the inherent limitations of these systems. In addition, they often create contact points rather than contact areas, making the marginal ridges more susceptible to fracture (Loomans *et al.*, 2008). Attempts to "shape" or burnish matrix bands with elliptical instrumentation to create an anatomic contact only "distort" or "indent" the band and do not recreate complete natural interproximal contours.

The best proximal contact areas in class II composite restorations were obtained using a sectional matrix system. The packability of the resin composite did not help to achieve better proximal contacts (Peumans

et al., 2001). Class II posterior composite resin restorations placed with a combination of sectional matrices and separation rings resulted in a stronger proximal contact than when a circumferential matrix system was used, due in part to the occlusal–gingival contour of the band that enhances proximal contact and contour (Loomans *et al.*, 2006, 2009). The use of circumferential bands paired with separating rings becomes more advantageous with larger restorations. A study (Loomans *et al.*, 2006) investigated the tightness of the proximal contact when placing posterior resin composite restorations with circumferential and sectional matrix systems in an in vitro model using a special measuring device (Tooth Pressure Meter). The use of sectional matrices combined with separation rings resulted in tighter proximal contacts compared to when circumferential (Tofflemire) systems were used. This new in vitro model, which uses the Tooth Pressure Meter to simulate clinical conditions when restoring class II resin composite restorations, seems to produce reliable, clinically representative results (Loomans *et al.*, 2008).

Inadequate finishing and polishing of the proximal restoration

After placing a class II composite restoration with an adequate contact, the restoration must be properly finished and polished. The posterior interproximal areas are particularly difficult to access, and special techniques must be employed to accomplish optimal restorations.

Prevention and management

After removal of the sectional matrix and BiTine (also called separating rings, G-Ring, and V-Rings) ring and wedge assembly, a sharp explorer may be used to assess the marginal integrity of the composite in the proximal areas. Dental floss is also very useful to evaluate the presence of overhanging composite material and BiTine (also called separating rings, G-Ring, and V-Rings) ring and wedge assembly, a sharp explorer may be used to assess the marginal integrity of effective in the removal of excess material interproximally. Following the gross removal step, the surface may be planed smooth with sequential (course to fine) composite finishing strips. Care must be exercised to avoid lacerating the gingival tissues and lips during this step. Ultrathin composite finishing disks may also achieve reasonable access to facial and lingual embrasures.

Overhanging margins
Prevention and management
Overhanging margins can be removed with interproximal gold knives or No. 12 scalpels. When overhangs cannot be removed, it is advised to replace the restoration. Finishing strips are usually unable to remove large overhangs.

Bulky indirect restorations with overhangs should be trimmed and polished to be flush with the tooth margins, without any overhangs prior to cementation. If not possible, a new restoration should be fabricated.

Poor registration of contacts on moist articulating paper
Prevention and management
To show occlusal contacts, tooth surfaces must be well isolated and dry (McCullock, 2003). Instructing the patient to bite on dry gauze may also further dry the teeth. Ink transfer to teeth and even highly polished restorations are facilitated with the use of even very thin articulating paper, if the paper is coated with a thin layer of petroleum jelly (Vaseline). The patient must also be positioned in the upright position in order to record more functional contacts typical with mastication.

Complications related to occlusal adjustments

False contacts on teeth caused by thick articulating paper
Prevention and management
When the excessive thickness of articulating paper exceeds the maximum recommended thickness of occlusal recording strips, it can result in false contacts (Sapkota and Gupta, 2014). To record the first point of contact, the author recommends thin strips lightly coated with Vaseline on dry teeth as noted earlier.

Perforation of crowns due to excessive occlusal grinding
Prevention and management
According to Wassell, Barker, and Steele (2002), the use of a Svensen gauge is invaluable for predicting areas vulnerable to perforation during occlusal adjustment of crowns.

A perforated crown must be sent back to the laboratory. Prevention of this complication is the only management. If the crown is perforated, the crown preparation should be reevaluated, and adequate clearance for the crown should be provided with a new crown fabricated and delivered for the best outcome.

Selecting best shaped and grit bur for occlusal adjustments with ceramics
Prevention and management
Wassell, Barker, and Steele (2002) suggest the use of a flame-shaped diamond in a high- or low-speed handpiece for occlusal adjustment. Other shapes may be employed as long as the diamond grit is 30μm (red striped diamonds, Brasseler USA) or less, as more course grits may lead to deep scratches and crack propagation of modern ceramic materials.

Infra-occlusion
If the tooth is out of occlusion (in hypo-occlusion), the opposing tooth will supra-erupt. After supra-eruption, the proximal contacts might be lost in the opposing arch, leading to a mesial drift, which might disturb occlusal stability. If a crown is infra-occluded, a new crown should be delivered with proper occlusal contacts. In the case of direct composite restorations, proper occlusion should be built by adding material on the deficient spots. Amalgam restorations which are in infra-occlusion should be removed and replaced if occlusal stability depends on the amalgam surface.

Difficult to be certain when the mandible is in centric relation
Prevention and management
According to Long (1973) and as cited by Golsen and Shaw (1984), the use of a leaf gauge aids significantly in positioning the mandible in centric relation. The leaf gauge technique involves inserting thin plastic leaves between the anterior teeth, having the patient bite normally, and then asking them to squeeze with a centric relation. The leaf gauge technique involves inserting thin plastic leaves between the anterior teeth till the first point of contact is identified (by the patient), after which a few more leaves are added back to keep the teeth separated. At this point, centric relation may be recorded with a rigid bite registration material or hard wax.

Abfraction lesions may be a result of occlusal discrepancies
Prevention and management

Occlusal splints have been recommended to prevent the initiation and progression of abfraction lesions (Perez *et al.*, 2012); however, it is generally believed that these lesions are most likely multifactorial and may also involve abrasion from tooth brushing with abrasive dentifrices and corrosion from either intrinsic or extrinsic acid sources (Grippo, Simring, and Schreiner, 2004).

Loss of vertical dimension due to injudicious occlusal grinding
Prevention and management

Maxillary lingual cusps and mandibular buccal cusps are essential to maintain vertical dimension. It's a rule that the centric holding cusps are not adjusted unless necessary to allow for maximum intercuspal position (MIP) (Patel and Tripathi 2014). When extensive occlusal discrepancies exist, it is recommended that a centric relation record be taken and the diagnostic casts mounted. The occlusion may then be evaluated and a trial equilibration completed on the casts to use vertical dimension changes.

Inordinate amount of time is often required to adjust the occlusion of a newly fabricated crown
Prevention and management

Management required to adjust the occlusion of a new unit cast restoration may significantly decrease the chance of a lengthy clinical occlusal adjustment (Boyarsky, Loos, and Leknius, 1999). Prior to waxing the crown, for example, the technician or dentist should perform a minor equilibration of the casts to insure accurate MIP.

Complications related to gold/ceramic: Inlay/onlays

The most common technical reason for failure is loss of retention. Other reasons could be:
- Inappropriate seating of cast restorations
- Visible cement margin (Hollenback, 1943)
- Improper function and esthetics after restoring

- Inaccurate seating or fit
- Improper function and esthetics after restoring
- Secondary caries due to poor marginal fit
- Crown failures due to caries and defective margins

Corrosion of gold and amalgam

There could be corrosion of gold and amalgam placed in contact with each other. Contact of a gold surface with freshly placed amalgam will produce a silver-colored stain on the contact area of the gold.

Prevention and management

Cast gold restorations may be placed next to old or freshly placed amalgams without significant permanent corrosion of the restorations.

When these restorations are placed next to each other, it does produce silver staining; this may be polished away with pumice or allowed to wear away over time (Fusayama, Katayori, and Nomoto, 1963).

Fractured ceramic inlays

In many cases, fractures take place during the initial trying-in and cementation stage and are probably caused by the formation of local stress zone in the inlay (Dérand, 1991). Thin inlays are far more sensitive to fracture than thicker ones. Other factors that contribute to inlay fracture are the production of defects such as pores, cracks, and poor fit, as well as an exaggerated fissure system, which constitutes crack initiators and reduces the thickness of inlays.

Prevention and management

The thickness of a ceramic inlay in the direction of a load should be 1.5 mm minimum, and if it is not 1.5 mm, there could be fractures. Certain defects like pores, cracks, and poor fit may affect the strength of inlays. The occurrence of smooth supporting surfaces and softly rounded contours reduces the degree of tensile and bending stress and thereby reduces the risk of local stress concentrations. The avoidance of thin inlay edges and restricting the occlusal dimension of the inlay address these risks. Reduction of weak cusps not only reduces the risk of ceramic fractures (Milleding, Ortengren, and Karlsson, 1995) but also with the intentional extension of an inlay to an onlay will reduce the wedging effect observed with large inlays.

Deep fissures in ceramic inlays

Overly deep fissures may be created in ceramic inlays by technicians, and reduced material thickness increases the risk of the inlay to fracture (Milleding, Ortengren, and Karlsson, 1995).

Polymerization shrinkage of luting agents may lead to stresses, and due to microcracks in the tooth, shooting pain may be elicited (Milleding, Ortengren, and Karlsson, 1995).

Prevention and management

It is important to inform lab technicians to maintain at least 1 mm of inlay thickness at the base of grooves. Obviously, the restorative dentist will need to provide preparations of adequate depth to afford the technician with a bulk of ceramic which is resistant to fracture.

Poorly adapted indirect restorations

Marginal adaptation (fit) is considered to be a primary and significant factor in the prevention of secondary caries and is an important indicator of the overall acceptability of the cast restoration.

Prevention and management

Methods of improving marginal adaptation and seating of restorations (Schwartz, 1986) include:
- Intentional over-waxing the margins of the wax pattern
- Removing wax from the internal surface of the wax pattern prior to fabrication
- Internal relief of the cast restoration by sandblasting
- Adjusting the intaglio with burs after using a disclosing technique (PVS or occlusal indicating sprays)
- Mechanical milling with burs with or without disclosing wax
- Internal relief of the ceramic restoration by acid etching
- Electrochemical milling (stripping, deplating) gold restorations
- Occlusal venting for escape of excess cement of fall gold crowns
- Devices to apply and maintain seating force (bite sticks)
- Vibration during cementation (with ultrasonics or hand malleting)
- Internal relief of wax by application of a die spacer to the die before fabrication of wax pattern

Inadequate retention and resistance form

What is the best method to mitigate inadequate retention and resistance form of the cavity preparation?

Prevention and management

The correction of inadequate retention and resistance form of cemented (not bonded) restorations may usually be addressed by decreasing taper and increasing preparation length. When neither of these modifications are possible, secondary fractures may be employed (Gilboe and Teteruck, 2005).

Secondary auxiliary retention features include proximal boxes, axial grooves, and the use of integral pins (parts of the casting). Adding proximal boxes will give superior results over grooves. Although cast pins are helpful, they require impression and waxing analogues, and these are difficult to locate today. An alternative to a pin is a slot, made into the pulpal or gingival walls with a 169 L bur to a depth of 1.5–2.0 mm. Impressions may be easy to obtain with slots by using a small instrument (or 30 gauge needle to vent out air) to adapt the PVS impression material to the internal retentive features during the impression making (Stevenson and Patrice, 2013) (Table 1.2).

Resistance to fully seating crowns against the prepared margin due to heavy proximal contacts
Prevention and management

Insert a precision single face diamond dental strip (ContacEZ diamond dental strip) into the distal interproximal space with the abrasive side facing the crown. Pass the strip buccolingually a few times to check interproximal pressure against the strip. Repeat this procedure in the mesial interproximal space.

When more pressure is detected in the mesial than the distal interproximal space, pass the strip buccolingually a few more times (5–6 times), through the mesial space until there is light resistance in the interproximal space.

When light resistance in both the mesial and distal interproximal spaces is equal, the ideal proximal contact adjustment of the crown is complete. The proximal surface may then be highly polished with a ceramic polishing wheel.

A finished crown from the dental laboratory may present with a heavy proximal contact. Dentist should test both contacts, with dental floss to determine which contact is heavier. Many times the assumption is wrong, causing an open proximal contact on one side with the heavy proximal contact left intact on the other side. The crown then has to be sent back to the dental laboratory for porcelain addition to the open contact, or sometimes, the restoration must be remade.

Table 1.2 Primary and secondary factors in retention and resistance form.

1. Primary factors:
    a. Parallelism
    b. Length
    c. Surface area
2. Secondary factors:
    a. Groove
    b. Box
    c. Pin hole
    d. Combination of a, b, and c

The application of principles and factors

Problem[a]	Correction	
Inadequate retention and resistance form	Compensatory principle (increase)	Compensatory factor (add)
Parallelism	Length	Groove
		Box
		Pin
Length	Parallelism	Pin
	Surface area	
Surface area	Surface area	Groove
		Box
		Pin

Gilboe and Teteruck (2005).
[a] Inadequate retention and resistance form.

Polishing

Damage to cementum at cervical area of restorations due to polishing
Prevention and management
Avoid rotary instruments over the cementum area as it may remove a layer of cementum at the cervical area (Carranza *et al.*, 2006).

The best method to avoid damage to the cementum is to control the restorative material during placement. If small amounts of composite resin extend on to the root surface, careful removal with a curette or scalpel is preferred to rotary instrumentation. Mopper recommends that finishing and polishing should be achieved with a low-speed, high-torque handpiece, typically anywhere from 7000 to 30000 rpm. A high-speed handpiece may be used to precontour, but using anything over 30000 rpm during finishing and polishing is too high. Low-speed, high-torque is preferable, because it gives the operator complete control and the side of a composite cup style polisher may be used to polish subgingival areas of class V restorations.

Dull finish on microfill composite restorations and nano-filled composite
Prevention and management
Diamond or aluminum oxide disks, rubber cups and points, and an aluminum oxide polishing paste are used to obtain the best polish on a microfill composite (Mopper, 2011; Türkün and Türkün 2004).

Finishing metal margins of porcelain fused to metal crowns
Prevention and management
Metal surfaces can be finished with finishing burs followed by rubber abrasive points (Kenda, Liechtenstein, and Shofu (brownie, greenie, and super greenie)). Abrasive disks (SofLex, 3M) are useful for flat areas such as proximal contact points and can be used on either metal or porcelain. Porcelain can also be finished with composite finishing diamonds (Premier: yellow and white stripe), but a light touch and water spray are needed to avoid stripping off the diamond coating. Further finishing is achieved with rubber abrasive points (Kenda: white) followed by a felt wheel or rubber cup with diamond polishing paste (Wassell, Barker, and Steele, 2002).

Polishing of gold restorations that appear to be dull
Prevention and management

Bruce (2008) advocates the use of a system of disks and powders. The three disks recommended are paper disks of medium garnet, fine sand, and fine cuttle grit on a slow-speed straight mandrel. According to Bruce (2008) "The powders are applied using a soft rubber cup that is ribbed, not webbed, to avoid scratching the gold using a slow-speed latch-type contra-angle. The first powder is a No. 4 flour of pumice used wet; the second a 15-μm alumin." Bruce (2008) states that this can be accomplished in small restorations using brownies, greenies, and super greenies with light pressure with higher speeds and always with an air stream to control heat.

Gingivally extensive composite restorations

Functional and esthetic failure due to inadequate contouring and polishing
Prevention and management

The initial contouring can be performed with a series of finishing burs to replicate the natural form of the tooth. For finishing the facial surface, a long, needle-shaped finishing bur is used to develop the proper anatomical contours of the facial aspect of the anterior tooth. To replicate natural form and texture, 16 and 30 fluted, needle-shaped finishing burs are used. These burs are used dry with light pressure to prevent heat buildup.

This short, tapered, needle-shaped finishing bur is used to develop the proper anatomical contours of the facial aspect of the anterior tooth. To replicate natural form and texture, 16 and 30 fluted, needle-shaped finishing burs are used. These burs are short, tapered, straight-edge finishing burs, which conforms to the straight emergence profile as the tooth emerges from the gingival sulcus. Care should be taken to avoid the cementum.

It is important to use a dry protocol and retract the gingiva with an instrument or placement of a cord, closely observing tooth structure and the gingival margin. It is important not to overheat the resin by using excessive pressure. It is also imperative not to ditch or scar the cementum at the gingival margin.

After the initial finishing procedure, the margins and surface defects are sealed. The restoration and all margins are re-etched for 15 s with a 35% orthophosphoric acid, rinsed for 5 s, and dried. A layer of composite surface sealant may be applied over the margins and the restoration. This will prevent leakage and seal any microfractures or microscopic porosities in the material that may have formed during finishing. The use of surface sealant has been shown to reduce the wear rate of posterior composite resins (Dickinson and Leinfelder, 1993), improve resistance to interfacial staining (Kemp-Scholte and Davidson, 1988), and decrease microleakage around class V composite resins (Estafan *et al.*, 2000). Any excess resin can be removed with a No. 12 scalpel.

Impression problems

Improper capture of margins due to various factors such as saliva, oral fluid, and bleeding
Prevention and management

This can be solved by using gingival displacement paste like Expasyl which has been shown to have a better response in achieving horizontal displacement of the gingival sulcus than gingival retraction cord (Prasanna *et al.*, 2013). Also, in cases of equigingival and subgingival (<2 mm) preparation margins, Magic FoamCord gingival retraction system is a less traumatic alternative method of gingival retraction than packing a retraction cord. However, when there are deep subgingival margins and a beveled preparation, the material is less effective than the single cord retraction technique (Beier, Kranewitter, and Dumfahrt, 2009). A two-cord technique works well in both vertical and horizontal retractions, with the top cord being removed prior to attempting the impression. One of the most important techniques is to dry the marginal area prior to injecting impression material in the sulcus.

There are three techniques for tissue displacement: mechanical, chemico-mechanical, and surgical. Mechanical displacement of the gingiva can be done either by the use of copper bands or with a plain retraction cord. By combining chemical action with packing of a retraction cord, a chemico-mechanical displacement of the tissue can take place. The surgical retraction is possible by laser, electrosurgery, or rotatory curettage (Levartovsky *et al.*, 2012), where excess tissue which impedes access to the finish line may be removed. Sulcular bleeding can be solved by using racemic epinephrine cord or aluminum sulfate cord, which are more effective than non-medicated cord. Hemorrhage control with a cord saturated in Hemodent is more effective than water-saturated or dry cords (Weir and Williams, 1984).

Voids and bubbles in the impression
Prevention and management
Addition of polyvinyl siloxane impression materials can solve this. They exhibit low contact angle values and the least number of voids in the die stone cast when compared with polysulfide impression materials (Reddy et al., 2012). A key principle in reducing voids is to thoroughly dry the teeth and preparations which will be impressed. The technique of impressing the preparation where every area of the surface is completely covered with a low-viscosity syringed material helps to reduce axial wall voids and creases caused from the difference in syringe and tray viscosities.

Gag reflex experienced by the patient during the impression taking
Prevention and management
If the patient has a gag reflex, try to mix thick alginate, so it does not flow in the sensitive area in the back of the throat and posterior aspects of the soft palate and faucial pillars. The patient should be made to sit upright, and legs should be raised. Salt on tongue has proven effective, while some indicate topical analgesia in the sensitive areas for the same (Farrier et al., 2011).

Audiotapes of relaxation procedures that include imagery, progressive muscle relaxation, and self-suggestion components should be given to the patient with instructions that the constant practice of listening to them might reduce his/her arousal level sufficiently to decrease or eliminate the gagging response (Neumann and McCarty, 2001). The use of acupuncture in controlling the gag reflex is an effective method of controlling severe gag reflex as well, during dental treatment including impression taking (Rosted et al., 2006). Also, the fears related to dental procedures should be discussed with the patient, and the patient should be advised to practice relaxation several times a week.

With routine single tooth posterior crowns/inlays/onlays, a double bite tray may often be used to eliminate gagging, versus using a full-arch impression technique.

Bleaching

More than 100 million Americans whiten and/or bleach their teeth and spend an estimated $15 billion (Krupp, 2008). Bleaching/whitening of teeth is a very demanding procedure now, and clinicians should be aware of the complications and challenges that might be attached to it.

Difficulties/challenges before beaching

Special cases
Tetracycline-stained teeth: Tetracycline is an antibiotic, which causes permanent discoloration of teeth which vary from yellow or gray to brown. Tooth staining/discoloration with tetracycline is influenced by the dosage used, length of treatment or exposure, stage of tooth mineralization (or calcification), and degree of activity of the mineralization process. It has been found in a study that "when used daily for 6 months, a 6.5% H_2O_2 bleaching strip can be effective in whitening tetracycline stains. The professional strip was well tolerated throughout the 6-month period" (Kugel et al., 2011).

Fluorosis: Endemic dental fluorosis is usually known as mottled enamel and can be defined as enamel hypoplasia characterized by moderate to severe staining of the tooth surface. Fluorosis becomes clinically significant when the patient has a prolonged history of ingesting water that contains more than 1.0 ppm of fluoride ion. The more the concentration of fluoride ion, the more severe the condition becomes (Bailey and Christen, 1968).

Sundfeld et al. indicate the use of enamel macroreduction, enamel microabrasion, followed by home bleaching with carbamide peroxide (Opalescence, Ultradent Products) to remove the texture of the intrinsic white enamel stain of hypoplastic areas and mild erosion due to dental fluorosis (Parinitha et al., 2014) (Table 1.3).

Complications during whitening treatment

Sensitivity
It has been found that the most common side effect of tooth bleaching is sensitivity of the teeth, and we can observe that in 15–78% of the patients (Dahl and Pallesen, 2003). If a patient experiences more than a

Table 1.3 Best bleaching practices for difficult cases.

S. no.	Condition	Bleaching
1	Enamel hypoplasia	Enamel macroreduction, enamel microabrasion followed by home bleaching with carbamide peroxide (Opalescence, Ultradent Products) to remove the texture of the intrinsic white enamel stain of hypoplastic areas and mild erosion due to dental fluorosis
2	Tetracycline	When used daily for 6 months, a 6.5% H_2O_2 bleaching strip can be effective in whitening tetracycline stains. The professional strip was well tolerated throughout the 6-month period
3	Restored teeth	Bleaching is contraindicated. If future trials and further research provide good results, new materials can be found promising, for example, chlorine dioxide (Agnihotry et al., 2014)

Gilboe and Teteruck (2005). Reproduced with permission from Elsevier.

moderate degree of tooth sensitivity, stop the treatment and place potassium nitrate as a desensitizing gel for about 20 min on the sensitive teeth (Zekonis et al., 2003).

Gingival irritation

High hydrogen peroxide concentrations are caustic to gingiva and oral mucosal tissues, which might cause burns and bleaching of the gingiva. To prevent an insult to the tissue, design a stiff tray that has contact solely with the teeth (Dahl and Pallesen, 2003).

Complications post whitening treatment

Posttreatment temperature sensitivity after bleaching is a common complication in up to half of vital tooth cases. However, the mechanism is not fully understood, but it is believed that the sensitivity results from pulp reaction to the bleaching agent in the early stages of treatment and it could last for 2–3 days (Li and Greenwall, 2013).

Prevention and management

To prevent this scenario, you should evaluate the tooth before bleaching by assessing the tooth vitality using the cold test and the electric pulp test; also looking at the periapical radiographs is important to rule out any possible sensitivity due to compromised situations (e.g., a cracked tooth) that already exist. If the teeth become sensitive after the treatment, the dentist can advise the patient to use a desensitizing toothpaste, and if this approach does not relieve the discomfort, after multiple applications, the dentist can start with the fluoride gel or any special desensitizing agent (Croll, 2003).

Postoperative hypersensitivity

Postoperative hypersensitivity (POH) refers to the pain associated with mastication or sensitivity to hot, cold, and/or sweet food or beverages, which is present from a few days to weeks after the tooth has undergone restoration. Pain that occurs during clenching only, indicating a restoration in hyperocclusion, usually is excluded from the definition of POH. Sensitivity can be measured clinically or by the participant's own report or both. (Strober et al., 2013).

Bonding failures

The longevity of resin-based composite restorations is compromised when bonding between the resin and interior cavity walls fails to prevent marginal microleakage. The passage of water and other species (microorganisms) into the space between the resin material and cavity wall may give rise to postoperative sensitivity, secondary caries, and further physical deterioration of the marginal seal (Christensen, 1996; Kohler, Rasmusson, and Odman, 2000; Van Nieuwenhuysen et al., 2003).

Inadequate air drying may also cause sensitivity after restoration. To be more precise, an explanation of the reduction in bond strengths seen with no air-drying was that solvents, such as water and ethanol, might act as inhibitors for the polymerization of resin components in adhesive (Cho, 2004).

Some self-etching primer bonding systems show dentin bond strengths that are less than adequate if the enamel surface was not air-dried or if air-drying was prolonged for more than 5 s after application of self-etching primer. Clinicians using these simplified systems must be aware of technique factors that can influence bond strengths (Chiba *et al.*, 2006).

Prevention and management

Apply two or more coats of bonding agent, air thinning, and curing each layer individually according to the manufacture instructions. Air thinning was advantageous with a 3 s blast of air as compared to 1 s (Bonilla *et al.*, 2003).

Changing material: The SE resins are the most foolproof way to eliminate postoperative sensitivity.

Large restorations can cause greater sensitivity

Al-Omari, Al-Omari, and Omar (2006) showed that short-term (2–30 days) postoperative sensitivity was affected by lesion depth (27% of the middle-third lesions, 58% of the inner third lesions), whereas medium-term (>30 days) postoperative sensitivity was affected neither by the method of cavity treatment nor by the depth of lesion. Furthermore, the larger the cavity preparation, the greater the area of dentinal tubules exposed. Likewise, the deeper the cavity, the wider are the dentinal tubules. These morphological factors could explain why deeper cavities had more reports of postoperative sensitivity and pain (Auschill *et al.*, 2009). This might also help to explain why class II cavities had more postoperative sensitivity than class I cavities.

Management

1 Sandwich technique (Figures 1.7 and 1.8):
   Resin-modified liner + glass ionomer as a body + layer of composite

2 Incremental layering of composite to rebuild the dentin and then place cusps individually to eliminate cross tooth shrinkage (Deliperi and Bardwell 2006a, b).

3 The use of indirect restorations in large restorations (inlay, onlay) or PFM:
   The indirect technique allows for the production of restorations in the laboratory after impression making. Appropriate proximal contour and contact and control of anatomic form can be easily achieved. In the direct inlay/onlay technique, the restoration is formed directly in the cavity; after an initial cure, it is removed from the cavity and post-cured in a heat and light oven. Improved mechanical and physical properties are expected, compared to the direct light-cured-onlay composite due to the overall increase in conversion (Wendt, 1987a, b).

   A higher stress relaxation and improved marginal adaptation are also expected. The amount of shrinkage is limited to the thin luting resin composite layer (Shortall and Baylis, 1991).

Miscellaneous complications in restorative dentistry

Overheating of pulp

The accidental overheating of the pulp during cavity preparation can cause sensitivity, especially when the remaining dentin thickness is less than 1.5 mm and when there is inadequate water coolant sprayed during cavity preparation with high and low torque handpieces.

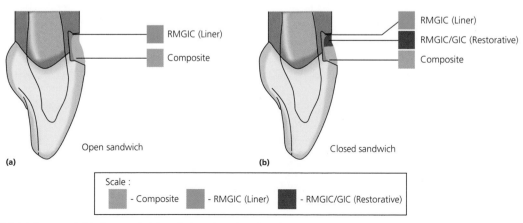

Figure 1.7 (a) Open and (b) close sandwich technique in a class V cavity.

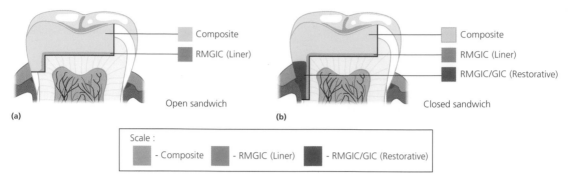

Figure 1.8 (a) Open and (b) close sandwich technique in a class II cavity.

Prevention and management

Sufficient water cooling is necessary, and if dry cutting is used, one must use it with light pressure and limit the bur-contact time to less than 20 s at a time during cavity preparation with high- and low-torque handpieces (Kwon *et al.*, 2013).

Thermal hazard to pulp

The following are the potential thermal hazard to the pulp and supporting tissue that might result from routine clinical procedures:

1 Tooth preparation
2 Light curing of composite resin
3 Fabrication of provisional crown
4 Thermoplasticized root canal obturation
5 The use of ultrasonic devices in post or file removal

Prevention and management

Clinical guidelines are summarized in the succeeding text:

Tooth preparation: Sufficient water cooling is necessary, and if dry cutting is used, one must use it with light pressure and limit the bur-contact time to less than 20 s at a time during cavity preparation with high- and low- torque handpieces.

Light curing of composite resin: A 1–2 mm thick insulation layer of glass ionomer in deep cavities with residual dentin thickness of 0.5 mm and two-step curing or ramp curing are recommended for complete polymerization and less heat generation.

Fabrication of provisional crowns: In vital crown preparation, air–water spray must be used as a cooling technique. One can also use the putty matrix as a heat sink, and depending on the situation, the putty matrix can be refrigerated.

Thermoplasticized root canal obturation: The heat source activation must be limited to 3 s, and efforts must be made to limit the amount of heated GP injected at one time, especially in dangerous zones where the dentin wall is very thin, such as the mandibular incisors and mesial canal of the lower molars.

The use of ultrasonic devices in post or file removal: One must use the smallest ultrasonic tips for the lowest power, together with at least 40 ml/min of water cooling. The tip-contact time must be limited to 60 s at a time.

Excess cement removal during crown cementation

Prevention and management

Lowe (2011) suggests that at the smallest ultrasonic tips of the lowest power, together with at least 40 ml/min of water, cooling spray should be used to remove excess cement. Furthermore, a sonic or piezo scaler with water spray can also be used carefully to ensure complete cement removal from the sulcular areas.

Resin cements prone to postoperative sensitivity

Prevention and management

Using self-etching primers before cementation and avoiding the total-etch procedure on teeth receiving resin-cemented restorations can reduce or eliminate this problem (Christensen, 2002).

Improper seating of restoration during cementation of a crown
Prevention and management

If a restoration has been seated incorrectly and this problem is determined almost immediately after cementation, gently tapping on the restoration may help remove it (Christensen, 2002). Unfortunately, the more common occurrence is that the restoration may not be easily dislodged from the tooth and will require bur sectioning to remove it, thereby requiring the fabrication of a new restoration. If care is taken not to damage the finish line area of the preparation during removal, the original die may be used to fabricate a new restoration without the need for a new impression, assuming the die itself is also undamaged.

Set cement in the contact area
Prevention and management

Remove the most coronal portion of cement between the observable occlusal contact areas. After clearing the most coronal aspect with a sharp instrument or an explorer, the next step would be to clean the area around the contract. Apply gentle force between the teeth with a blunt instrument such as a beaver-tail burnisher and push waxed dental floss through the partially open contact area to remove the cement (Christensen, 2002). Another technique is to use any of the interproximal stripping materials, like diamond-coated finishing strips. Some of these are available with serrated edges to facilitate cement removal.

References

Accorinte, M., Loguercio, A., Reis, A. and Costa, C. (2007) Response of human pulps capped with different self-etch adhesive systems. *Clinical Oral Investigations*, **12** (2), 119–127.

Accorinte, M., Loguercio, A., Reis, A., Carneiro, E., Grande, R., Murata, S. and Holland, R. (2008) Response of human dental pulp capped with MTA and calcium hydroxide powder. *Operative Dentistry*, **33** (5), 488–495.

Agnihotry, A., Gill, K.S., Singhal, D., Fedorowicz, Z., Dash, S. and Pedrazzi, V. (2014) A comparison of the bleaching effectiveness of chlorine dioxide and hydrogen peroxide on dental composite. *Brazilian Dental Journal*, **25** (6), 524–527.

Akkayan, B. and Gülmez, T. (2002) Resistance to fracture of endodontically treated teeth restored with different post systems. *The Journal of Prosthetic Dentistry*, **87** (4), 431–437.

Alleman, D. and Mange, P. (2012) A systematic approach to deep caries removal end points: the peripheral seal concept in adhesive dentistry. *Quintessence International*, **43** (3), 197–208.

Al-Omari, W., Al-Omari, Q. and Omar, R. (2006) Effect of cavity disinfection on postoperative sensitivity associated with amalgam restorations. *Operative Dentistry*, **31** (2), 165–170.

Arora, R., Kapur, R., Sibal, N. and Juneja, S. (2012) Evaluation of microleakage in class II cavities using packable composite restorations with and without use of liners. *International Journal of Clinical Pediatric Dentistry*, **5**, 178–184.

Asmussen, E., Peutzfeldt, A. and Sahafi, A. (2005) Finite element analysis of stresses in endodontically treated, dowel-restored teeth. *The Journal of prosthetic dentistry*, **4** (94), 321–329.

Auschill, T., Koch, C., Wolkewitz, M., Hellwig, E. and Arweiler, N. (2009) Occurrence and causing stimuli of postoperative sensitivity in composite restorations. *Operative Dentistry*, **1** (34), 3–10.

Bailey, R. and Christen, A. (1968) Bleaching of vital teeth stained with endemic dental fluorosis. *Oral Surgery, Oral Medicine, Oral Pathology*, **26** (6), 871–878.

Bateman, G., Ricketts, D. and Saunders, W. (2003) Fibre-based post systems: a review. *British Dental Journal*, **195** (1), 43–48.

Beier, U., Kranewitter, R. and Dumfahrt, H. (2009) Quality of impressions after use of the Magic FoamCord gingival retraction system—a clinical study of 269 abutment teeth. *International Journal of Prosthodontics*, **22** (2), 143–147.

Bjørndal, L., Reit, C., Bruun, G., Markvart, M., Kjaeldgaard, M., Näsman, P., Thordrup, M., Dige, I., Nyvad, B., Fransson, H., Lager, A., Ericson, D., Petersson, K., Olsson, J., Santimano, E.M., Wennström, A., Winkel, P. and Gluud, C. (2010) Treatment of deep caries lesions in adults: randomized clinical trials comparing stepwise vs. direct complete excavation, and direct pulp capping vs. partial pulpotomy. *European Journal of Oral Sciences*, **118** (3), 290–297.

Bonilla, E., Stevenson, R., Yashar, M. and Caputo, A. (2003) Effect of application technique and dentin bonding agent interaction on shear bond strength. *Operative Dentistry*, **5** (28), 568–573.

Boyarsky, H., Loos, L. and Leknius, C. (1999) Occlusal refinement of mounted casts before crown fabrication to decrease clinical time required to adjust occlusion. *The Journal of Prosthetic Dentistry*, **82** (5), 591–594.

Braga, N., Paulino, S., Alfredo, E., Sousa-Neto, M. and Vansan, L. (2006) Removal resistance of glass-fiber and metallic cast posts with different lengths. *Journal of Oral Science*, **48** (1), 15–20.

Carranza, F., Newman, M., Takei, H. and Klokkevold, P. (2006) *Carranza's Clinical Periodontology*, Saunders Elsevier, St. Louis, MO.

Chacko, V. and Kurikose, S. (2006) Human pulpal response to mineral trioxide aggregate (MTA): a histologic study. *Journal of Clinical Pediatric Dentistry*, **30** (3), 203–209.

Chen, R., Liuiw, C., Tseng, W., Hong, C., Hsieh, C. and Jeng, J. (2001) The effect of curing light intensity on the cytotoxicity of a dentin-bonding agent. *Journal of Operative Dentistry*, **26** (5), 505–510.

Chiba, Y., Yamaguchi, K., Miyazaki, M., Tsubota, K., Takamizawa, T. and Moore, B. (2006) Effect of air-drying time of single-application self-etch adhesives on dentin bond strength. *Operative Dentistry*, **2** (31), 233–239.

Cho, B. (2004) Effects of the acetone content of single solution dentin bonding agents on the adhesive layer thickness and the microtensile bond strength. *Dental Materials*, **20** (2), 107–115.

Christensen, G. (1996) The bonding evolution in dentistry continues. *Journal of the American Dental Association*, **127** (7), 1114–1116.

Christensen, G. (2002) Preventing postoperative tooth sensitivity in class I, II and V restorations. *Journal of the American Dental Association*, **2** (133), 229–231.

Christensen, G. (2012) Advantages and challenges of bulk fill resins. *Clinicians Report*, **5** (1), 1–6.

Cohen, B., Pagnillo, M., Musikant, B. and Deutsch, A. (1999) Comparison of the retentive and photoelastic properties of two prefabricated endodontic post systems. *Journal of Oral Rehabilitation*, **26** (6), 488–494.

Cooney, J., Caputo, A. and Trabert, K. (1986) Retention and stress distribution of tapered-end endodontic posts. *The Journal of Prosthetic Dentistry*, **55** (5), 540–546.

Corralo, D. and Maltz, M. (2013) Clinical and ultrastructural effects of different liners/restorative materials on deep carious dentin: a randomized clinical trial. *Caries Research*, **47** (3), 243–250.

Croll, T.P. (2003) Bleaching sensitivity. *The Journal of the American Dental Association*, **134** (9), 1168.

Dahl, J. and Pallesen, U. (2003) Tooth bleaching—a critical review of the biological aspects. *Critical Reviews in Oral Biology and Medicine*, **4** (14), 292–304.

Deliperi, S. and Bardwell, D. (2006a) Clinical evaluation of direct cuspal coverage with posterior composite resin restorations. *Journal of Esthetic and Restorative Dentistry*, **18** (5), 256–265.

Deliperi, S. and Bardwell, D. (2006b) Direct cuspal-coverage posterior resin composite restorations: a case report. *Operative Dentistry*, **31** (1), 143–150.

Dérand, T. (1991) Stress analysis of cemented or resin-bonded loaded porcelain inlays. *Dental Materials*, **7** (1), 21–24.

Dickinson, G. and Leinfelder, K. (1993) Assessing the long-term effect of a surface penetrating sealant. *Journal of American Dental Association*, **124** (7), 68–72.

Dietrich, T., Lösche, A.C., Lösche, G.M. and Roulet, J. (1999) Marginal adaptation of direct composite and sandwich restorations in class II cavities with cervical margins in dentin. *Journal of Dentistry*, **27** (2), 119–128.

Dietschi, D., Romelli, M. and Goretti, A. (1998) Adaptation of adhesive posts and cores to dentin after fatigue testing. *The International Journal of Prosthodontics*, **6** (10), 498–507.

El-Mowafy, O., El-Badrawy, W., Lewis, D.W., Shokati, B., Soliman, O., Kermalli, J., Encioiu, A., Rajwani, F. and Zawi, R. (2005) Intensity of quartz–tungsten–halogen light-curing units used in private practice in Toronto. *Journal of the American Dental Association*, **136** (6), 766–773.

Estafan, D., Dussetschleger, F., Miuo, L. and Kondamani, J. (2000) Class V lesions restored with flowable composite and added surface sealing resin. *General Dentistry*, **40** (1), 78–80.

Farrier, S., Pretty, I.A., Lynch, C.D. and Addy, L.D. (2011) Gagging during impression making: techniques for reduction. *Dental Update*, **38** (3), 171–172 174–176.

Ferracane, J., Berge, H. and Condon, J. (1998) In vitro aging of dental composites in water—effect of degree of conversion, filler volume, and filler/matrix coupling. *Journal of Biomedical Materials Research*, **42** (3), 465–472.

Ford, H.P., Ford, T.P. and Rhodes, J. (2004) *Endodontics: Problem-Solving in Clinical Practice*, CRC Press, London.

Fusayama, T., Katayori, T. and Nomoto, S. (1963) Corrosion of gold and amalgam placed in contact with each other. *Journal of Dental Research*, **42** (5), 1183–1197.

Galhano, A.G., Felipevalandro, L., Marquesdemelo, R., Scotti, R. and Antoniobottino, M. (2005a) Evaluation of the flexural strength of carbon fiber-, quartz fiber-, and glass fiber-based posts. *Journal of Endodontics*, **31** (3), 209–211.

Galhano, G.A., Valandro, L.F., de Melo, R.M., Scotti, R. and Bottino, M.A. (2005b) Evaluation of the flexural strength of carbon fiber-, quartz fiber-, and glass fiber-based posts. *Journal of Endodontics*, **3** (31), 209–211.

Gandolfi, M., Siboni, F. and Prati, C. (2012) Chemical-physical properties of TheraCal, a novel light-curable MTA-like material for pulp capping. *International Endodontic Journal*, **45** (6), 571–579.

Gilboe, D.B. and Teteruck, W.R. (2005) Fundamentals of extracoronal tooth preparation. Part I. Retention and resistance form. *The Journal of Prosthetic Dentistry*, **94** (2), 105–107.

Golsen, L. and Shaw, A. (1984) Use of leaf gauge in occlusal diagnosis and therapy. *Quintessence International*, **15**, 611–621.

Goracci, C. and Ferrari, M. (2011) Current perspectives on post systems: a literature review. *Australian Dental Journal*, **56**, 77–83.

Grippo, J., Simring, M. and Schreiner, S. (2004) Attrition, abrasion, corrosion and abfraction revisited: a new perspective on tooth surface lesions. *Journal of the American Dental Association*, **8** (135), 1109–1118.

Hagge, M., Wong, R. and Lindemuth, J. (2002) Retention strengths of five luting cements on prefabricated dowels after root canal obturation with a zinc oxide/eugenol sealer: 1. Dowel space preparation/cementation at one week after obturation. *Journal of Prosthodontics Implant, Esthetic and Reconstructive Dentistry,* **11** (3), 168–175.

Hammouda, I. (2010) Effect of light-curing method on wear and hardness of composite resin. *Journal of the Mechanical Behavior of Biomedical Materials,* **3** (2), 216–222.

Harper, R., Schnell, R., Swartz, M. and Phillips, R. (1980) In vivo measurements of thermal diffusion through restorations of various materials. *The Journal of Prosthetic Dentistry,* **43** (2), 180–185.

Heintze, S. and Rousson, V. (2012) Clinical effectiveness of direct class II restorations—a meta-analysis. *Journal of Adhesive Dentistry,* **14** (5), 407–431.

Hilton, T., Ferracane, J., Mancl, L., Baltuck, C., Barnes, C., Beaudry, D., Shao, J., Lubisich, E., Gilbert, A. and Lowder, L. (2013) Comparison of CaOH with MTA for direct pulp capping: a PBRN randomized clinical trial. *Journal of Dental Research,* **92** (7 Suppl), S16–S22.

Hochman, N. and Zalkind, M. (1999) New all-ceramic indirect post-and-core system. *The Journal of Prosthetic Dentistry,* **81** (5), 625–629.

Hollenback, G.M. (1943) Precision gold inlays made by a simple technic. *The Journal of the American Dental Association,* **30** (1), 99–109.

Hunter, A., Feiglin, B. and Williams, J. (1989) Effects of post placement on endodontically treated teeth. *The Journal of Prosthetic Dentistry,* **62** (2), 166–172.

Jandt, K. and Mills, R. (2013) A brief history of LED photopolymerization. *Dental Materials,* **29** (6), 605–617.

Kemp-Scholte, C. and Davidson, C. (1988) Marginal sealing of curing contraction gaps in class V composite resin restorations. *Journal of Dental Research,* **67** (5), 841–845.

Kinney, J., Marshall, S. and Marshall, G. (2003) The mechanical properties of human dentin: a critical review and re-evaluation of the dental literature. *Critical Reviews in Oral Biology & Medicine,* **14** (1), 13–29.

Kohler, B., Rasmusson, C. and Odman, P. (2000) A five-year clinical evaluation of Class II composite resin restorations. *Journal of Dentistry,* **28** (2), 111–116.

Krupp, C. (2008) *How Not To Look Old,* Grand Central Publishing, New York, p. 94.

Kugel, G., Gerlach, R., Aboushala, A., Ferriera, S. and Magnuson, B. (2011) Long-term use of 6.5% hydrogen peroxide bleaching strips on tetracycline stain: a clinical study. *Compendium of Continuing Education in Dentistry,* **32** (8), 50–56.

Kwon, S.-J., Park, Y.-J., Jun, S.-H., Ahn, J.-S., Lee, I.-B., Cho, B.-H., Son, H.-H. and Seo, D.-G. (2013) Thermal irritation of teeth during dental treatment procedures. *Restorative Dentistry & Endodontics,* **38** (3), 105–112.

Lacy, A.M. (1987) A critical look at posterior composite restorations. *Journal of American Dental Association,* **114** (3), 357–362.

Leary, J., Aquilino, S. and Svare, C. (1987) An evaluation of post length within the elastic limits of dentin. *The Journal of Prosthetic Dentistry,* **57** (3), 277–281.

Leprince, J., Devaux, J., Mullier, T., Vreven, J. and Leloup, G. (2010) Pulpal-temperature rise and polymerization efficiency of LED curing lights. *Operative Dentistry,* **35** (2), 220–230.

Levartovsky, S., Masri, M., Alter, E. and Pilo, R. (2012) Refu'at ha-peh yeha-shinayim [Tissue displacement and impression techniques—part 1]. *XX,* **1993** (29), 19–27.

Li, Y. and Greenwall, L. (2013) Safety issues of tooth whitening using peroxide-based materials. *British Dental Journal,* **1** (215), 29–34.

Liebenberg, W. (1995) An innovative method of cushioning metal clamp jaws during rubber dam isolation. *Journal of Canadian Dental Association,* **61** (10), 876–881.

Long, J.H. (1973) Locating centric relation with a leaf gauge. *The Journal of Prosthetic Dentistry,* **29** (6), 608–610.

Loomans, B., Opdam, N., Roeters, F., Bronkhorst, E. and Burgersdijk, R. (2006) Comparison of proximal contacts of class II resin composite restorations in vitro. *Operative Dentistry,* **31** (6), 688–693.

Loomans, B., Opdam, N., Roeters, E., Bronkhorst, F. and Dörfer, C. (2007) A clinical study on interdental separation techniques. *Operative Dentistry,* **32** (3), 207–211.

Loomans, B.A.C., Roeters, F.J.M., Opdam, N.J.M. and Kuijs, R.H. (2008) The effect of proximal contour on marginal ridge fracture of class II composite resin restorations. *Journal of Dentistry,* **36** (10), 828–832.

Loomans, B., Opdam, N., Roeters, F., Bronkhorst, E. and Huysmans, M. (2009) Restoration techniques and marginal overhang in Class II composite resin restorations. *Journal of Dentistry,* **37** (9), 712–717.

Lowe, R. (2011) Dental cements: an overview. *Dentistry Today,* **10** (30), 140–143.

Macedo, V., Faria e Silva, A. and Marcondes Martins, L. (2010) Effect of cement type, relining procedure, and length of cementation on pull-out bond strength of fiber posts. *Journal of Endodontics,* **36** (9), 1543–1546.

Madison, S., Jordan, R. and Krell, K. (1986) The effects of rubber dam retainers on porcelain fused-to-metal restorations. *Journal of Endodontics,* **12** (5), 183–186.

Maltz, M. and Alves, L. (2013) Incomplete caries removal significantly reduces the risk of pulp exposure and post-operative pulpal symptoms. *Journal of Evidence Based Dental Practice,* **13** (3), 120–122.

Maltz, M., Garcia, R., Jardim, J., de Paula, L., Yamaguti, P., Moura, M., Garcia, F., Nascimento, C., Oliveira, A. and Mestrinho, H. (2012a) Randomized trial of partial vs. stepwise caries removal: 3-year follow-up. *Journal of Dental Research,* **91** (11), 1026–1031.

Maltz, M., Henz, S., de Oliveira, E. and Jardim, J. (2012b) Conventional caries removal and sealed caries in permanent teeth: a microbiological evaluation. *Journal of Dentistry*, **40** (9), 776–782.

Marangos, D. (2006) *The Direct Posterior Composite Restoration—Solving Everyday Clinical Problems* [online]. Available at: http://www.oralhealthgroup.com/news/the-direct-posterior-composite-restoration-solving-everyday-clinical-problems/1000204908/?&er=NA (accessed on December 21, 2014).

Matsuo, T., Nakanishi, T., Shimizu, H. and Ebisu, S. (1996) A clinical study of direct pulp capping applied to carious-exposed pulps. *Journal of Endodontics*, **22** (10), 551–556.

McCullock, A. (2003) Making occlusion work: I. Terminology, occlusal assessment and recording. *Dental Update*, **30** (3), 150–157.

Meyenberg, K., Lüthy, H., & Schärer, P. (1995). Zirconia posts: A new all-ceramic concept for nonvital abutment teeth. *Journal of Esthetic Dentistry*, **7** (2), 73–80.

Michalakis, K., Hirayama, H., Sfolkos, J. and Sfolkos, K. (2004) Light transmission of posts and cores used for the anterior esthetic region. *The International Journal of Periodontics & Restorative Dentistry*, **24** (5), 463–469.

Milleding, P., Ortengren, U. and Karlssan, S. (1995) Ceramic inlay systems: some clinical aspects. *Journal of Oral Rehabilitation*, **22** (8), 571–580.

Mjör, I. (2005) Clinical diagnosis of recurrent caries. *Journal of the American Dental Association*, **10** (136), 1426–1433.

Mopper, K. (2011) Contouring, finishing, and polishing anterior composites. *Inside Dentistry*, **7**, 62–70.

Morgan, L.A. and Marshall, J.G. (1990) Solving endodontic isolation problems with interim buildups of reinforced glass ionomer cement. *Journal of Endodontics*, **16** (9), 450–453.

Murray, P. and Garcia-Godoy, F. (2006) The incidence of pulp healing defects with direct capping materials. *American Journal of Dentistry*, **19** (3), 171–177.

Neumann, J. and McCarty, G. (2001) Behavioral approaches to reduce hypersensitive gag response. *The Journal of Prosthetic Dentistry*, **85** (3), 305.

Oberholzer, T., Makofane, M., du Preez, I. and George, R. (2012) Modern high powered led curing lights and their effect on pulp chamber temperature of bulk and incrementally cured composite resin. *European Journal of Prosthodontics and Restorative Dentistry*, **20** (2), 50–55.

Ona, M., Wakabayashi, N., Yamazaki, T., Takaichi, A. and Igarashi, Y. (2013) The influence of elastic modulus mismatch between tooth and post and core restorations on root fracture. *International Endodontic Journal*, **46** (1), 47–52.

Oshida, Y., Munoz, C., Winkler, M., Hashem, A. and Itoh, M. (1993) Fractal dimension analysis of aluminum oxide particle for sandblasting dental use. *Biomedical Materials and Engineering*, **3** (3), 117–126.

Ozel, E. and Soyman, M. (2009) Effect of fiber nets, application techniques and flowable composites on microleakage and the effect of fiber nets on polymerization shrinkage in class II MOD cavities. *Operative Dentistry*, **34** (2), 174–180.

Parinitha, M.S., Annapoorna, B.M., Tejaswi, S., Shetty, S. and Sowmya, H.K. (2014) Effect of power bleaching on the fluorosis stained anterior teeth case series. *Journal of Clinical and Diagnostic Research*, **8**, ZJ01–ZJ03.

Parirokh, M., Eskandarizadeh, A., Shahpasandzadeh, M., Shahpasandzadeh, M. and Torabi, M. (2011) A comparative study on dental pulp response to calcium hydroxide, white and grey mineral trioxide aggregate as pulp capping agents. *Journal of Conservative Dentistry*, **14** (4), 351.

Patel, M. and Tripathi, G. (2014) Guiding intellect for occlusal errors. *Journal of Clinical and Diagnostic Research*, **7** (11), 2619–2622.

Perez, C. (2010) Alternative technique for class V resin composite restorations with minimum finishing/polishing procedures. *Operative Dentistry*, **35** (3), 375–379.

Perez, C., dos, R., Gonzalez, M.R., Prado, N.A.S., de Miranda, M.S.F., Macêdo, M.d.A. and Fernandes, B.M.P. (2012) Restoration of Noncarious cervical lesions: when, why, and how. *International Journal of Dentistry*, **2012**, 1–8.

Peumans, M., Van Meerbeek, B., Asscherickx, K., Simon, S., Abe, Y., Lambrechts, P. and Vanherle, G. (2001) Do condensable composites help to achieve better proximal contacts? *Dental Materials*, **17** (6), 533–541.

Prasanna, G., Reddy, K., Kumar, R. and Shivaprakash, S. (2013) Evaluation of efficacy of different gingival displacement materials on gingival sulcus width. *The Journal of Contemporary Dental Practice*, **14** (2), 217.

Price, R.B. (2014) Light curing guidelines for practitioners: a consensus statement from the 2014 symposium on light curing in dentistry, Dalhousie University, Halifax, Canada. *Journal of Canadian Dental Association*, **80**, e-61.

Price, R. and Ferracane, J. (2012) Effect of energy delivered on the shear bond strength to dentin. *Canadian Journal of Restorative Dentistry & Prosthodontics*, **5**, 48–55.

Price, R., Fahey, J. and Felix, C. (2010) Knoop microhardness mapping used to compare the efficacy of LED, QTH and PAC curing lights. *Operative Dentistry*, **35** (1), 58–68.

Prithviraj, D., Soni, R., Ramaswamy, S. and Shruthi, D. (2010) Evaluation of the effect of different surface treatments on the retention of posts: a laboratory study. *Indian Journal of Dental Research*, **21** (2), 201.

Rada, R.E. (2013) New Options for Restoring a Deep Carious Lesion. Available at: http://www.dentistrytoday.com/dental-materials/8820-new-options-for-restoring-a-deep-carious-lesion (accessed on January 20, 2016).

Reddy, G., Reddy, N., Itttigi, J. and Jagadeesh, K. (2012) A comparative study to determine the wettability and castability of different elastomeric impression materials. *The Journal of Contemporary Dental Practice*, **3** (13), 356–363.

Roberson, T., Heymann, H., Swift, E. and Sturdevant, C. (2006) *Sturdevant's Art and Science of Operative Dentistry*, Mosby, St. Louis, MO.

Rosted, P., Bundgaard, M., Fiske, J. and Pedersen, A. (2006) The use of acupuncture in controlling the gag reflex in patients requiring an upper alginate impression: an audit. *British Dental Journal*, **201** (11), 721–725.

Rueggeberg, F. (2013) Cure times for contemporary composites. *Journal of Esthetic and Restorative Dentistry*, **25** (1), 3–3.

Saber, M., El-Badrawy, W., Loomans, B., Ahmed, D., Dörfer, C., A. C. and El Zohairy, A. (2011) Creating tight proximal contacts for MOD resin composite restorations. *Operative Dentistry*, **36** (3), 304–310.

Santos, M. (2015) A restorative approach for class II resin composite restorations: a two-year follow-up. *Operative Dentistry*, **40** (1), 19–24.

Sapkota, B. and Gupta, A. (2014) Pattern of occlusal contacts in lateral excursions (canine protection or group function). *Kathmandu University Medical Journal*, **12** (45), 43–47.

Schwartz, I. (1986) A review of methods and techniques to improve the fit of cast restorations. *The Journal of Prosthetic Dentistry*, **56** (3), 279–283.

Schwartz, J., Anderson, M. and Pelleu, G. (1990) Reducing microleakage with the glass-ionomer/resin sandwich technique. *Operative Dentistry*, **15** (5), 186–192.

Segerström, S., Astbäck, J. and Ekstrand, K.D. (2006) A retrospective long term study of teeth restored with prefabricated carbon fiber reinforced epoxy resin posts. *Swedish Journal*, **30** (1), 1–8.

Shortall, A.C. and Baylis, R.L. (1991) Microleakage around direct composite inlays. *Journal of Dentistry*, **19** (5), 307–311.

Shortall, A., El-Mahy, W., Stewardson, D., Addison, O. and Palin, W. (2013) Initial fracture resistance and curing temperature rise of ten contemporary resin-based composites with increasing radiant exposure. *Journal of Dentistry*, **41** (5), 455–463.

Silva, A., Tarquinio, S., Demarco, F., Piva, E. and Rivero, E. (2006a) The influence of haemostatic agents on healing of healthy human dental pulp tissue capped with calcium hydroxide. *International Endodontic Journal*, **39** (4), 309–316.

Silva, G., Lanza, L., Lopes-JÃ°nior, N., Moreira, A. and Alves, J. (2006b) Direct pulp capping with a dentin bonding system in human teeth: a clinical and histological evaluation. *Operative Dentistry*, **31** (3), 297–307.

Small, B. (2008). Cast Gold: The standard of care for operative dentistry. *Inside Dentistry*, **4** (2), [E–pub].

Standlee, J. and Caputo, A. (1993) Effect of surface design on retention of dowels cemented with a resin. *The Journal of Prosthetic Dentistry*, **70** (5), 403–405.

Standlee, J., Caputo, A. and Hanson, E. (1978) Retention of endodontic dowels: effects of cement, dowel length, diameter, and design. *The Journal of Prosthetic Dentistry*, **39** (4), 401–405.

Stevenson, R. and Patrice, F. (2013) Cast gold restorations, in *Summitt's Fundamentals of Operative Dentistry. A Contemporary Approach*, 4th edn (eds T.J. Hilton, J.L. Farrance and J. Boome), Quintessence Publishers, Hanover Park, IL.

Stockton, L. (1999) Vital pulp capping: a worthwhile procedure. *Journal of Canadian Dental Association*, **65** (6), 328–331.

Strober, B., Veitz-Keenan, A., Barna, J., Matthews, A., Vena, D., Craig, R., Curro, F. and Thompson, V. (2013) Effectiveness of a resin-modified glass ionomer liner in reducing hypersensitivity in posterior restorations. *The Journal of the American Dental Association*, **144** (8), 886–897.

Strydom, C. (2006) Handling protocol of posterior composites—part 3: matrix systems. *South African Dental Association Journal*, **61**, 18–21.

Sunnegårdh-Grönberg, K., van Dijken, J.W., Funegård, U., Lindberg, A. and Nilsson, M. (2009) Selection of dental materials and longevity of replaced restorations in public dental health clinics in northern Sweden. *Journal of Dentistry*, **37** (9), 673–678.

Taylor, M. and Lynch, E. (1993) Marginal adaptation. *Journal of Dentistry*, **21** (5), 265–273.

Toksavul, S., Turkun, M. and Toman, M. (2004) Esthetic enhancement of ceramic crowns with zirconia dowels and cores: a clinical report. *The Journal of Prosthetic Dentistry*, **92** (2), 116–119.

Türkün, L.S. and Türkün, M. (2004) The effect of one-step polishing system on the surface roughness of three esthetic resin composite materials. *Operative Dentistry*, **29** (2), 203–211.

Van Nieuwenhuysen, J., D'Hoore, W., Carvalho, J. and Qvist, V. (2003) Long-term evaluation of extensive restorations in permanent teeth. *Journal of Dentistry*, **31** (6), 395–405.

Wakabayashi, H., Ochi, K., Tachibana, H. and Matsumoto, K. (1986) A clinical technique for the retention of a rubber dam clamp. *Journal of Endodontics*, **12** (9), 422–424.

Wassell, R., Barker, D. and Steele, J. (2002) Crowns and other extra-coronal restorations: try-in and cementation of crowns. *British Dental Journal*, **193** (1), 17–28.

Weir, D. and Williams, B. (1984) Clinical effectiveness of mechanical-chemical tissue displacement methods. *The Journal of Prosthetic Dentistry*, **51** (3), 326–329.

Wendt, S. (1987a) The effect of heat used as a secondary cure upon the physical properties of three composite resins. I. Diametral tensile strength, compressive strength, and marginal dimensional stability. *Quintessence International*, **4** (18), 265–271.

Wendt, S. (1987b) The effect of heat used as secondary cure upon the physical properties of three composite resins. II. Wear, hardness, and color stability. *Quintessence International*, **5** (18), 351–356.

Xu, X., Sandras, D. and Burgess, J. (2006) Shear bond strength with increasing light-guide distance from dentin. *Journal of Esthetic and Restorative Dentistry*, **18** (1), 19–28.

Yang, H., Lang, L., Molina, A. and Felton, D. (2001) The effects of dowel design and load direction on dowel-and-core restorations. *The Journal of Prosthetic Dentistry*, **6** (85), 558–567.

Yeo, I., Yang, J. and Lee, J. (2003) In vitro marginal fit of three all-ceramic crown systems. *The Journal of Prosthetic Dentistry*, **90** (5), 459–464.

Zekonis, R., Matis, B., Cochran, M., Al Shetri, S., Eckert, G. and Carlson, T. (2003) Clinical evaluation of in-office and at-home bleaching treatments. *Operative Dentistry*, **28** (2), 114–121.

CHAPTER 2

Periodontal complications

Deborah A. Termeie and Paulo M. Camargo

Section of Periodontics, Clinical Dental Sciences, UCLA School of Dentistry, Los Angeles, CA, USA

Complications of periodontitis

Periodontal abscess

A periodontal abscess is an acute inflammatory reaction to the bacterial biofilm and dental calculus. It is important to understand the difference between periodontal, gingival, and pulpal (endodontic) abscesses. Gingival abscesses are confined to the soft gingival tissues and do not involve loss of attachment; they are usually caused by the accidental inclusion of foreign bodies into the soft tissues. Pulpal abscesses can drain through the periodontal ligament space causing a localized pocket but are associated with a necrotic pulp. Hence, testing tooth vitality is crucial in differentiating between a periodontal and a pulpal abscess.

Prevention

Because a periodontal abscess (Figure 2.1) is essentially initiated by bacteria accumulation, it is of utmost importance for patients to have good oral hygiene habits to prevent inflammation. Patients with poorly controlled or noncontrolled diabetes should be monitored because they tend to develop periodontal abscesses with high frequency and greater numbers than controlled or nondiabetics.

Treatment

Figure 2.2 describes the treatment for periodontal abscess.

Pericoronitis

Pericoronitis occurs around the crown of a partially erupted tooth due to the accumulation of bacteria and/or foreign bodies under the gingiva (Hupp, Ellis, and Tucker, 2008). Partially erupted mandibular third molars are commonly involved.

Clinical signs and symptoms (Juniper and Parkins, 1990):

1 Severe pain radiating from the tooth (can spread to the ear or throat).
2 Fever and malaise.
3 Gingiva may be ulcerated and reddish in color.
4 Suppuration.
5 Swelling at the angle of the mandible.
6 Trismus.
7 Lymphadenitis.
8 May progress to Ludwig angina.

Prevention

Removal of the partially impacted tooth (Hupp, Ellis, and Tucker, 2008) and good oral hygiene

Treatment

The treatment includes irrigating the site under local anesthesia, draining the acute inflammatory process, and often extracting the affected tooth (Topazian, Goldberg, and Hupp, 2001). If the tooth is salvageable and space exists for its eruption, the tissue covering the tooth may be excised (operculectomy). It may be prudent to adjust the occlusal surface of the opposing tooth so the gingiva is no longer injured. Antibiotics may be prescribed if there are systemic signs present (Serio and Hawley, 2002). Studies have found that patients improved the periodontal status of the distal second molars and teeth more anterior in the mouth with removal of the third molars with mild pericoronitis (Dicus-Brookes *et al.*, 2013).

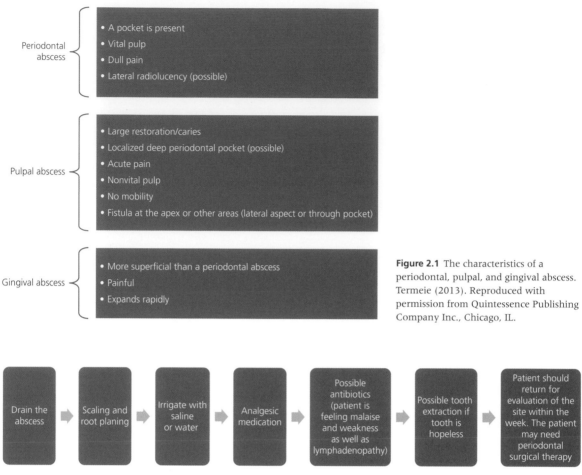

Periodontal abscess
- A pocket is present
- Vital pulp
- Dull pain
- Lateral radiolucency (possible)

Pulpal abscess
- Large restoration/caries
- Localized deep periodontal pocket (possible)
- Acute pain
- Nonvital pulp
- No mobility
- Fistula at the apex or other areas (lateral aspect or through pocket)

Gingival abscess
- More superficial than a periodontal abscess
- Painful
- Expands rapidly

Figure 2.1 The characteristics of a periodontal, pulpal, and gingival abscess. Termeie (2013). Reproduced with permission from Quintessence Publishing Company Inc., Chicago, IL.

Drain the abscess → Scaling and root planing → Irrigate with saline or water → Analgesic medication → Possible antibiotics (patient is feeling malaise and weakness as well as lymphadenopathy) → Possible tooth extraction if tooth is hopeless → Patient should return for evaluation of the site within the week. The patient may need periodontal surgical therapy

Figure 2.2 Treatment of a periodontal abscess.

Gingival enlargement

Gingival enlargement may be secondary to biofilm-induced inflammation, genetics (hereditary gingival fibromatosis), systemic disorders (leukemia, granulomatous diseases, diabetes, vitamin C deficiency, plasma cell gingivitis, and pregnancy), puberty, developmental deformities (tumors), mouth breathing, or medications (see Figure 2.3).

Prevention

Biofilm control through proper oral hygiene is of utmost importance to help prevent gingival enlargement, even in cases where the primary offending agent is a systemic medication. The incidence of gingival enlargement (Figure 2.4) in kidney transplant patients taking cyclo-sporine A was reduced with intensive motivation of patients to maintain good oral hygiene (Reali *et al.*, 2009). It should be remembered that drug-induced gingival enlargement can be minimized, but not fully prevented, by meticulous oral hygiene, regular periodontal recalls, and elimination of local irritants (Hall, 1997). Patients may also prevent gingival enlargement caused by drugs by ceasing drug therapy or substituting the offending medication by another drug; this approach is not always an option, and patients should always speak to their medical care provider before changing medication regimens.

Treatment

If gingival enlargement hinders function, esthetics, speech, or oral hygiene, tissue reduction can be achieved by a flap procedure or gingivectomy (Hall, 1997).

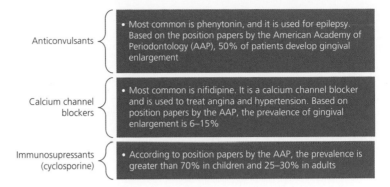

Anticonvulsants
- Most common is phenytonin, and it is used for epilepsy. Based on the position papers by the American Academy of Periodontology (AAP), 50% of patients develop gingival enlargement

Calcium channel blockers
- Most common is nifidipine. It is a calcium channel blocker and is used to treat angina and hypertension. Based on position papers by the AAP, the prevalence of gingival enlargement is 6–15%

Immunosupressants (cyclosporine)
- According to position papers by the AAP, the prevalence is greater than 70% in children and 25–30% in adults

Figure 2.3 Medications causing gingival enlargement. Adapted from Dongari-Bagtzoglu (2004) in Termeie 2013.

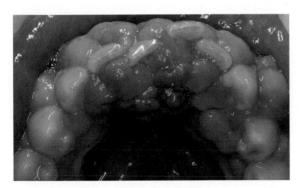

Figure 2.4 Drug-induced gingival hyperplasia.

Recurrent periodontitis

Recurrent periodontitis is defined as disease that has not responded to treatment. This can be caused by inadequate home care, inadequate maintenance, or poor response to therapy (recalcitrant disease) (Novak, 2006). The bacteria flora associated with recurrent disease include higher counts of *Tannerella forsythia*, *Prevotella intermedia*, and *Porphyromonas gingivalis*. It has also been shown that 90% of patients with recurrent disease are smokers (Johnson and Slach, 2001). The effect of smoking on the lack of response to therapy and/or disease recurrence may be associated to modifications in neutrophil phagocytosis and altered production of cytokines.

Prevention

Patients who have had periodontal therapy, both non-surgical and surgical for the treatment of periodontitis, should have maintenance visits at least four times a year (Schallhorn and Snider, 1981; Cohen, 2003). The shorter the recall interval for maintenance visits

following periodontal surgery, the greater the likelihood of the long-term benefits of periodontal therapy (Westfelt *et al.*, 1983). Good oral hygiene should be maintained to aid in preventing recurrent disease.

Treatment

In cases of recurrent disease due to persistent pathogens and possibly weakened host resistance (recalcitrant disease), systemic antibiotics can be helpful (Slots, 2004). It has been shown (Serino *et al.*, 2001) that patients with recurrent disease and who received retreatment with scaling and root planing, comprehensive supragingival plaque removal, and systemic administration of antibiotics showed improved periodontal conditions in the short term (3 years). However, even though some patients and most sites remained free of disease progression, only 5 of the 17 patients had fully stable periodontal attachment levels at 5 years after retreatment.

Tooth loss due to periodontitis

Periodontitis may result in tooth loss due to progressive destruction of the attachment and supporting bone. Long-term studies have examined the effects of periodontal treatment in preventing tooth loss. Hirschfeld and Wasserman (1978) followed 600 patients over 22 years and found a rate of 7.1% overall tooth loss (0.08 teeth per patient per year), and 31% of the teeth that were lost had furcation invasions at baseline. Another study (McFall, 1982) observing 100 patents over 19 years found 9.8% of all surgically treated teeth were lost, while 7.1% of nonsurgically treated teeth were lost. Based on the aforementioned studies, the following conclusions can be made (Termeie, 2013):

1 Furcation-involved teeth are lost 3–5 times as often as other teeth.
2 Maxillary molars are the most often lost teeth, while lower canines are the least often lost teeth.
3 Periodontal disease tends to be bilateral and symmetrical.
4 Periodontal therapy has 87–92% tooth retention over prolonged periods of time.

It is also known that slightly less than 20% of all tooth extractions are caused by periodontitis (Brown, Oliver, and Löe, 1989), making it still a fairly common reason to perform extractions.

Prevention

Oral hygiene and periodic recalls combined with frequent professional examinations are the best way to prevent tooth loss. A study by Becker, Becker, and Berg (1984) examined patients who did not comply with recommended periodontal treatment and found the following after an average of 3.7 years:

0.36 teeth lost per patient per year in patients who were not treated
0.22 teeth lost per patient per year in patients who were treated but not maintained
0.11 teeth lost per patient per year in patients who were treated and maintained

Furcation involvement

Attachment and bone loss in furcation areas are more challenging to arrest and maintain than flat surfaces on molar and other teeth. Hence, early furcation diagnosis and treatment enhance the long-term prognosis of molars. There is a greater prevalence of furcation involvement in maxillary molars (distal aspect of the maxillary first molar) than in mandibular molars (Svärdström and Wennström, 1966). Studies have shown a higher percentage of furcation involvement but no greater mobility in molars with a crown or proximal restoration when compared with nonrestored molars (Wang, Burgett, and Shyr, 1993). The anatomical factors associated with furcation lesions are shown in Figure 2.5.

Classification

The Glickman (1953) classification is as follows:

1 Grade I: Incipient suprabony lesion. Radiographic changes are rarely found.

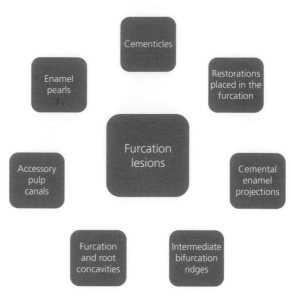

Figure 2.5 Anatomical factors associated with furcation lesions. Termeie (2013). Reproduced with permission from Quintessence Publishing Company Inc., Chicago, IL.

2 Grade II: Furcation bone loss with a horizontal component. Radiographs may not show bone loss in the furcation.
3 Grade III: A through and through lesion (bone is not attached to the fornix of the furcation) that is not clinically visible because it is filled with soft tissue.
4 Grade IV: A through and through lesion that is clinically visible. The soft tissue has receded apically. Radiolucency is clearly visible in the furcation area.

Prevention

Tooth-related local factors should be corrected when possible and routine professional cleanings.

Treatment

1 Nonsurgical debridement
2 Surgical debridement
3 Surgical exposure of the furcation
4 Regeneration (bone grafts, GTR, and biologicals)
5 Root resection
6 Tunnel preparation
7 Extraction

A review of 50 papers evaluating 1016 grade II furcations showed that regenerative treatment only resulted in complete closure of the furcation in 20% of the lesions and an improvement from grade II to a grade I furcation in 33% of the cases. In general, there was a 50% improvement in pocket depth reduction and clinical attachment gain with regenerative treatment of grade II furcations. The most effective treatment was a GTR combined with a bone graft (Evans *et al.*, 1996).

The following were found to reduce the frequency of clinical closure of class II defects when attempting to perform regenerative therapy (Bowers *et al.*, 2003):

1 Increased distance between the roof of the furcation and the crest of the bone
2 Increased distance between the roof of the furcation and the base of the defect
3 The depth of the horizontal defect
4 Increased divergence of roots at the crest of the bone
5 Smoking

Suppuration

Suppuration is a clinical sign of infection and inflammation. Increased levels of gingival inflammation and a slight increase in connective tissue neutrophils have been observed histologically in sites with suppuration (Passo *et al.*, 1988). Because suppuration is found in only 3–5% of sites with periodontal disease, by itself, it is not a reliable predictor of periodontal disease progression. Suppuration with other clinical parameters such as bleeding on probing and increased probing depth increases the positive predictive value of disease progression (Lang *et al.*, 2008). Periodontal health should include the absence of suppuration.

Prevention

Decreasing and maintaining low levels of bacterial biofilm result in the elimination of gingival suppuration. Good oral hygiene and frequent recalls can help in preventing suppuration following the active phase of treatment.

Treatment

Scaling and root planing, reevaluation, and a decision about surgical treatment are the options to eliminate suppuration. Kaldahl *et al.* (1990) looked at the effect of modified Widman flap surgery, osseous resective surgery, scaling and root planing, and coronal scaling in the treatment of periodontitis, including the elimination of gingival suppuration. Modified Widman flap surgery, osseous resective surgery, and scaling and root planing were more effective than coronal scaling in reducing suppuration in pockets greater than or equal to 5 mm.

Complications of periodontal treatment

Postoperative bleeding

Excessive bleeding following periodontal surgery can be a result of an overlooked medical condition (i.e., uncontrolled hypertension) or a medication taken by the patient (antiplatelet aggregation agents such as aspirin or other anticoagulant agents such as warfarin).

Bleeding after surgery can also be a result of other local and general factors, like mechanical trauma to the area, ingestion of hot liquids (coffee, soup, etc.), or extensive physical activities.

Flap preparation and suturing are important factors in preventing postoperative bleeding. Poor adaptation of the flap to the underlying bone where "dead" spaces are created can result in postoperative hemorrhage. The blood clot that often forms in such spaces and its dislodgment may initiate bleeding in the course of healing. Proper flap preparation, suturing, and digital pressure application immediately after surgery will minimize the possibility of such "dead" spaces to develop.

Prevention

1 Thorough examination of the patient's medical history
2 Knowledge of nonprescription and prescription medications that the patient may be taking
3 Achievement of hemostasis at the end of the surgery and before the patient is dismissed
4 Proper postoperative instructions

Treatment

Removal of the blood clot by the patient is necessary. If bleeding is indeed active, digital pressure with a 2×2 gauze compress or a black tea bag for an uninterrupted period of 10 min is the first step. Should it not be effective, the dental professional must assess the patient for emergency treatment.

In-office management of postoperative bleeding includes identification of the bleeding area, injection of the anesthetic solution that contains vasoconstrictor, removal of any blood clot present in the area, and possible resuturing of the surgical area. The aforementioned steps can be combined with the application of local clot formation-enhancing agents such as oxidized cellulose polymer (polyanhydroglucuronic acid), which can be cut in different shapes and placed over the affected area. Microfibrillar collagen is another effective hemostatic agent. It is delivered to the bleeding site with the use of a forceps, and it attracts and immobilizes platelets efficiently.

If the patient fails to respond to in-office treatment, referral to an emergency room for further management is recommended.

Nerve injury

Please see section "Implant Hits a Nerve" in Chapter 7.

Postsurgical inflammation/edema/pain/infection

The signs of inflammation include rubor (redness), tumor (swelling), calor (heat), dolor (pain), and loss of function. Edema or gingival swelling can be found in inflamed gingival tissues. There is an accumulation of fluids in the connective tissue due to increased permeability as a result of inflammation. Edema causes the gingival margins to be more rounded, puffy, and enlarged. Periodontal therapy, whether surgical or nonsurgical, is associated with systemic inflammation (Graziani *et al.*, 2010).

There are two reasons why edema may occur. It may occur due to inflammation or infection. When edema is caused by inflammation, the edema peaks at the third day and subsides thereafter as opposed to when the edema is associated with an infection and the edema increase after the third day. Table 2.1 discusses the differences.

It is expected for a patient to have pain following periodontal surgery; however, severe pain may indicate abnormal healing. Curtis, McLain, and Hutchinson (1985) evaluated pain with flap surgery, mucogingival surgery, and osseous surgery and reported 5.5% (304 patients) of cases had moderate to severe pain. Mucogingival surgery was 3.5 times more likely to cause pain than osseous surgery.

Prevention

1 Reduce surgical time.
2 Clean incisions, gentle handling of flaps, avoiding temperatures to exceed 47°C (to prevent necrosis) and flaps healing by primary intention can help prevent pain (Greenstein *et al.* 2008)
3 Offering long-lasting analgesia right after surgery (bupivacaine)
4 Place cold ice packs for the first couple of hours
5 Patients should take nonsteroidal anti-inflammatory drugs even if they have no pain

The principles of asepsis must be followed to prevent infection. It is also prudent to do scaling and root planing before periodontal surgery to mechanically decrease the bacterial load. The data suggests that there is no benefit to prophylactic antibiotics to prevent infection (Pack and Haber, 1983; Callis, Lemmer, and Touyz, 1996). Routine prescription of antibiotics following periodontal surgery is not recommended (Tseng, Huang,

Table 2.1 Difference between edema associated with infection and inflammation.

Edema	Associated with inflammation	Associated with infection
Cause	Normal healing response	Mostly unknown
		Contamination during surgery
Time of onset	Increase till about the third day	Worsens after the third day
Pain	Discomfort for the first couple of days	Increased pain after a couple of days
Discharge	No	Yes
Common	Yes	Rare after periodontal therapy
		Found about 2% after periodontal surgery and 6% when surgery was done without osteoplasty or ostectomy (Powell *et al.*, 2005; Pack and Haber, 1983)
Treatment	Cold compresses	Systemic antibiotics

and Tseng, 1993). Lastly, it is of importance to debride the surgical site before suturing the flaps to remove loose debris.

Treatment

When treating pain, it is important to understand the cause of the pain before deciding to use drugs (see Table 2.2) to get rid of it. If fever and lymphadenopathy are present, antibiotics may be needed. The clinician should consider prescribing narcotics when nonsteroidal drugs are not working:

1 Inquire about the patient's medical and dental history (e.g., trauma from brushing or chewing food, temperature stimulus, mouth opening, lying down, presence of pulpal or periapical pathologies or caries, or root fracture on treated teeth or teeth adjacent to the surgical area, which may lead to a diagnosis of reversible or irreversible pulpitis and dentinal hypersensitivity)

2 Inquire about the patient's analgesic intake and compliance to postoperative instructions

3 Assess the presence of abnormal healing which may be due to an infection, flap dehiscence, or a bone sequestrum. If an infection is present, systemic antibiotics should be prescribed. For flap dehiscence, the dentist should mitigate the pain and give it adequate time to heal. A bone sequestrum should be removed

4 Assess radiographic enlargement of the periodontal ligament of teeth involved in the surgical area and the sensitivity to percussion, which may lead to a diagnosis of trauma from occlusion

Investigation of Pain (Durand *et al.*, 2013)

Table 2.2 Drug options for pain.

Drug and dosage	Frequency
Ibuprofen: 800 mg	Take one tablet every 8 h (may interfere with hypertensive drugs)
Acetaminophen: 300 mg Codeine: 30 mg	Take one tablet every 8 h
Hydrocodone: 7.5 mg Ibuprofen: 200 mg	Take one tablet every 6 h (q6h)
Hydrocodone: 5 mg Acetaminophen: 325 mg	Take one tablet every 6 h (q6h)
Oxycodone: 5 mg Acetaminophen: 325 mg	Take one tablet every 6 h (q6h)
Oxycodone: 4.88 mg Aspirin: 325 mg	Take one tablet every 6 h (q6h)

CASE: PATIENT DEVELOPS AN INFECTION

- A 40-year-old healthy patient calls her surgeon a week after she has pocket reduction complaining that she feels weak and feverish. The surgeon schedules her that day and finds (Figures 2.6 and 2.7) that the left side of her face is swollen and the surgical site is red, swollen, and erythematous.

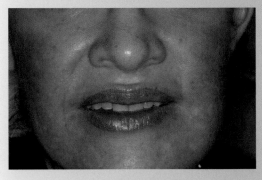

Figure 2.6 Patient presentation to the office (swelling on the left side).

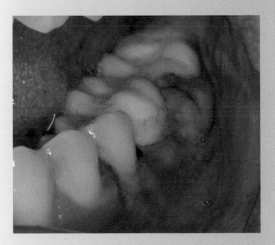

Figure 2.7 Infection at post-op (swollen and inflamed tissue).

- The patient has an infection. She was placed on clindamycin 300 mg three times a day for 8 days (she is allergic to penicillin). She was also put on a soft diet and was seen every other day for debridement of the area with saline and minocycline. The patient healed after 2 weeks and had no other complications.

Tooth/root sensitivity

Dentinal hypersensitivity is common in patients who have attrition, abrasion, erosion, and gingival recession of teeth. It usually affects individuals in between the ages of 20 and 50 years. The most common sites are the buccal-cervical regions of the canine and premolar teeth. Patients feel a short and sharp pain triggered by exposed dentinal tubules as a consequence to tactile, chemical, thermal, osmotic, or evaporative stimuli (Samuel, Khatri, and Acharya, 2014).

Management/treatment

The two most important points in the management of dentinal sensitivity are plaque control and patient education. Dental sensitivity is transient and may be resolved in 8 weeks following surgery (Trowbridge and Silver, 1990).

If the patient continues to complain of dentin hypersensitivity, there are several products available that can be applied either at home or in the office. The products that are available for home use take time to take effect. Patients should not eat or drink for 1 h following treatment with the agent.

Mobility of the teeth after surgery

Tooth mobility may be increased postsurgery, but it goes back to pretreatment levels by the fourth week (Klokkevold, Takei, and Carranza, 2006). It has been shown (Kerry *et al.*, 1982) that tooth mobility did not change following scaling and root planing, curettage, or modified Widman flap; however, mobility increased temporarily after surgery involving an apically positioned flap combined with osseous surgery. However that increased mobility returns to presurgical levels within 6 months.

Prevention

The clinician should exercise judgment in the amount of ostectomy performed because it can lead to permanent tooth mobility.

Treatment

Treatment is not recommended for this complication. Splinting may be necessary when the teeth do not return to presurgical levels or have increasing mobility.

Ecchymosis

Ecchymosis, a nonelevated hemorrhagic patch greater than 10 mm (Greenstein *et al.*, 2008), may result from bleeding into the tissue planes of the neck, injury to small capillaries, reflection of large flaps, and incomplete hemostasis. It is more common in the elderly and is of concern when infection is present. The ecchymosis may be tender at first, but it disappears rapidly. The bruise may take several days to get better. It may initially appear as a deep blue-black color to a lighter shade of purple and then green (Killey and Kay, 1977).

Prevention

Ecchymosis can be reduced with gentle soft tissue management. When elevating a flap, elevators should be placed on bone, and when flaps are repositioned, it is essential to place pressure for several minutes to allow the bleeding to cease. Lastly, the suction tip should be placed on bone and not on the soft tissue (Greenstein *et al.*, 2008).

Treatment

A comprehensive informed consent would educate and reassure the patient that the condition does not require any treatment and resolves by itself overtime.

Flap necrosis/wound dehiscence/flap tears or perforations

Flap necrosis is also referred to as sloughing, and it is a consequence of compromised blood supply to the flap. Healing occurs by secondary intention through the development of granulation tissue.

During the first 10 days following suturing, the wound may become dehisced and heal by secondary intention. This can be caused by poor suturing, flap tension, poor flap design (see the following text under the section "Prevention"), trauma, dead space, radiation therapy, and flap perforation at the base (Greenstein *et al.*, 2008).

Flap tears can be a major complication and may occur because the tissue is thin, there are exostosis present that make it more difficult to reflect the tissue, or an incomplete incision (do not use a dull blade) was made and reflection causes a tear.

Prevention

Proper flap design and management are important in preventing necrosis. Specific factors are:

1 Flap wider at the base
2 Flap thicker at the base
3 Overall flap thickness
4 Avoidance of flap perforations
5 Flap adaptation

Wound dehiscence can be prevented if there is adequate extension and reflection of the flaps (tension-free closure). Proper suturing techniques including a minimal amount of sutures are used (to prevent an ischemic incident) (Fugazzotto, 1999), and the flaps are sutured without tension. Dentures should be relined and relieved to prevent any trauma to the surgical site. Smokers should refrain from smoking after surgery to prevent wound dehiscence. To prevent pull from muscles, interrupted sutures with mattress sutures should be used (Greenstein *et al.*, 2008).

Flap perforation can be prevented with careful planing and reflection of an adequately sized flap and employing a gentle surgical technique to prevent too much tension. Adequate flap release is important to prevent flap perforation, and that can be achieved via vertical incisions and mesial–distal extension of the surgical area to avoid tension on the flap. It is also important to place the surgical suction away from the thin tissue to prevent a tear in the flap. Cortellini and Tonetti (2001) found that microsurgery can limit soft tissue damage, improve soft tissue healing, and limit recession.

Management

Time is the most important factor when managing flap necrosis. Since the bone becomes exposed following soft tissue necrosis, its outermost layers also become nonviable. Osteoclasts have to migrate from underlying viable bone in order to resorb the necrotic portion of it. It is only after the completion of the resorption process that new soft tissue will develop in the area. This process is long and uncomfortable for the patient. Analgesic medication is usually necessary for prolonged periods of time. Chlorhexidine and/or antibiotics should also be prescribed for the patient to avoid secondary infection. In order to accelerate necrotic bone resorption, its mechanical removal can be performed with rotary instruments under local anesthesia. In certain cases, particularly those of overall thin bone, flap and bone necrosis can lead to permanent deformities of the alveolar house and result in tooth loss.

If a perforation occurs, the flaps should be cautiously repositioned and sutured first, and then the tear should be sutured with 6.0 absorbable sutures.

CASE

- A 63-year-old patient with mild hypertension and high cholesterol presented to the office with generalized 4–6 mm pockets on the lower left side. She had osseous surgery on #17–#21. After surgery there was necrosis of the lingual flap (Figure 2.8). Ibuprofen 800 mg 3×/day for 1 week was prescribed with chlorhexidine rinses. The soft tissue healed after 2.5 months.

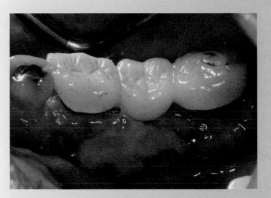

Figure 2.8 A case of necrosis on the lingual flap.

Suture abscess

This complication is often caused when a part of the suture is not removed at the postoperative appointment.

Prevention

Sharp surgical scissors should be utilized for suture removal. The number of sutures placed at the time of surgery should be documented in the notes and then checked at the time of suture removal (Killey and Kay, 1977). The use of resorbable sutures would avoid the need to remove the suture, and thus prevent a possible suture abscess.

Treatment

The patient may need to be given local anesthesia, and the suture must be recovered. An incision is made in the mucosa and the abscess is drained, and the area is curetted. The area can remain unsutured to allow drainage. The patient may also be given a course of antibiotics (Vastardis and Yukna, 2003).

Loss of the interdental papilla

Inappropriate flap design and diminished blood supply to the papilla can cause it to be lost. The effect of papilla loss includes phonetic problems, esthetic impairment, and interproximal food entrapment. The treatment plan depends on whether the interdental papilla loss has occurred in an esthetic area.

Prevention

Because it is extremely difficult to reconstruct papillae, they must be preserved. When planing flap design and the teeth are not too close interproximally, a papilla preservation flap may be used. The papilla is incorporated into the lingual or facial flap.

Treatment

Esthetic: The success of papillae reconstruction depends on the distance between the bone crest and the interproximal contact point (Tarnow, Magner, and Fletcher, 1992). According to many studies, predictable reconstruction of lost interproximal papillae is not yet possible. Forced eruption may be the best way to bring tissue down to support the interdental papilla. The entire attachment of a tooth will follow the root of the tooth as it is moved coronally. Restorative materials (pink acrylic or porcelain) can also be used to enhance the esthetics in the area. The patient should be educated on proper oral hygiene as well.

Procedure specific complications

Free gingival graft
Bleeding from the donor site (palate)

The area of most concern is the posterior palate. It is important to understand the average distances from the greater palatine foramen (should be avoided) to the cementoenamel junction (CEJ). Guidelines for average distances have been described as follows (Reiser *et al.*, 1996):

- Deep palate: 17 mm
- Average depth palate: 12 mm
- Shallow palate: 7 mm

Bleeding following a free gingival graft may be caused by severing the vessel. All attempts should be made to achieve hemostasis before the palate is resutured. This should be done to prevent bleeding into the tissue planes of the neck (Killey and Kay, 1977).

Prevention

1 Knowledge of key anatomical landmarks and avoiding an incision at or around the greater palatine foramen.
2 Locate the greater palatine foramen with tactile pressure around the first, second, or third molar.
3 The graft should be between 0.75 and 1.25 mm in thickness so that enough connective tissue is obtained and no deeper to prevent injuring branches of the greater palatine foramen.
4 Instructions after surgery play an important role in preventing postoperative bleeding.
5 A surgical stent should be made for the patient to prevent bleeding by protecting the surgical wound in the donor area.

Management

1 Remove the clot and identify the area of bleeding.
2 Apply pressure at the site for at least 10 min with a 2 × 2 gauze.
3 If bleeding has not stopped, infiltrate anesthetic with epinephrine 1 : 50 000 (depending on patient's medical history) for vasoconstriction and temporarily stop the bleeding.
4 The blood vessel may be clamped with a hemostat to prevent further bleeding.
5 The application of a topical hemostatic agent, such as Surgicel or Avitene (Davol), can be delivered to the site to enhance the formation and stabilization of a clot.
6 If none of the above work, ligation of the bleeding area with a suture can be attempted.

Free gingival graft detachment postoperatively

A free gingival graft is sutured to the recipient site using a variety of suturing techniques (i.e., sling, interrupted sutures). There are several reasons why a free gingival graft becomes detached, and this can be due to poor adaptation (i.e., the graft is too big for the site), inadequate suturing technique, or the use of the wrong suture material.

Prevention

Suturing of a free gingival graft should be conducted with sutures that have a small needle and thin thread (i.e., 5.0 or 6.0). Synthetic materials such as monofilament are hydrophobic, less subject to bacterial contamination, and result in less tissue marks along the incision lines. It is particularly indicated for microsurgical procedures. It has been shown that the use of ethyl cyanoacrylate did not alter the graft healing process when compared to using sutures (Barbosa *et al.*, 2009).

Suturing technique is essential to prevent graft detachment. The graft needs to be sutured along the horizontal incision and vertical incision, if used. Periosteal sutures anchored around the treated teeth are useful in eliminating spaces between the underlying tissue and the graft which may lead to poor vascularization. Digital pressure should also be applied to the graft to prevent dead space.

Management

A new graft has to be done in 4–6 weeks after the donor site and recipient site have healed.

CASE

- A 50-year-old healthy male comes to the office for a free gingival graft on the lower anterior teeth. The graft is sutured with gut (Figure 2.9), and the patient leaves the office. That night the patient calls the surgeon complaining that the graft has come out. When the patient presents to the office the next day, it is obvious that the graft has detached. Minimal keratinized attached tissue is found a month later (Figure 2.10). The graft was not sutured correctly (the graft was not sutured to the periosteum or the lateral borders), and a better suture material should have been used (polypropylene 6.0). There is also a visible dead space beneath the graft. The patient will have to receive a new graft.

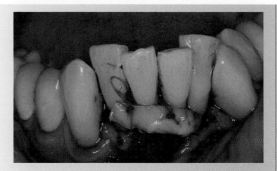

Figure 2.9 The graft was sutured inappropriately.

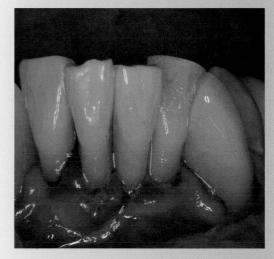

Figure 2.10 One month after graft detachment.

Graft shrinkage

Free gingival grafts can shrink as much as 45% for very thin, 44% for thin, and 38% for intermediate grafts as compared to their original dimension (Mormann, Schaer, and Firestone, 1981). It is prudent to prepare a recipient site that is 50% larger than the intended result would be. After treatment the surgical objections are achieved.

Management

Although some shrinkage is expected, it is prudent to have a graft thickness between 0.75 and 1.25 mm (a thinner graft can lead to more shrinkage). If there is excessive shrinkage, then the dentist needs to assess the site for further mucogingival surgical treatment.

Connective tissue graft
Failure to cover the root

The mean expected root coverage by a connective tissue graft is 84% (Greenwell *et al.*, 2005). There are many reasons why connective tissue grafts may fail or only partially succeed:

1 Smoking: Root coverage procedures are less predictable and successful in smokers than in nonsmokers (58.02% versus 83.35% respectively) (Souza *et al.*, 2008).
2 Full coverage of connective tissue grafts with a flap improves blood supply and decreases the possibility of dieback.
3 The defect is too deep and/or wide.
4 Mobility of the graft postoperatively.
5 Increased flap tension because of improper periosteal release at the base.

Prevention

Refraining from smoking to the extent possible is beneficial for healing. It is also important to be able to stabilize the graft (without tension) with sutures to prevent its movement during healing. Vertical incisions should be used cautiously as they tend to cause more pain, swelling, and decreased blood circulation. The flap should have a broad base, and the length to width ratio should not exceed 2 : 1.

Treatment

Depending on the amount of root coverage already obtained (if any) and the esthetic concerns of the patient, a second procedure may need to be done.

Shallow vestibule following surgery

A shallow vestibule may be a consequence of a connective tissue graft that is combined with coronal advancement of the flap. This can lead to difficulty in

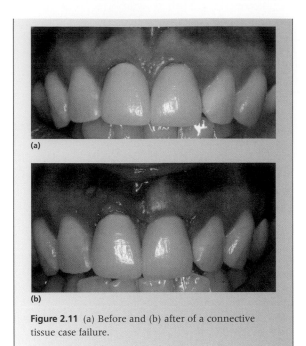

Figure 2.11 (a) Before and (b) after of a connective tissue case failure.

following proper oral hygiene measures and prosthetic problems (especially in patients that use partial or full dentures) (Ho, Elangovan, and Shih, 2012).

Prevention

If the vestibule is too shallow at baseline, then the area should be treated with a free gingival graft to increase the vestibular depth prior to placement of the connective tissue graft.

Treatment

The patient may need to get vestibuloplasty or a free gingival graft (if there is a lack of keratinized attached gingiva). Studies on deepening the vestibule found that they were not effective unless a free gingival graft (or a variant) was used (Takei, Azzi, and Han, 2006).

Flap surgery for pocket reduction or crown lengthening

The principles of flap preparation and osseous resection in surgeries for pocket reduction or crown lengthening are similar. Therefore, the complications associated with both procedures are alike.

CASE

- A 40-year-old patient presented for a connective tissue graft on #8 and #9. She did not like the gingival recession on #8 and #9. She wanted the teeth to look even and the roots to be covered. A connective tissue procedure was performed (Figure 2.11a and b), but the roots were not evenly covered. A second procedure is necessary to address the patients' concerns.

Nicking the adjacent tooth/root

Prevention

The use of instruments, rotary or manual, that are adequate in size combined with magnification are the most effective techniques to avoid unintended tooth damage. If root proximity is severe, consideration can be given to orthodontic treatment prior to surgical therapy.

It is important to note that when performing crown lengthening, it is recommended to use end-cutting burs for ostectomy to prevent nicking an adjacent tooth.

Treatment

Root damage can only be remediated with odontoplasty, restoration, or, in extreme cases, extraction.

Furcation defect while trying to maintain positive architecture

It is important to have knowledge of the association between furcations and the anatomy in the area when performing osseous surgery.

The differences in the position of the furcation entrance are as follows (Bower, 1979):

Mandibular molars: Buccal furcation opening is more coronal than lingual furcation entrance.

Maxillary molars: Mesial entrance width is bigger than the distal entrance width which is greater than the buccal entrance width.

The longer the root trunk, the easier it would be for the clinician to perform osseous surgery and maintain positive architecture without creating furcation involvement. In the process of osseous surgery, the clinician needs to be cautious of protecting bone in the furcation. If the establishment of positive architecture requires bone removal in furcations that are otherwise closed, resection is contraindicated.

Prevention

The palatal approach is advocated when performing osseous surgery on maxillary molars because the surgeon can avoid exposure of the buccal furcation (Ochsenbein and Bohannan, 1963). A lingual approach is recommended for the mandibular molars because the furcation on the lingual aspect is in a more apical position than the buccal, the bottom of the crater is usually located more lingually because of the natural lingual incline of the bicuspids and molars, the root length is shorter on the facial, and the buccal furcation is avoided (Tibbettes, Ochsenbein, and Loughlin, 1976).

If creating positive architecture would compromise the prognosis of the tooth/teeth in the surgical area by creating iatrogenic furcation lesions and/or creating poor crown to root ratio, it may be more prudent to adopt the regenerative approach, leave residual negative architecture, or consider extracting the tooth and replacing it.

Treatment

Figure 2.12 depicts treatment options for furcation involvement.

Recession following surgery

There is a tendency for recession after periodontal surgery because the bone supports the soft tissue. Studies have shown that following periodontal therapy the gingival margin often shifts an apical direction (Lindhe and Nyman, 1980; Gupta and Vandana, 2009). This may lead to dental sensitivity and esthetic issues. The greatest change occurs in the first 6 months following therapy with 29% of sites experiencing an apical shift (Isidor, Karring, and Attstrom, 1984). Performing surgery in the anterior region may create an esthetic compromise (Figure 2.13) particularly if the patient has a high smile line. The patient must know that esthetics can be compromised and be informed of all risks and alternatives. In cases that combine periodontal surgery and restorative dentistry, it is important to wait 6–12 months for the gingival margin to stabilize (Pontoriero and Carnevale, 2001).

Prevention

There is no way to prevent recession in the periodontal area. If surgery must be done, conservative therapy is preferred. Therefore, when considering surgery in the anterior segment, consideration should be given to perioscopy and the papilla preservation technique:

1 Perioscopy: Allows real-time indirect visualization of the root during scaling and root planing. According to Stambaugh (2002), it "can offer many patients an alternative to periodontal surgery in carefully selected sites."

2 Papilla preservation flap, as described by Takei *et al.* (1985), where a palatal incision is made to allow the papilla to move in a buccal direction. However, adequate width (>2 mm) of the papilla is necessary as well as a sufficient embrasure space.

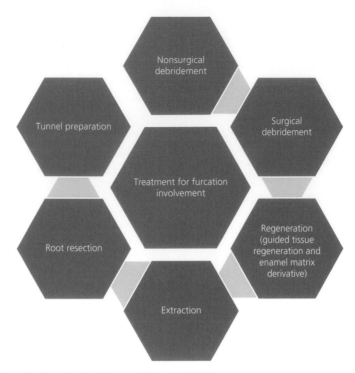

Figure 2.12 Treatment options for furcation involvement. Termeie (2013).

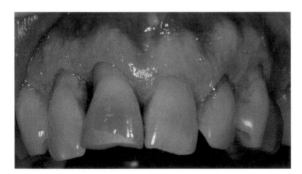

Figure 2.13 Recession after pocket reduction surgery.

Treatment

The patient may complain of sensitivity (please see complication tooth/root dental sensitivity in this chapter) following surgery. The only method of improving the esthetic concerns of a patient of recession following surgery is restorative dentistry (e.g., bonding).

According to many studies, reconstruction of lost interproximal papillae is not yet predictable. The success depends on the distance between the bone crest and the interproximal contact point (Tarnow, Magner, and Fletcher, 1992). Hirsch *et al.* (2004) found that flap debridement with a subepithelial connective tissue graft (with maintenance therapy) was effective in preventing mandibular anterior tooth recession. Lastly, restorative techniques (pink acrylic) can mask some of the recession.

Sequestrum formation postoperatively

Very rarely, a small sharp area of the bone can perforate through the gingival tissues and occasionally detach from the bone. This is called a sequestrum and occurs when gingival tissues are very thin and the bone becomes sharp during the remodeling that occurs with this type of surgery. It may also occur after the surgeon recontours the bone but fails to smooth the sharp areas that can poke through the soft tissue.

Management

The sequestrum will usually take care of itself. Unfortunately, this can take several weeks and the area can cause discomfort while it is healing. The sequestrum will usually exfoliate on its own which is usually followed by soft tissue healing.

Regenerative therapy

Membrane exposure during regeneration

Table 2.3 describes the characteristics of two types of membranes.

There is a 96.1% success rate for the maintenance of primary soft tissue closure which means that there is a premature membrane exposure 3.9% of the time in 695 cases studied (Fugazzotto, 1999). Machtei (2001) found that nonabsorbable and absorbable membrane exposure during healing had a minimal effect on GTR around natural teeth.

Another study (De Sanctis, Zucchelli, and Clauser, 1996) following patients with chronic periodontitis found that exposed areas of membranes had bacterial colonization in all the microscopic fields. Although no bacteria-positive field was observed in the most apical portion of the membranes, the middle portion of many of the membranes (16 of 39 (41%)) demonstrated microbial colonization.

Prevention

The patient should take antibiotics for at least 1 week postoperatively and rinse with 0.12% chlorhexidine for 12 weeks after guided bone regeneration to reduce postoperative infection and ensure optimal clinical results (Villar and Cochran, 2010). The flap should be designed to allow adequate blood flow and flap closure (adequate release of the flaps is essential). The flaps should be

sutured together with a horizontal mattress and then single interrupted sutures (Fontana, Rocchietta, and Simion, 2010).

A study by Nowzari, Matian, and Slots (1995) had the experimental group receive Augmentin (GlaxoSmithKline) and GTR while the control group only had GTR. A significantly higher gain in mean probing attachment was found at 6 months in the test group (36.5% of potential gain to the cementoenamel junction) compared with the control group (22.4% of potential gain). When the membranes were removed, significantly fewer organisms were found in the test group ($52.2 \times 10(6)$) compared with the control group ($488.6 \times 10(6)$).

Lastly, smoking has an effect on membrane exposure. One paper (Lindfors *et al.*, 2010) found that bone grafts covered with a nonabsorbable membrane in smokers were successful in 63% of cases, whereas the success rate in nonsmokers was 95%.

Treatment

Figure 2.14 presents the steps involved in postoperative management of membrane exposure. The membrane should be monitored, and if infection is evident, it should be removed.

If the antibiotic prescribed fails to eradicate the infection, a broader spectrum antibiotic can be prescribed (Amoxicillin can be changed to Augmentin). When the infection persists after the antibiotic treatment, the site needs to be reopened and debrided.

Failure to regenerate the periodontal unit

It is important to allow selective cells to repopulate the wound.

As suggested by Melcher (1976), the repopulation of the defect by cells that originate from the Periodontal ligament and bone will improve predictability of the surgical procedure.

Table 2.3 Characteristics of resorbable and nonresorbable membranes.

Resorbable	Nonresorbable
• Removal is not necessary	• First to be developed
• Collagenases break down the collagen membrane	• Another surgery is needed to remove it

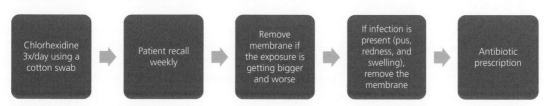

Figure 2.14 Postoperative management of membrane exposure. Termeie (2013). Reproduced with permission from Quintessence Publishing Company Inc., Chicago, IL.

Melcher believed that it was important to exclude epithelium and allow selective repopulation of the wound.

Additionally, there are other factors that can negatively impact periodontal regeneration:

1 Anatomy of the defect: There are greater linear gains in deeper pockets, and a site with an angle of 25° or less (bony wall to long axis of the tooth) had 1.6 mm more attachment than in defects with an angle of 37° or more (Tonetti, Pini-Prato, and Cortellini, 1993). The greater the number of walls, the better the regenerative outcome (Kim *et al.*, 2004). Another study found that the intrabony defect has to be at least 4 mm deep to benefit from GTR procedures (Laurell *et al.*, 1998).
2 Poor oral hygiene.
3 Inflammation: It should be controlled as much as possible before surgery as well as after surgery for more effective flap management and minimal swelling.
4 Poor technique: Inadequate soft tissue to cover the defect because of poor flap design.
5 Hypermobility of the teeth: Severe hypermobility can negatively impact the clinical outcome of regeneration (Cortellini, Labriola, and Tonetti, 2007). If needed, teeth should be splinted.
6 Smoking: Studies have shown that smokers have less pocket reduction than nonsmokers in bone regeneration studies (Tonetti, Pini-Prato, and Cortellini, 1995; Stravropoulos *et al.*, 2004).
7 Systemic issues (e.g., poorly controlled diabetes and immune suppression).

Prevention

Good defect selection and oral hygiene with proper maintenance, proper flap design, tooth splinting, and elimination of smoking can lead to more favorable outcomes. Adequate presurgical therapy can reduce tissue trauma.

Treatment

The surgeon may decide that due to anatomical factors or social behaviors (for instance, smoking) regeneration was not ideal for the patient. Osseous surgery or more frequent scaling and root planing appointments may be an alternative approach. However, if the cause of the first failed regenerative attempt is understood and can be avoided, regeneration may be attempted again.

Insufficient keratinized tissue to cover the defect and regenerative devices

It is important for the surgeon to plan the flap design and predict the need to cover the bone graft and barrier membranes. If the membrane or graft becomes exposed, it can compromise the outcome (Rose and Minsk, 2004).

Management

It is important for the surgeon to design a flap with tension-free closure. Vertical incisions, coronal advancement, and periosteal releasing incisions (at the base of the flap) may be required to allow the flap to cover the surgical site. Horizontal mattress sutures and interrupted sutures allow the flap to be stabilized (Rose and Minsk, 2004). If the lack of keratinized attached tissue appears critical, a free gingival graft should be done as a separate procedure.

Complications to the periodontium influenced by trauma from occlusion

Clinical signs of trauma include wear facets, tooth fracture, increased tooth mobility, loss of the lamina dura and increased periodontal ligament (pdl) space (radiographically), tooth migration, pain on chewing, occlusal prematurities, fremitus, hypertrophy of muscles of mastication, and temporomandibular joint dysfunction.

Occlusion can impact periodontitis in two important ways:

1 Trauma in the absence of inflammation
2 Trauma in the presence of inflammation induced by the bacterial biofilm

Trauma in the absence of inflammation

Trauma from occlusion in the absence of biofilm-induced inflammation will change bone levels, but it will not induce apical migration of the junctional epithelium. In these cases, if trauma from occlusion is treated, bone changes are reversible. Trauma from occlusion combined with biofilm-induced inflammation may accelerate the rate of attachment loss.

Treatment

In areas where occlusal forces are necessary, therapy can be performed by occlusal adjustment, splining, and fabrication of an occlusal appliance. Splint therapy has been found to be harmless (Gümüş *et al.*, 2013) and effective. Patients who have had implant therapy and found to have bruxism should use a rigid occlusal stabilization appliance alleviated in the region of implants (Sarmento *et al.*, 2012).

Inflammation of the supporting tissues in the presence of occlusal trauma

One proposed theory is that inflammation of the supporting tissues in the presence of occlusal trauma alters the alignment of the transseptal fibers allowing inflammation to spread to the periodontal ligament (pdl) space with resultant intrabony pocket formation (Glickman, 1963). Another theory is that traumatic occlusion does not initiate or aggravate gingivitis or initiate pockets, but it can increase mobility and may

accelerate bone loss and pocket formation, depending on the presence of inflammation (Ramfjord and Ash, 1981). Others believe that bacterial plaque in conjunction with local anatomy is the primary cause of intrabony defect formation, not occlusal trauma (Waerhaug, 1979). Trauma from occlusion may constitute an additional risk factor for severity and progression of the disease, but it does not cause periodontal pockets or gingivitis (Carranza, 2006). Tooth mobility may be initiated by inflammation as well as other causes (Figure 2.15).

Prevention

It is important to prevent biofilm inflammation by instructing patients on proper oral hygiene and having a regular maintenance schedule for each patient.

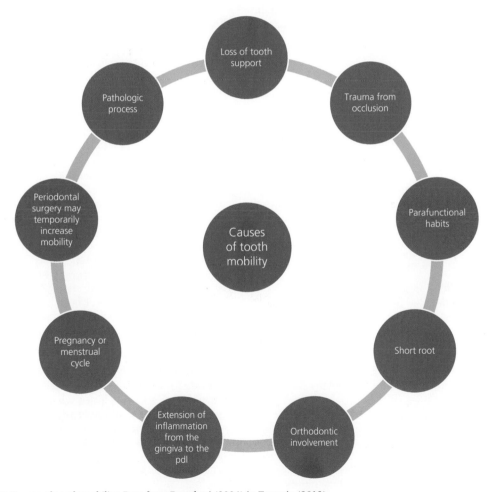

Figure 2.15 Causes of tooth mobility. Data from Donghari (2004) in Termeie (2013).

Treatment

It is vital to remove the inflammation in patients with trauma from occlusion because it has been shown that in regions that are kept healthy and clean after preexisting inflammation, trauma from occlusion did not induce progressive destruction of the periodontal tissues (Ericsson and Lindhe, 1977).

Periodontitis can be treated and periodontal health maintained in the presence of traumatic occlusal forces without occlusal adjustment. When occlusal adjustment was incorporated as a component of periodontal therapy, statistically greater gains in clinical periodontal attachment level have been reported. The extent is currently unclear. Once periodontal health is determined, occlusal therapy can be employed to regain bone lost due to traumatic occlusal forces, to reduce mobility, and to alleviate an assortment of clinical problems related to occlusal instability and restorative needs (Gher, 1998). This indicates that the role played by trauma from occlusion in progression of periodontitis is secondary.

Occlusal adjustment is effective in reducing tooth mobility when mobility is caused by increased width of pdl (Lindhe, Nyman, and Ericsson, 2008). Burgett *et al.* (1992) found that there is a significant gain of 0.4 mm in attachment in patients who receive occlusal adjustment. There was no effect of occlusal adjustment on the response in pocket depth, nor did initial tooth mobility or initial periodontal disease severity influence the response to occlusal adjustment. Splinting teeth is indicated in the following situations (Lemmerman, 1976):

1 To prevent drifting of the teeth
2 For comfort
3 To prevent mobility
4 Following trauma

Lastly, an interocclusal appliance (a reversible way of redistributing force) for the maxilla with full palatal coverage helps tighten teeth with its increased surface area compared to an appliance that only covers the occlusal surfaces (McDevitt and Bibb, 2006).

References

Barbosa, F.I., Corrêa, D.S., Zenóbio, E.G., Costa, F.O. and Shibli, J.A. (2009) Dimensional changes between free gingival grafts fixed with ethyl cyanoacrylate and silk sutures. *J Int Acad Periodontol.*, **11**, 170–176.

Becker, W., Becker, B.E. and Berg, L.E. (1984) Periodontal treatment without maintenance. A retrospective study in 44 patients. *J Periodontol*, **55**, 505–509.

Bower, R.C. (1979) Furcation morphology relative to periodontal treatment. Furcation root surface anatomy. *J Periodontol*, **50**, 366–374.

Bowers, G.M., Schallhorn, R.G., McClain, P.K., Morrison, G.M., Morgan, R. and Reynolds, M.A. (2003) Factors influencing the outcome of regenerative therapy in mandibular class II furcations: Part 1. *J Periodontol*, **74**, 1255–1268.

Brown, L.J., Oliver, R.C. and Löe, H. (1989) Periodontal diseases in the U.S. in 1981: Prevalence, severity, extent, and role in tooth mortality. *J Periodontol*, **60**, 363–370.

Burgett, F.G., Ramfjord, S.P., Nissle, R.R., Morrison, E.C., Charbeneau, T.D. and Caffesse, R.G. (1992) A randomized trial of occlusal adjustment in the treatment of periodontitis patients. *J Clin Periodontol*, **19**, 381–387.

Callis, S., Lemmer, J. and Touyz, L.Z. (1996) Antibiotic prophylaxis in periodontal surgery. A retrospective study. *J Dent Assoc S Afr*, **5**, 1806–1809.

Carranza, F.A. (2006) Periodontal response to external forces, in *Carranza's Clinical Periodontology*, 10th edn (eds M.G. Newman, H. Takei, P.R. Klokkevold and F.A. Carranza), Elsevier Saunders, St. Louis, MO, p. 474.

Cohen, R.E. (2003) Research, Science and Therapy Committee of the American Academy of Periodontology. Position paper: Periodontal maintenance. *J Periodontol*, **74**, 1395–1401.

Cortellini, P. and Tonetti, M.S. (2001) Microsurgical approach to periodontal regeneration. Initial evaluation in a case cohort. *J Periodontol*, **72**, 559–569.

Cortellini, P., Labriola, A. and Tonetti, M.S. (2007) Regenerative periodontal therapy in intrabony defects: state of the art. *Minerva Stomatol*, **56**, 519–539.

Curtis, J.W., Jr, McLain, J.B. and Hutchinson, R.A. (1985) The incidence and severity of complications and pain following periodontal surgery. *J Periodontol*, **56**, 597–601.

De Sanctis, M., Zucchelli, G. and Clauser, C. (1996) Bacterial colonization of bioabsorbable barrier material and periodontal regeneration. *J Periodontol*, **67**, 1193–1200.

Dicus-Brookes, C., Partrick, M., Blakey, G.H., 3rd, Faulk-Eggleston, J., Offenbacher, S., Phillips, C. and White, R.P., Jr (2013) Removal of symptomatic third molars may improve periodontal status of remaining dentition. *J Oral Maxillofac Surg.*, **71**, 1639–1646.

Dongari-Bagtzoglu, A. (2004) Research, Science and Therapy Committee of the American Academy of Periodontology. Drug-assisted gingival enlargement. *J Periodontol*, **75**, 1424–1431.

Durand, R., Tran, S.D., Mui, B. and Voyer, R. (2013) *Managing Postoperative Pain Following Periodontal Surgery*, http://www.jcda.ca/article/d66 (assessed November 14, 2013).

Ericsson, I. and Lindhe, J. (1977) Lack of effect of trauma from occlusion on the recurrence of experimental periodontitis. *J Clin Periodontol*, **4**, 115.

Evans, G.H., Yukna, R.A., Gardiner, D.L. and Cambre, K.M. (1996) Frequency of furcation closure with regenerative periodontal therapy. *J West Soc Periodontol Abstr*, **44**, 101–109.

Fontana, F., Rocchietta, I. and Simion, M. (2010) Complications in guided bone regeneration, in *Dental Implant Complications Etiology, Prevention, and Treatment* (ed S. Froum), John Wiley & Sons, Chichester, p. 271.

Fugazzotto, P.A. (1999) Maintenance of soft tissue closure following guided bone regeneration: technical considerations and report of 723 cases. *J Periodontol.*, **70**, 1085–1097.

Gher, M.E. (1998) Changing concepts. The effects of occlusion on periodontitis. *Dent Clin North Am*, **42**, 285–299.

Glickman, I. (1953) *Clinical Periodontology: The Periodontium in Health and Disease; Recognition, Diagnosis and Treatment of Periodontal Disease in the Practice of General Dentistry*, Saunders, Philadelphia, PA.

Glickman, I. (1963) Inflammation and trauma from occlusion. Co-destructive factors in chronic periodontic disease. *J Periodontol*, **34**, 5–10.

Graziani, F., Cei, S., Tonetti, M., Paolantonio, M., Serio, R., Sammartino, G., Gabriele, M. and D'Aiuto, F. (2010) Systemic inflammation following non-surgical and surgical periodontal therapy. *J Clin Periodontol*, **37**, 848–854.

Greenstein, G., Cavallaro, J., Romanos, G. and Tarnow, D. (2008) Clinical recommendations for avoiding and managing surgical complications associated with implant dentistry: a review. *J Periodontol*, **79**, 1317–1329.

Greenwell, H., Fiorellini, J., Giannobile, W., Offenbacher, S., Salkin, L., Townsend, C., Sheridan, P., Genco, R. and Research, Science and Therapy Committee (2005) Oral reconstructive and corrective considerations in periodontal therapy. *J Periodontol*, **76**, 1588–1600.

Gümüş, H.Ö., Kılınç, H.İ., Tuna, S.H. and Ozcan, N. (2013) Computerized analysis of occlusal contacts in bruxism patients treated with occlusal splint therapy. *J Adv Prosthodont.*, **5**, 256–261.

Gupta, I. and Vandana, K.L. (2009) Alterations of the marginal soft tissue (gingival margin) following periodontal therapy: a clinical study. *J Indian Soc Periodontol.*, **13**, 85–89.

Hall, E.E. (1997) Prevention and treatment considerations in patients with drug-induced gingival enlargement. *Curr Opin Periodontol*, **4**, 59–63.

Hirsch, A., Brayer, L., Shapira, L. and Goldstein, M. (2004) Prevention of gingival recession following flap debridement surgery by subepithelial connective tissue graft: consecutive case series. *J Periodontol.*, **75** (5), 757–761.

Hirschfeld, L. and Wasserman, B. (1978) A long-term survey of tooth loss in 600 treated periodontal patients. *J Periodontol*, **49**, 225–237.

Ho, D.K.T., Elangovan, S. and Shih, S.D. (2012) Frenectomy and vestibuloplasty, in *Clinical Cases in Periodontics* (ed N. Karimbux), John Wiley & Sons, Chichester, p. 201.

Hupp, J.R., Ellis, E. and Tucker, M.R. (2008) *Contemporary Oral and Maxillofacial Surgery*, 5th edn, Mosby, St. Louis, MO, p. 153.

Isidor, F., Karring, T. and Attstrom, R. (1984) The effect of root planing as compared to that of surgical treatment. *J Clin Periodontol.*, **11**, 669–681.

Johnson, G.K. and Slach, N.A. (2001) Impact of tobacco use on periodontal status. *J Dent Educ*, **65**, 313–321.

Juniper, R.P. and Parkins, B.J. (1990) *Emergencies in Dental Practice*, Heinemann Professional Publishing, Oxford Ltd, p. 19.

Kaldahl, W.B., Kalkwarf, K.L., Patil, K.D. and Molvar, M.P. (1990) Evaluation of gingival suppuration and supragingival plaque following 4 modalities of periodontal therapy. *J Clin Periodontol*, **17**, 642–649.

Kerry, G.J., Morrison, E.C., Ramfjord, S.P., Hill, R.W., Caffesse, R.G., Nissle, R.R. and Appleberry, E.A. (1982) Effect of periodontal treatment on tooth mobility. *J Periodontol*, **53**, 635–638.

Killey, H.C. and Kay, L.W. (1977) *The Prevention of Complications in Dental Surgery*, Churchill Livingstone, Edinburgh, p. 48.

Kim, C.S., Choi, S.H., Chai, J.K., Cho, K.S., Moon, I.S., Wikesjö, U.M. and Kim, C.K. (2004) Periodontal repair in surgically created intrabony defects in dogs: influence of the number of bone walls on healing response. *J Periodontol*, **75**, 229–235.

Klokkevold, P.R., Takei, H.H. and Carranza, F.A. (2006) General principles of periodontal surgery, in *Carranza's Clinical Periodontology*, 10th edn (eds M.G. Newman, H.H. Takei, P.R. Klokkevold and F.A. Carranza), Elsevier Saunders, St. Louis, MO, p. 894.

Lang, N.P., Brägger, U., Salvi, G.E. and Tonetti, M. (2008) Supportive periodontal therapy, in *Clinical Periodontology and Implant Dentistry*, 5th edn (ed J. Lindhe), Blackwell Publishing, Oxford, p. 1310.

Laurell, L., Gottlow, J., Zybutz, M. and Persson, R. (1998) Treatment of intrabony defects by different surgical procedures. A literature review. *J Periodontol*, **69**, 303–313.

Lemmerman, K. (1976) Rationale for stabilization. *J Periodontol*, **47**, 405–411.

Lindfors, L.T., Tervonen, E.A., Sándor, G.K. and Ylikontiola, L.P. (2010) Guided bone regeneration using a titanium-reinforced ePTFE membrane and particulate autogenous bone: the effect of smoking and membrane exposure. *Oral Surg Oral Med Oral Pathol Oral Radiol Endod.*, **109**, 825–830.

Lindhe, J. and Nyman, S. (1980) Alterations of the position of the marginal soft tissue following periodontal surgery. *J Clin Periodontol.*, **7**, 525–530.

Lindhe, J., Nyman, S. and Ericsson, I. (2008) Trauma from occlusion: periodontal tissues, in *Clinical Periodontology and Implant Dentistry*, 5th edn (eds J. Lindhe, T. Karring and N.P. Lang), Blackwell Munksgaard, Oxford, p. 359.

Machtei, E.E. (2001) The effect of membrane exposure on the outcome of regenerative procedures in humans: a meta-analysis. *J Periodontol*, **72**, 512–516.

McDevitt, M.J. and Bibb, C.A. (2006) Occlusal evaluation and therapy, in *Carranza's Clinical Periodontology*, 10th edn (eds M.G. Newman, H. Takei, P.R. Klokkevold and F.A. Carranza), Elsevier Saunders, St. Louis, MO, p. 851.

McFall, W.T., Jr (1982) Tooth loss in 100 treated patients with periodontal disease. A long-term study. *J Periodontol*, **53**, 539–549.

Melcher, A.H. (1976) On the repair potential of periodontal tissues. *J Periodontol*, **47**, 256–260.

Mormann, W., Schaer, F. and Firestone, A.R. (1981) The relationship between success of free gingival grafts and transplant thickness. Revascularization and shrinkage. A one year clinical study. *J Periodontol*, **52**, 74–80.

Novak, M.J. (2006) Classification of diseases affecting the periodontium, in *Carranza's Clinical Periodontology*, 10th edn (eds M.G. Newman, H. Takei, P.R. Klokkevold and F.A. Carranza), Elsevier Saunders, St. Louis, MO, p. 104.

Nowzari, H., Matian, F. and Slots, J. (1995) Periodontal pathogens on polytetrafluoroethylene membrane for guided tissue regeneration inhibit healing. *J Clin Periodontol*, **22**, 469–474.

Ochsenbein, C. and Bohannan, H.M. (1963) The palatal approach to osseous surgery. I. Rationale. *J Periodontol*, **34**, 60.

Pack, P.D. and Haber, J. (1983) The incidence of clinical infection after periodontal surgery. A retrospective study. *J Periodontol*, **54**, 441–443.

Passo, S.A., Reinhardt, R.A., DuBois, L.M. and Cohen, D.M. (1988) Histological characteristics associated with suppurating periodontal pockets. *J Periodontol*, **59**, 731–740.

Pontoriero, R. and Carnevale, G. (2001) Surgical crown lengthening: a 12-month clinical wound healing study. *J Periodontol.*, **72**, 841–848.

Powell, C.A., Mealey, B.L., Deas, D.E., McDonnell, H.T. and Moritz, A.J. (2005) Post-surgical infections: prevalence associated with various periodontal surgical procedures. *J Periodontol*, **76**, 329–333.

Ramfjord, S.P. and Ash, M.M., Jr (1981) Significance of occlusion in the etiology and treatment of early, moderate, and advanced periodontitis. *J Periodontol*, **52**, 511–517.

Reali, L., Zuliani, E., Gabutti, L., Schönholzer, C. and Marone, C. (2009) Poor oral hygiene enhances gingival overgrowth caused by calcineurin inhibitors. *J Clin Pharm Ther.*, **34**, 255–260.

Reiser, G.M., Bruno, J.F., Mahan, P.E. and Larkin, L.H. (1996) The subepithelium connective tissue graft palatal donor site: anatomic considerations for surgeons. *Int J Periodontics Restorative Dent*, **16**, 130–137.

Rose, L.F. and Minsk, L. (2004) Dental implants in the periodontally compromised dentition, in *Periodontics Medicine, Surgery, and Implants* (eds L.F. Rose and B.L. Mealey), Elsevier Mosby, St. Louis, MO, p. 644.

Samuel, S.R., Khatri, S.G. and Acharya, S. (2014) Clinical evaluation of self and professionally applied desensitizing agents in relieving dentin hypersensitivity after a single topical application: a randomized controlled trial. *J Clin Exp Dent.*, **6**, 339–343.

Sarmento, H.R., Dantas, R.V., Pereira-Cenci, T. and Faot, F. (2012) Elements of implant-supported rehabilitation planing in patients with bruxism. *J Craniofac Surg*, **23**, 1905–1909.

Schallhorn, R.G. and Snider, L.E. (1981) Periodontal maintenance therapy. *J Am Dent Assoc*, **103**, 227–231.

Serino, G., Rosling, B., Ramberg, P., Hellström, M.K., Socransky, S.S. and Lindhe, J. (2001) The effect of systemic antibiotics in the treatment of patients with recurrent periodontitis. *J Clin Periodontol*, **28**, 411–418.

Serio, F.G. and Hawley, C. (2002) *Manual of Clinical Periodontics*, Lexi-Comp, Hudson, OH.

Slots, J. (2004) Research, Science and Therapy Committee. Systemic antibiotics in periodontics. *J Periodontol*, **75**, 1553–1565.

Souza, S.L., Macedo, G.O., Tunes, R.S., Silveira e Souza, A.M., Jr Novaes, A.B., Grisi, M.F., Jr Taba, M., Palioto, D.B. and Correa, V.M. (2008) Subepithelial connective tissue graft for root coverage in smokers and non-smokers: a clinical and histologic controlled study in humans. *J Periodontol.*, **79**, 1014–1021.

Stambaugh, R.V. (2002) A clinician's 3-year experience with perioscopy. *Compend Contin Educ Dent*, **23**, 1061–1070.

Stravropoulos, A., Mardsas, N., Herrero, F. and Karring, T. (2004) Smoking affects the outcome of guided tissue regeneration with bioresorbable membranes: a retrospective analysis of intrabony defects. *J Clin Periodontol*, **31**, 945–950.

Svärdström, G. and Wennström, J.L. (1966) Prevalence of furcation involvement in patients referred for periodontal treatment. *J Clin Periodontol*, **23**, 1093–1099.

Takei, H.H., Han, T.J., Carranza, F.A., Jr, Kenney, E.B. and Lekovic, V. (1985) Flap technique for periodontal bone implants. Papilla preservation technique. *J Periodontol*, **56**, 204–210.

Takei, H.H., Azzi, R.R. and Han, T.J. (2006) Periodontal plastic and esthetic surgery, in *Carranza's Clinical Periodontology*, 10th edn (eds M.G. Newman, H. Takei, P.R. Klokkevold and F.A. Carranza), Elsevier Saunders, St. Louis, MO.

Tarnow, D.P., Magner, A.W. and Fletcher, P. (1992) The effect of the distance from the contact point to the crest of bone on the presence or absence of the interproximal dental papilla. *J Periodontol*, **63**, 995–996.

Termeie, D. (2013) *Periodontal Review*, Quintessence Publishing Co., Chicago, IL.

Tibbettes, L.S., Jr, Ochsenbein, C. and Loughlin, D.M. (1976) Rationale for the lingual approach to mandibular osseous surgery. *Dent Clin North Am*, **20**, 61–78.

Tonetti, M.S., Pini-Prato, G. and Cortellini, P. (1993) Periodontal regeneration of human intrabony defects. IV. Determinants of healing response. *J Periodontol*, **64**, 934–940.

Tonetti, M.S., Pini-Prato, G. and Cortellini, P. (1995) Effect of cigarette smoking on periodontal healing following GTR in infrabony defects. A preliminary retrospective study. *J Clin Periodontol*, **22**, 229–234.

Topazian, R.G., Goldberg, M. and Hupp, J.R. (2001) *Oral and Maxillofacial Infections*, 4th edn, Saunders, Philadelphia, PA, p. 144.

Trowbridge, H.O. and Silver, D.R. (1990) A review of current approaches to in-office management of tooth hypersensitivity. *Dent Clin North Am*, **34**, 561–581.

Tseng, C.C., Huang, C.C. and Tseng, W.H. (1993) Incidence of clinical infection after periodontal surgery: a prospective study. *J Formos Med Assoc.*, **92**, 152–156.

Vastardis, S. and Yukna, R.A. (2003) Gingival/soft tissue abscess following subepithelial connective tissue graft for root coverage: report of three cases. *J Periodontol*, **74**, 1676–1681.

Villar, C.C. and Cochran, D.L. (2010) Regeneration of periodontal tissues: guided tissue regeneration. *Dent Clin North Am*, **54**, 73–92.

Waerhaug, J. (1979) The infrabony pocket and its relationship to trauma from occlusion and subgingival plaque. *J Periodontol*, **50**, 355–365.

Wang, H.L., Burgett, F.G. and Shyr, Y. (1993) The relationship between restoration and furcation involvement on molar teeth. *J Periodontol*, **64**, 302–305.

Westfelt, E., Nyman, S., Socransky, S. and Lindhe, J. (1983) Significance of frequency of professional tooth cleaning for healing following periodontal surgery. *J Clin Periodontol*, **10**, 148.

CHAPTER 3

Endodontic complications

Shane N. White and Daniel J. Boehne

Section of Endodontics, Clinical Dental Sciences, UCLA School of Dentistry, Los Angeles, CA, USA

Introduction

Endodontic pathology

Patients frequently present with endodontic pathoses, sometimes requiring emergency endodontic treatment. The keys to successful resolution without complication are in understanding the disease process, diagnostic methods, and application of appropriate clinical technique. In this chapter, we break the endodontic treatment process into its various steps and their common complications. We explain how to avoid potential complications and how to manage those that may occur.

Endodontics is a complex discipline, often underestimated by clinicians and patients. The first step to providing high-quality, predictable endodontic care is to realize that the process requires a mind-set of thoroughness and precision. Root canal treatment is best thought of as a biologic process where bacteria, their toxins and metabolites, inflamed or necrotic tissue, and debris are removed and excluded from a root canal system. It is a mistake to think of endodontic therapy as a series of mechanical or procedural goals. A clinician's endodontic skills are not measured by how quickly they can complete a case but on what their long-term success rates are. In fact, endodontists spend considerable time, often over multiple appointments, to ensure that the biologic goals of treatment are met.

Pulpal and periapical disease are generally sequelae of caries and its restorative treatment; it is primarily bacterial in origin (Kakehashi, Stanley, and Fitzgerald, 1965; Sundqvist *et al.*, 1979). Endodontic pathology depends on the mix of involved bacterial species, the condition of the pulpal tissues, and the host defense or immunological factors. Invading bacteria cause pulpal inflammation; this may progress to pulpal death, inflammation of the supporting tissues, and infection. Although it is tempting to think of this as a continuous linear process, the reality is not so simple. Additionally, we are limited to indirect clinical testing of the inaccessible pulpal and periradicular tissues. Therefore, we use clinical diagnoses, not histological diagnoses to classify pulps and periapical tissues; these diagnostic classifications help us to make treatment decisions and to estimate prognosis.

Preventing disease of pulpal origin

Caries is the primary causes of pulpal disease, but complications or consequences of its restorative treatment may run a close second. Preventing caries, or treating it early and conservatively, would prevent most disease of pulpal origin. Conservative tooth preparation, use of copious water spray, use of antimicrobials (e.g., Consepsis, Ultradent, South Jordan, Utah), rubber dam isolation, minimizing tooth drying, using dentin sealers (e.g., Gluma Desensitizer), and minimizing leakage of temporary restorations will all protect the pulp. It used to be believed that absolutely all caries had to be removed, but it is now known that the cariostatic indirect pulp cap, with incomplete caries removal, has a reasonable long-term prognosis for the pulp, much better than stepwise caries removal or direct pulp capping (Mertz-Fairhurst *et al.*, 1988; Maltz *et al.*, 2012). Stepwise caries removal is no longer indicated and direct pulp caps or pulpotomies are only indicated in immature teeth.

Avoiding and Treating Dental Complications: Best Practices in Dentistry, First Edition. Edited by Deborah A. Termeie.
© 2016 John Wiley & Sons, Inc. Published 2016 by John Wiley & Sons, Inc.

Occasionally, trauma can expose pulps or damage the tooth's supporting structures. Preventive measures include using mouthguards during sports. In young patients with open apices, pulpotomy is the treatment of choice for preserving the vitality of injured pulp and allowing completion of root formation. In an injured tooth with a normal response to vitality testing, the removal of the injured coronal portion of pulp tissue may increase the chances that the remaining pulp will survive. As with other traumas, pulpectomy or complete extirpation of the pulp is indicated with large exposures, pain, or mobility or if the patient is not seen until several days after injury.

Diagnosis

A decision on how, or even whether, to treat a particular clinical situation cannot be made unless a proper diagnosis is made first. "Root canal treatment" is not a diagnosis; it is a treatment plan arrived at through a thorough diagnosis and prognostic assessment. Neither a simple finding of deep caries nor a radiolucency on a radiograph alone can provide a diagnosis. Separate pulpal and periapical diagnoses must be reached before treatment can be initiated.

A careful diagnosis consists of a thorough medical, dental, and pain history; examination of the supporting tissues (palpation, percussion, mobility, and periodontal probing); pulp testing (primarily cold, but electric and heat may be needed); and radiography (Figure 3.1). All of the endodontic tests are somewhat relative, so at least two control teeth are needed. Reproducing the patient symptoms are a hallmark of a successful endodontic diagnosis. Endodontic diagnoses can change overnight, so current findings are necessary.

Radiographic images help to identify etiology for bacterial ingress to the pulp (deep caries, deep restorations, coronal fractures, etc.) and changes that occur in periradicular tissues in response to pulp infection (widened periodontal ligament space, periapical radiolucencies, condensing osteitis, etc.) (Figure 3.2). A straight-on periapical view should be supplemented by an off-angle view for all teeth that may have more than a single canal, for example, lower anterior teeth, to build a three-dimensional (3-D) understanding of the anatomy. Usually, a couple of carefully read periapical views and a bite-wing view are sufficient to tell the story, but in complex or perplexing cases, cone beam computed tomography can assist in visualizing 3-D anatomy.

Misdiagnosis, or the absence of a diagnosis, means that teeth that do not require RCT are treated and many teeth that require RCT go untreated. Both situations have potential risks and complications. Importantly, many systemic or non-endodontic conditions can also cause radiographic periapical radiolucencies. These are mistaken for conditions that require root canal therapy. Misdiagnosing a periapical lesion from metastatic carcinoma as endodontic disease is a preventable and tragic complication. A thorough evaluation must always be used to arrive at a correct diagnosis.

Antibiotic use in endodontics

Antibiotics do not cure disease of endodontic origin. Furthermore, antibiotics cannot reach the source of the problem; a necrotic pulp inside a root canal is not served by the body's circulatory or immune systems. Antibiotics cannot be a substitute for pulpectomy and chemo-mechanical debridement. Antibiotics do not treat pulpal or periapical inflammation (Fedorowicz et al., 2013). Antibiotics are reserved for acute apical abscesses and then only when there is systemic involvement or spread (Cope et al., 2014). Penicillin VK is the choice for endodontic infections due to its appropriate spectrum, low toxicity, and low cost (Baumgartner and Xia, 2003). Penicillin VK should be administered orally with a loading dose of 1000 mg, followed by 500 mg every 4–6 h for 5–7 days in adults. Clindamycin is the antibiotic of choice for those with penicillin allergies. Clindamycin should be administered orally every 6 h, with a loading dose of 600 mg, followed by 300 mg for 5–7 days in adults. Conditions not requiring antibiotics include pulpitis, necrotic pulps, radiolucencies, draining chronic abscesses, and local fluctuant swellings. Excessive and inappropriate use of antibiotics has resulted in widespread antibiotic resistance and exposes patients to unnecessary risk.

Common endodontic conditions causing complications

Pain

Patients frequently present with endodontic emergencies. Pain is usually the major complaint. Contrary to popular belief, pain of endodontic origin is generally of moderate severity (Pak and White, 2011). Pain is best managed using nonsteroidal anti-inflammatory (NSAID) drugs,

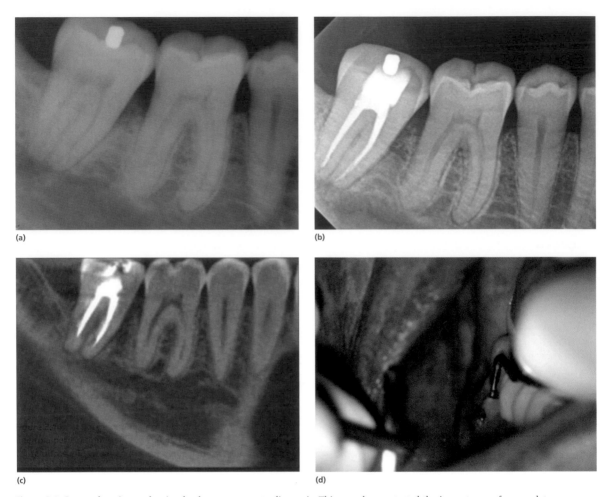

Figure 3.1 Comprehensive evaluation leads to an accurate diagnosis. This case demonstrated the importance of a complete endodontic workup including thorough medical, dental, and pain histories and examination. Non-odontogenic problems can masquerade as endodontic disease. This patient was referred for retreatment of the second molar, with a suspected vertical fracture in the mesial root. (a) Historic preop periapical (PA) radiograph from 3 months prior; although no caries, deep restorations, or unusual pulpal symptoms were present, root canal treatment was provided. (b) PA radiograph upon referral showing radiolucency along the mesial surface of the mesial root and loss of the lamina dura. (c) Cone beam computed tomograph (CBCT) showing mesial bone loss. (d) Localized swelling and localized narrow deep 10 mm probing along the mesial root. Although the history, examination, and radiography suggested a failing root canal treatment associated with a vertical root fracture, the medical history revealed that the patient had received a weekly IV infusion of Aredia for the last 5 years to treat multiple myeloma. As part of a thorough dental history, historic preop radiographs and pulp testing results were requested from the previous dentist; the radiographs failed to show an obvious etiology for pulpal disease and the pulp tests were within normal limits. Rather than performing endodontic retreatment, a biopsy was taken that confirmed a diagnosis of bisphosphonate-related osteonecrosis of the jaws (BRONJ/ARONJ).

such as ibuprofen. Pain is caused by inflammation or infection of bacterial origin; these bacteria must be removed. The comprehensive diagnostic evaluation must be performed, as described earlier, and the causal condition must be diagnosed, as described later, and the cause must be treated. For all pulpal conditions (except normal pulp and reversible pulpitis) and for all apical conditions, the primary treatment is simply nonsurgical root canal treatment. At the emergency appointment, any remaining pulpal tissue, vital or nonvital, must be removed, pulpectomy performed, and the canals chemomechanically cleaned using appropriate files and copious gentle sodium hypochlorite irrigation to remove bacteria and their products. A nonsetting calcium

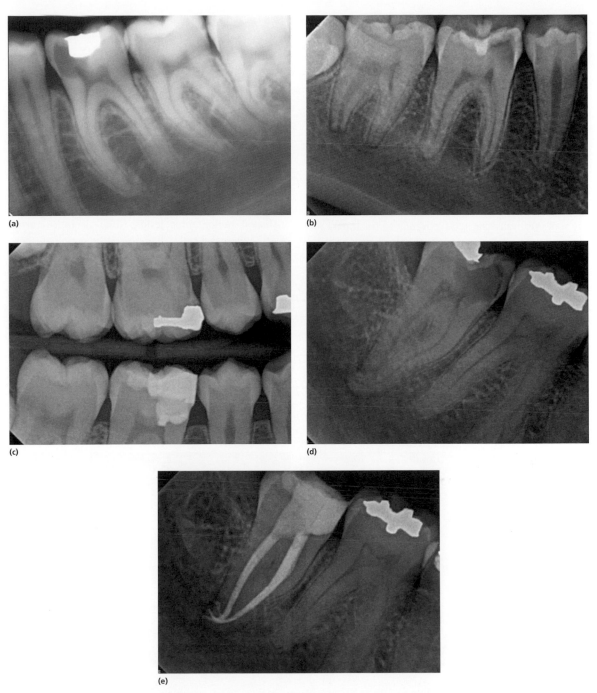

Figure 3.2 Radiography complements history and examination. These three cases with deep caries demonstrate how similar radiographic appearances can have different diagnoses requiring different treatments. (a) Case 1 presented with a caries-free cusp fracture; the pulp was superimposed over the fracture (a), and the pulp was normal upon testing; root canal treatment was not indicated and restoration was completed. (b and c) Case 2 presented with a carious pulp exposure (b), but pain history and pulp testing indicated reversible pulpitis, so vital pulp therapy, apexogenesis, was completed (c). (d and e) Case 3 presented with a carious pulp exposure (d) and complaints of lingering cold sensitivity, spontaneous pain, and pain on chewing; a pain history and pulpal and periradicular testing indicated irreversible pulpitis with symptomatic apical periodontitis, and root canal treatment was provided (e).

hydroxide intracanal medicament should be placed within the root canal to help kill any remaining bacteria. Placement of a durable leak-proof temporary restoration is essential; oral bacteria must not be allowed to enter or reenter the root canal system. After intervention, endodontic pain decreases to minimal levels of severity and incidence over the following week.

Cracked teeth

Many teeth have superficial cracks, infractions, in their coronal enamel; some of these extend a short way into superficial dentin, but they are of little consequence unless they extend past the pulpal floor vertically into the root. Vertically cracked teeth may be frustrating for patients and dentists (Lubisich, Hilton, and Ferracane, 2010). Some indicators of a crack include isolated vertical probing defects; J-shaped radiographic lesions, running alongside the root and around the apex; sensitivity on biting; pain on release; pain on jiggling a Tooth Slooth; and overly wide posts, but these findings may not be pathognomonic in and of themselves (Figure 3.3). Cracks can often be visualized using transillumination, using methylene blue stain, and using the endodontic microscope after accessing the pulp chamber and viewing internally or using surgical exploration externally. The diagnostic hallmark of a vertical root fracture is direct visualization of the fracture under the microscope. The prognosis is variable: a partial crack limited to the crown of a vital tooth may have a fair prognosis; an infected crack extending below the pulpal floor of a long necrotic tooth may have a guarded prognosis; and a through-and-through crack is hopeless.

Treatment considerations

Treatment or extraction will depend on the extent of the crack. A shallow superficial crack in a vital tooth will likely not necessitate root canal treatment. A crack that extends across the pulpal floor, and down the canals, represents a hopeless situation, as do some, but not all, J-shaped radiographic lesions in a necrotic cracked tooth, whereas a crack that crosses the marginal ridges, but not the pulpal floor, may have a good prognosis. After accessing the pulp chamber, the extent of the crack can be judged by using methylene blue stain, transillumination, and a microscope. Cracked posterior teeth should receive coronal coverage, an onlay, or a full crown.

Traumatic injury

Emergency treatments for traumatic fractures involving the pulp in permanent teeth with mature roots include direct pulp capping, which will generally need to be

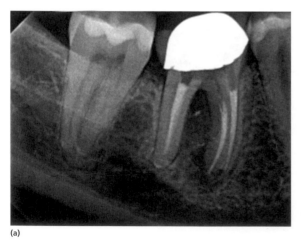

(a)

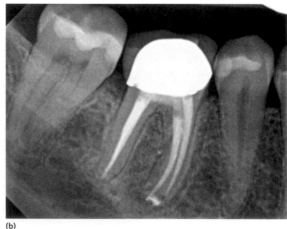

(b)

Figure 3.3 Microscopy assists in cracked root diagnosis. This patient was told by her dentist that her first molar needed to be extracted due to a vertical root fracture. (a) Circumstantial evidence suggesting a vertical root fracture included prior root canal treatment, a J-shaped radiolucency, and deep isolated probing along the mesial root. (b) After examining the root internally by accessing and removing the buildup and gutta-percha and using methylene blue stain and transillumination, direct visualization through the dental operating microscope found no crack. Retreatment gained patency on all canals and achieved appropriate flare; a buildup without voids was placed. The symptoms, periodontal probing defect, and the periradicular radiolucencies had resolved at the 3-month recall.

followed by root canal treatment; pulpectomy, which will need to be followed by root canal treatment; and root canal treatment at the initial visit (American Association of Endodontists (AAE), 2004; Krastl *et al.*, 2011; DiAngelis *et al.*, 2012). The best prognosis for a direct pulp cap is for a small traumatic exposure, without contamination, without pain, and which is performed immediately after the traumatic accident; but in the long term, the prognosis for pulpal survival in mature teeth is poor. Rubber dam isolation must be used for any procedures involving the pulp and is strongly recommended whenever traumatically exposed dentin is encountered or when adhesive procedures are being performed.

Treatment considerations

For permanent teeth with immature roots, the goal is to maintain pulpal vitality through vital pulp therapy or apexogenesis, at least until the formation of the entire root has been completed (American Academy of Pediatric Dentistry (AAPD) Council on Clinical Affairs, 2010). In this situation, a high or shallow pulpotomy, the Cvek technique, is usually used. The tooth is isolated, and pulpal tissue is gently removed to approximately 2 mm below the exposure using a small water-cooled round diamond bur. The pulp is rinsed with sterile saline, hemostasis is achieved, the clot is gently rinsed away, and a hard calcium hydroxide liner is placed, followed by a glass ionomer or resin-modified glass ionomer base, and then by a bonded composite restoration. Alternatively, mineral trioxide aggregate (MTA, Dentsply) or other inorganic materials can be placed over the pulp instead of a hard-setting calcium hydroxide liner. MTA has advantages in that it can be used in a damp field, seals well against the dentin, and is bacteriostatic. However, because it sets slowly, its manufacturer recommends checking at a subsequent appointment prior to restoration. Staining has sometimes been observed following the use of MTA materials. It is likely that quicker setting variants of MTA will soon be introduced. Although traumatized teeth with pulpal exposures should be seen within 24 h, the shallow pulpotomy may still be successful even after a week.

If the pulp in an immature permanent tooth becomes necrotic, or is already necrotic, then nonvital therapy, apexification, is performed (AAE, 2004; AAPD Council on Clinical Affairs, 2010). The tooth is isolated, carefully and thoroughly debrided, a nonsetting bactericidal

calcium hydroxide paste placed, and a durable provisional restoration made. Typically, after 3–6 months, a delicate calcific barrier is formed across the root apex, but root formation remains incomplete. Then, the calcium hydroxide is carefully removed, a conventional gutta-percha obturation performed, and the access closed and a definitive coronal restoration made. Alternatively, an apical plug of MTA can be placed after brief placement of calcium hydroxide for 1 week to 1 month, and after setting has been checked, a conventional gutta-percha obturation can be performed. Revascularization and regenerative endodontics hold future promise.

Procedural endodontic complications

Tooth isolation

Rubber dam isolation is an absolute necessity for root canal treatment (Ahmed *et al.*, 2014). The key to successful root canal treatment is removing oral bacteria from the root canal system and keeping them out. Ingress of saliva during or after root canal treatment will contaminate the root canal system and is a common cause of failure. The absence of a rubber dam is also considered to be an ethical failure because patients are at risk of inhaling or ingesting endodontic files and contaminated debris.

Treatment considerations

Single tooth isolation is simple, fast, and appropriate for endodontics. A tight well-fitting clamp that engages the tooth root with all four tines will be stable. A rubber dam can be placed on a winged clamp before the clamp is placed on the tooth. If the tooth is broken down, it can be restored before endodontics using a glass ionomer (e.g., Fuji IX, GC, Tokyo, Japan) or a resin-modified glass ionomer (e.g., Fuji II LC, GC). In cases where the tooth lacks coronal undercuts to retain a clamp, an "A" clamp with downturned tines will engage the root surface. A minor leak in a rubber dam can be sealed using caulking or putty (e.g., OraSeal, Ultradent).

Access cavity preparation

Access is driven by the individual tooth's root canal anatomy; the canals must be located; files must reach the canals with constraint occlusally; and the pulp horns must be removed or cleaned. If caries, pulp, or bacteria are allowed to remain, root canal treatment cannot be successful. Missed canals are a major cause of end-odontic failure. However, the access cavity should be as small as conservative as possible in reaching these aims (Gluskin, Peters, and Peters, 2014).

Treatment considerations

Canals should be identified radiographically and projected back up to the occlusal surface and the occlusal outline form visualized. As well as a straight-on view, an off-angle view will help to identify multiple canals and build a 3-D understanding of pulpal anatomy and the necessary access cavity. The depths to the roof and floor of the pulp chamber should be measured on the preoperative radiograph, so that one will know the expected depth for the bur to reach the roof of the pulp chamber and fall into the pulp chamber and so that one will definitely not let a bur extend beyond the floor of the pulp chamber. If the bur does not fall into the pulp chamber at the expected depth, then one should stop, reassess, and make an additional radiograph before proceeding. A periodontal probe should be used to sound the angle and shape of the root subgingivally. This will provide information about the inclination, position, and shape of the root so that the access bur can be appropriately aligned, reducing the risk of perforation. For example, the width and shape of mesio-buccal roots in upper molars and mesial and distal concavities in lower incisors, premolars, and molars will indicate whether one or two canals are present. After all caries is first removed, an ideal access should be established. Access to the pulp chamber is first established in the center of the visualized cavity using a small round number 2 carbide bur. Indirect vision should be used so that the alignment of the bur can be related to the tooth in all three dimensions. Next, the sides of the cavity should be extended and refined to allow unconstrained access of the files to the canals using a gentle side-cutting bur with a noncutting tip (e.g., Endo-Z Bur, Dentsply, York, Philadelphia).

Insufficient access can prevent canals from being located; prevent canals from being adequately cleaned; stress files; and prevent pulp horns from being located, removed, or cleaned. Files must be able to stand up in their canals without contacting the cavosurface margins when they are being used to clean and shape.

Excessively large access cavities greatly weaken the tooth; the prognosis for the tooth is directly related to the amount of remaining tooth structure (Figure 3.4).

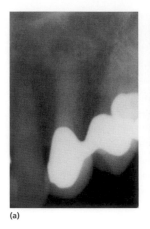 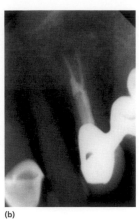

(a)   (b)

Figure 3.4 Excessive removal of dentin during access weakens teeth. (a) Thorough assessment of the preoperative off-angle periapical radiograph revealed multiple periodontal ligament outlines, two apices, calcified canals, and an obliterated pulp: an extremely difficult case. (b) Drilling to the apical third was required to locate both canals. Although both canals were located and treated, this tooth is at risk of fracture due to excessive removal of tooth structure during access and canal location.

Only structure that must be removed to facilitate the files being used for cleaning and shaping should be removed. If a canal cannot be located, it is wise to stop and take a radiograph. Often a bite-wing view provides the best view of the neck of a tooth; the clamp may be removed, but the rubber dam must remain in place, retained by ligatures.

Gouges or perforations both weaken teeth and may permit microbial ingress and endodontic failure. Careful planning, as described earlier, will prevent their occurrence. Should a perforation occur, the patient should be informed, the area gently disinfected, the canal system packed with nonsetting calcium hydroxide paste (e.g., UltraCal XS, Ultradent), and the patient referred to an endodontist for nonsurgical internal perforation repair (Figure 3.5). In upper central incisors, most perforations or gouges occur to the buccal, just below the CEJ, because the bur is often mistakenly tilted toward the buccal. Upper first premolars and mandibular incisors have pronounced mesial and distal concavities just below the gumline; the margin of error is small. In all posterior teeth, care must be taken not to advance the bur below the floor of the pulp chamber. Sometimes, an overly vigorous search for a mesiobuccal-2 canal can result in perforation in the mesial concavity of an upper molar.

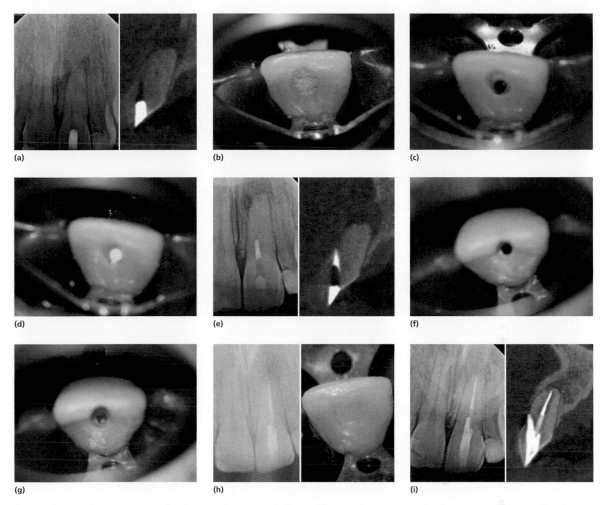

Figure 3.5 Managing an access perforation. The bucco-cervical area of incisors is a common site of access gouging or perforation. A small access bur must be carefully aligned to the long axis of the root in both bucco-lingual and mesio-distal planes and indirect vision used. (a and b) An access perforation was created, recognized, and temporized and the patient was referred. This tooth was extremely calcified; careful preoperative assessment of the tooth angulation, depth of the pulp chamber, and an operating microscope would be helpful. (c and d) Buccally oriented views: treatment included removing the provisional restoration, locating and disinfecting the perforation (c), and sealing with mineral trioxide aggregate (MTA) (d). (e) PA and CBCT views of the repaired perforation. (f and g) Axially oriented views: at the next visit, after the MTA had set, the canal was located and treated. A wider access cavity was not necessary; axial reorientation toward the canal was all that was required to find the canal. (h) Completed case, including perforation repair, obturation with gutta-percha, bonded fiber post, and conservative resin-composite restoration. (i) Recall PA and CBCT images show bony healing.

Missed canals

Unidentified and hence uncleaned canals are a major source of endodontic failure (Witherspoon, Small, and Regan, 2013). Knowledge of root canal anatomy and its variants is essential. Many lower anterior teeth will have 2 canals; the lingual ones are most likely to be missed. Most first molars, upper or lower, will have 4 canals. The mesiobuccal-2 canal is notoriously difficult to locate in upper molars. The distobuccal canal is most likely to be missed in lower molars. Premolars generally have 1 or 2 canals, but sometimes 3 are present (Figure 3.6). Sometimes a single large canal branches into several narrow ones, a fast break; originally, this was a UCLA basketball term but is now used by

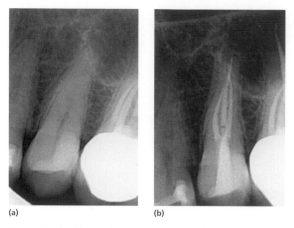

(a)　　　　　(b)

Figure 3.6 Identifying a fast break. (a) A single large coronal canal disappears where branches into three narrow fine canals that are too small to be visualized on the PA. (b) The completed case reveals that this premolar canal anatomy was like a mini-molar with 2 buccal canals and 1 palatal canal.

endodontists. Chemo-mechanical debridement cannot be successful unless all the canals are located.

Treatment considerations
Careful radiographic imaging using multiple views at different angles will help to build a 3-D map. Searching for double periodontal ligament outlines on the sides of roots will reveal the presence of concavities, "figure-8" root cross sections, and multiple canals. A canal that moves off-center in an off-angle film likely has a twin at the other side of the root (Figure 3.7). Reading the dentinal map, grooves or color changes on the floor of the pulp chamber often connect canals.

Length control
Good length control is a hallmark of precise, thoughtful, and careful endodontic treatment. Treatment that is too short will leave the critical apical parts of canals

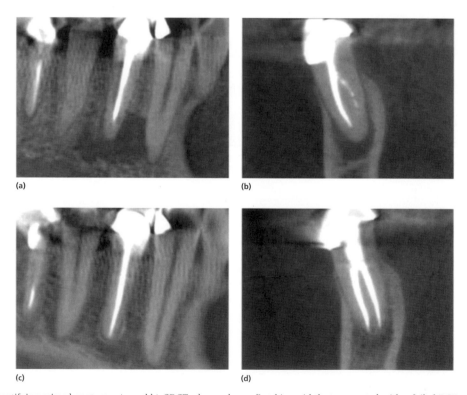

(a)　　　　　(b)

(c)　　　　　(d)

Figure 3.7 Identifying missed anatomy. (a and b) CBCTs show a lower first bicuspid that presented with a failed RCT and symptomatic apical periodontitis; a missed canal and a short treatment in the other caused failure. If a single canal is off-center, there is usually a twin hiding at the other side of the root. (c and d) CBCTs at 3-year recall, healing after an appropriate access led to the missed canal, and both canals were treated to their apices.

uncleaned and unfilled, harboring bacteria and causing failure. Complex anatomy, sharp curves, and bifurcations are common in the apical area, often making it difficult to reach an appropriate working length. The aim is to treat to the apical constriction, which is, on average, half a millimeter shorter than the radiographic root end (Kuttler, 1955). Treatment that is even 1 mm too short will allow bacteria to remain and the treatment will be likely to fail (Sjogren *et al.*, 1990) (Figure 3.8). Careful analysis of a preoperative radiograph and the use of an electronic apex locator and a file radiograph will assure that the appropriate working length is reached (Figure 3.9). Treatment that is too long will traumatize the apical tissues and make obturation control more difficult. Usually, a little puff of sealer is of no consequence.

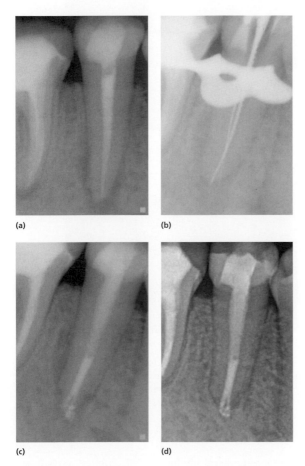

(a)   **(b)**

(c)   **(d)**

Figure 3.8 Untreated minor anatomy can prevent healing. (a–c) An apical bifurcation was located, shaped, cleaned, and obturated. (d) Eight-month recall shows that retreatment healed the large apical lesion.

A larger amount of sealer, or a nonresorbing resinous sealer, or a little gutta-percha may delay healing (Sjogren *et al.*, 1990; Molven *et al.*, 2002). Should sealer or gutta-percha enter a nerve canal or the maxillary sinus, referral to an oral surgeon or endodontist is needed.

Treatment considerations

Length estimates should be made using preoperative X-ray images, then using an apex locator, and using the initial apical file. Working lengths should be rechecked and refined using the apex locator during treatment and always prior to fitting gutta-percha cones. This is important because it will refine the accuracy of the original estimate, accommodate to small length changes as the canals become flared, and alert the dentist to loss of length or loss of patency. An X-ray image is only a two-dimensional (2-D) representation, whereas the apex locator tells you when the file tip reaches conductive apical tissues, right at the apical constriction. These techniques are complementary. In times of conflict, we give more weight to the apex locator. If a large adjustment is made, an additional file film is needed.

In narrow or calcified canals, length is reached using small flexible stainless steel K-files with the quarter-turn-and-pull or watch-winding technique. After working length is reached, files are used in an up and down motion. Care must be taken with length control; a secure finger rest and frequent checking of the rubber stopper are needed.

A master gutta-percha cone film further assures length accuracy before obturation. Slightly crimping the master cone at the reference point provides additional information during obturation. Should the crimp mark slip deeper into the tooth than the reference point, the cone is long. The cone is best trimmed by placing it on a stainless steel ruler and making a precise cut with a disposable scalpel while wearing magnifying loupes. Should the crimp mark remain coronal to the reference point, one should return to the files to regain lost length and recheck a master cone before beginning obturation. Losing length, or losing the ability to get the master cone all the way to the apical constriction, can result from debris being packed apically; an inaccurate length estimate; or from an inadequate, misplaced, or ledged apical preparation, resulting from poor technical length control during cleaning and shaping. An initial condensation film will reveal any problems in time for adjustments or even repreparation to be completed before finishing obturation.

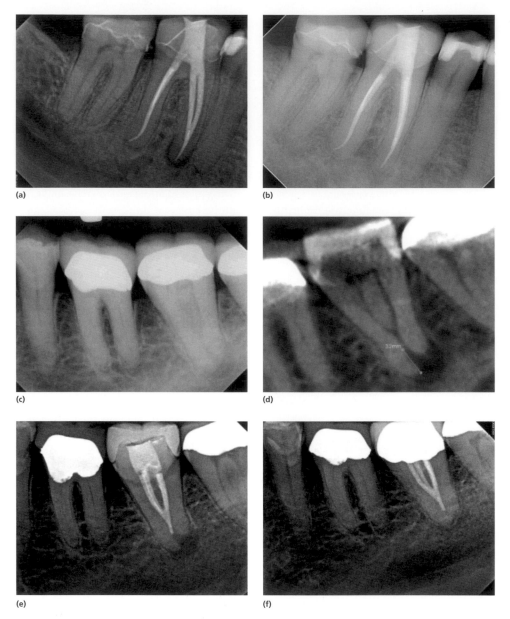

Figure 3.9 Locating the apical constriction, determining working length. (a and b) Case 1. Working length is on average 0.5 mm short of the root end. Radiographs and apex locators were used to determine working length before obturation and immediate restoration (a); healing at recall (b). (c–f) Case 2. In this case, the constriction was found to be 3.2 mm short of the radiographic root end terminus. PA (c), CBCT (d), and apex locater were used to locate the apical constriction before obturation (e). A 1-year recall PA shows complete healing (f).

Cleaning and shaping

Chemo-mechanical debridement is absolutely critical to removing bacteria, pulpal debris, and contaminated dentin to achieve successful healing (Siqueira, 2001).

The master apical file must be big enough to clean the critical apical area; the minimum size is #30 or at least three sizes bigger than the first file to feel snug at length, the initial apical file. An unnecessarily large file may be more likely to remove the apical constriction and make obturation control more difficult, as well as ledging or transporting. A narrow canal in a thin root may need less flaring than average; a wide canal in a wide root may need more flaring than average. So, the amount of flare must be chosen on a case by case basis.

Canals are rarely circular in cross section, so care must be taken to clean all the canal walls using circumferential filing, actively pressing the files against all the walls of the canal, one by one, in a brushing motion. Enough shaping must be done to adequately clean the canal, but too much dentin removal is also detrimental. Removing too much tooth structure can immediately cause perforation or weakening of the root and eventual root fracture.

Root walls are not of uniform thickness, and the root walls closest to the furcation tend to be the thinnest and most susceptible to strip perforation. This area is referred to as the "danger zone." The furcation walls of the mesial roots of mandibular molars are highly susceptible to strip perforation due a root concavity in this location and pronounced root curvature (Figure 3.10). Strip perforations can be avoided by understanding the anatomy and refraining from over-enlarging canals in this area. When using the anticurvature filing technique, as popularized by Dudley Glick, files are pressed away from the furcation and worked to preferentially remove tooth structure from the walls opposite of the danger zone.

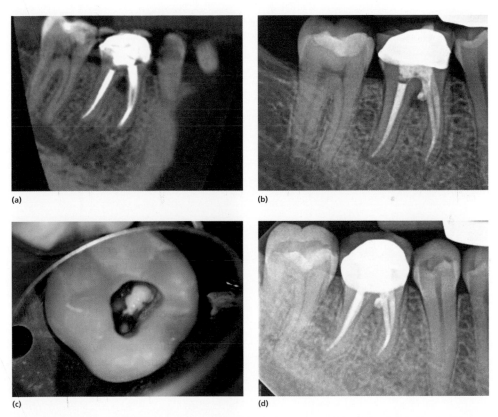

(a)   (b)   (c)   (d)

Figure 3.10 Management of a furcal strip perforation. (a) CBCT of previously treated lower first molar; the hygienist discovered a localized probing defect. The furcal side of the mesial root of mandibular molars is susceptible to strip perforation; this can be prevented by using precurved files and an anticurvature filing technique. (b) Immediate postoperative PA. The perforation was cleaned using a vacuum irrigation system with sodium hypochlorite and then repairing the perforation with MTA before recleaning and shaping and obturation. (c) View of MTA repair through microscope. (d) A 1-year recall PA showing healed periradicular tissues, and the periodontal probing depths had returned to 2 mm.

Transportation, ledging, and apical perforation

One must precurve stainless steel files and ensure that each file is loose and floating before moving on to the next file. Files should be precurved a little more than the natural curve of the canal, generally with a steeper curve at the apical end of the file (Figure 3.11). Files can be precurved by bending around a mirror handle, teasing them through the beaks of a cotton pliers, or using a file bender. If one does not precurve the files, moves up the sequence too quickly, uses force, or unknowingly loses length, transportation, blocking, or ledging may occur. If one ledges and then applies force in attempt to regain length, an apical perforation may occur. Patient gentle passive negotiation using copious irrigation and small stainless steel hand files until they are loose and floating will prevent transportation and ledging (Figure 3.12).

Management of transportation, ledging, and apical perforation

Should length be lost, or if a ledge is formed, one should return all the way back to the small precurved number 10 or 15 stainless steel K-files, gently negotiating a pathway back to the apical constriction of the original canal, maybe using the quarter-turn-and-pull technique, and then continuing through the usual file sequence slowly (AAE, 2008) (Figure 3.13).

File separation

File separation is unfortunate; critically, it can prevent the key goals of cleaning, shaping, and obturating the

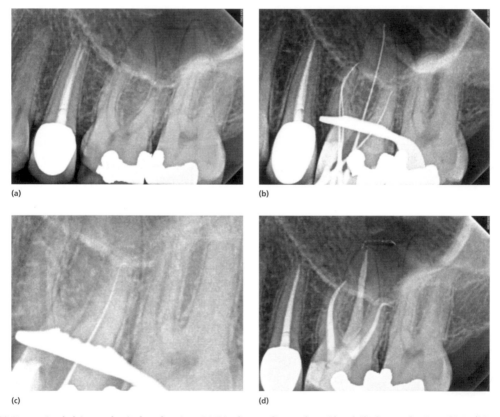

Figure 3.11 Preventing ledging and apical perforation. (a) PA of upper first molar with calcified curved apices. (b) In this working length film, the file in the DB root is short. The file hit a "hard stop" and would not progress apically. (c) Instead of applying excessive pressure, the canal was gently shaped to just above the hard stop, taking care not to create a false canal path or a ledge. Opening the canal body allowed a small precurved #6 K-file to negotiate the severe apical dilaceration, thus following and preserving the natural canal anatomy. (d) Postoperative PA.

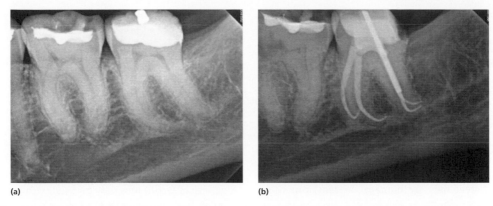

(a)   (b)

Figure 3.12 Preventing transportation, ledging, and perforation. (a) This lower molar has sharply curved narrow canals. (b) Gentle, passive canal negotiation, using small precurved stainless steel K-files, patience, and copious irrigation allowed these canals to be treated without complication.

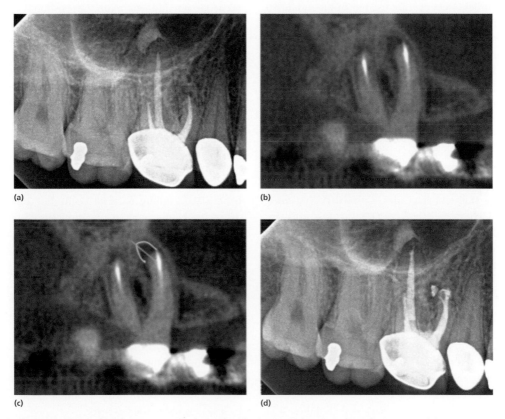

(a)   (b)

(c)   (d)

Figure 3.13 Managing an apical perforation. (a) PA shows that the lesion at the mesio-buccal root apex of this previously treated case did not heal, resulting in symptomatic apical periodontitis. (b and c) CBCT reveals that the true canal path was not followed and that an apical perforation was created; bacteria remain in the apical part of the true canal. A stiff, uncurved file had been forcefully applied. Lesions are usually centered on the portal of exit; note that the position of the radiolucency tells us the location of the true apical foramen. (d) The true canal path was recovered by passively scouting using small precurved files, and the canals were cleaned, shaped, and obturated using a warm gutta-percha technique.

entire canal to the apical constriction. However, if the biological aims of cleaning, shaping, and obturation to the apical constriction can be met, particularly in a previously uncontaminated vital tooth, a separated file may have little impact on prognosis (Crump and Natkin, 1970; Hansen, Beeson, and Ibarrola, 2013). When a file segment separates and remains inside a canal, the actual file fragment is of no consequence by itself. The separated fragment may become a problem if it interferes with the ability of cleaning and shaping to remove bacteria from the entire root canal system.

Stainless steel files are damage tolerant, but they should be repeatedly cleaned and inspected for unwinding or kinking during use (Madarati, Watts, and Qualtrough, 2008). Each stainless steel file should be loose and floating before the next file in the sequence is used. Stainless steel files are used in an up and down motion to clean and shape canals; if they are spun or rotated more than a quarter turn, they are at risk of breaking.

Rotary nickel titanium, or NiTi, files deserve special care (Madarati, Watts, and Qualtrough, 2008). NiTi is weaker than stainless steel, is subject to cyclic fatigue, and can fracture without warning. Although NiTi has superelasticity, meaning that it bends easily, it also has shape memory, meaning that it always wants to straighten out. First, the access must not constrain the file. A glide path to the apex must have already been made using stainless steel files. Coronal flaring must have been completed before NiTi shaping files are used. NiTi files must be used in accordance with the manufacturers' recommended sequence, torque, and speed. Alternating between files of different flare (e.g., 0.04 and 0.06 mm/mm) will reduce contact area and reduce file stress. Frequent irrigation and file cleaning are critically important. A gentle pecking or pumping motion should be used, rather than continuous engagement. The pressure applied should be no more than writing with a fine pencil, and each file should only be engaged for 6 or 7 s before moving on to the next one. It is recommended that NiTi files be used for only a single case and then discarded. Smaller NiTi files may fracture early in the preparation sequence if excessive force is used. Larger NiTi files may fracture later in the sequence when the canal shape approximates the file shape allowing too much surface area of the file to engage the canal walls.

Management of file separation

Should file separation occur, the patient must be immediately informed so that they can make the choice of continuing treatment, requesting an extraction or a referral to continue treatment elsewhere (AAE, 2008). Frequently, the broken fragment can be bypassed using small precured stainless steel K-files, with a quarter-turn-and-pull or watch-winding technique, and the instrumentation sequence completed with or without file removal. Sometimes a stainless steel fragment may simply float out during continuing instrumentation. A variety of techniques may be used with visualization and lighting from an endodontic microscope to remove separated fragments. NiTi fragments may be more difficult to remove because their shape memory may lock them into the canal. Nonetheless, healing generally occurs despite file separation. Cases should be followed for healing; should healing not occur, referral to a specialist is advised—if not already made, for assessment, possible retreatment or apical surgery.

Prevention of hypochlorite accidents

Removal of bacteria, tissue remnants, and toxic debris from root canal systems requires chemo-mechanical debridement. Physical removal of debris by filing alone will not adequately clean the root canal system. In fact, files only remove debris from parts of the canal walls (Paqué et al., 2010). Sodium hypochlorite is extremely beneficial in killing bacteria (Zehnder, 2006) and in dissolving biofilm and tissue remnants (Stojicic et al., 2010). For optimal effectiveness, sodium hypochlorite must reach all aspects of the pulpal system, including apical parts of the canal.

If sodium hypochlorite is expressed beyond the root apex, it will cause severe damage to the periapical tissues and beyond. It can cause severe damage if it drips into a patient's eyes (AAE, 2008). Commercially available sodium hypochlorite bleaches are sold in concentrations from 2 to 8%. Immediate sharp pain, during irrigation, despite anesthesia, is a hallmark of a hypochlorite accident. Substantial diffuse swelling occurs, followed by bruising and tissue necrosis.

Hypochlorite accidents are best prevented by careful technique. A safety-tipped, side-vented, or perforated irrigation needle should be used. Light pressure and slow delivery should be used. The tip should be kept moving so as to assure that it has not become wedged or bound. Alternatively, a negative-pressure irrigation system can be used (e.g., EndoVac, SybronEndo, Orange, CA). Hypochlorite can also be expressed through iatrogenic perforations or through-and-through resorption. Special care should be taken with open apices. Nerve injury and damage to the maxillary sinus can occur if hypochlorite is expressed into these areas.

Management of a hypochlorite accident

Palliative treatment including an ice pack and non-steroidal anti-inflammatory medications, such as ibuprofen, are used (Hülsmann and Hahn, 2000). Tissue damage from any substantial accident should be immediately assessed and followed by an oral surgeon. Resolution can take from weeks to months, depending on severity.

Temporization

Durable and leak-resistant provisional or temporary restorations must be used to prevent leakage of saliva and microbial ingress. Coronal microleakage is thought to be one of the commonest causes of endodontic failure (Swanson and Madison, 1987; Gillen *et al.*, 2011). Intra-appointment medication, nonsetting calcium hydroxide paste, has excellent antimicrobial properties, killing remaining bacteria over the week or two between treatment appointments. It is recommended that non-setting calcium hydroxide paste be routinely placed between treatment appointments; not only will it kill existing bacteria in the canal, but it also offers some protection should the provisional restoration leak.

Inter-appointment coronal leakage

Coronal leakage through a poorly sealed access cavity allows new pathogenic oral bacteria to enter and colonize the root canal system, even before treatment has been completed. A durable thick temporary filling should be placed between appointments or after obturation and before definitive restoration. If temporary restoration is extensive or will be in service for more than a week or two, glass ionomer (e.g., Ketac Bond, 3M ESPE, St. Paul, Minnesota) or a resin-modified glass ionomer (e.g., Vitremer, 3M ESPE) temporary restoration is recommended. The thickness of the restorative material should be maximized, and the thickness of any underlying cotton or foam pellet should be minimized. A reinforced zinc oxide eugenol temporary restorative material (e.g., IRM) can be used for shorter periods. It is

critically important that any underlying cotton pellet is not forgotten and removed at definitive restoration—damp cotton is an excellent culture material. Soft temporary materials are easily damaged by normal mastication and tend to be unstable over time; they must only be used for very short periods in small cavities and must then be completely removed.

Management of inter-appointment coronal leakage

Should gutta-percha become exposed to the oral environment for more than a few days, retreatment, recleaning, and reshaping and chemo-mechanical debridement may be indicated.

Inter-appointment medication

Calcium hydroxide paste is used to kill bacteria remaining in the root canal system and to prevent the growth of any new bacteria that may enter through coronal leakage. Calcium hydroxide has an excellent therapeutic index but should be used with care because it can be toxic to periapical tissues and can damage nerves and the maxillary sinuses if misplaced (Sjögren *et al.*, 1991; Mohammadi and Dummer, 2011). If it is to be effective, it must reach the canal apex. Extrusion beyond the apex will not assist healing but is generally of little consequence unless a large amount is extruded and it reaches a nerve or enters the maxillary sinus. Calcium hydroxide owes its substantivity to it low solubility in water; unlike previously used phenolic medicaments, it stays where it is placed and has much lower toxicity.

Calcium hydroxide can be placed using a capillary tip, but care must be taken to avoid binding the tip and gently backfilling not extruding material. Calcium hydroxide can then be carried to the apex, by spinning the largest file that you have brought to the apex anti-clockwise, using it as an Archimedes screw.

Calcium hydroxide can be removed, using the biggest file that went to working length along with copious gentle irrigation. Calcium hydroxide is relatively insoluble, so it has excellent substantivity and stays where it is placed but can be difficult to remove. The use of sodium hypochlorite followed by EDTA can help in removing this paste.

Obturation

Obturation problems typically follow problems in cleaning and shaping.

Long obturations typically occur when the apical constriction is damaged, enlarged, or removed due to an incorrect, long, working length estimate; inadequate length control during filing; or to an immature tooth with an open apex.

Short obturations typically occur when an incorrect, short, working length estimate was used; when ledging, apical transportation, or apical perforation occurred; or when debris was packed into the canal apex.

Voids typically occur when part of the canal preparation has uneven taper, a constriction, no taper, or even reverse taper. Voids are generally located just apical to a taper problem.

Prevention of obturation complications

Obturation problems are best prevented by careful attention to length control, using carefully precurved files, and attaining smooth even taper and flare during cleaning and shaping, as described earlier. Checking file length frequently will prevent and quickly identify length errors. Likewise, confirming the exact length with an apex locator and making gutta-percha cone and/or an initial condensation radiographs will also identify problems before obturation is completed.

Management of obturation complications

Generally, the gutta-percha should be removed, any cleaning and shaping errors addressed as earlier, and the canal reobturated. Voids can be corrected during obturation if they are noticed on initial condensation radiographs or final obturation radiographs, and additional gutta-percha can be brought to their depth through the addition of accessory cones or through warm gutta-percha techniques.

Flare-up following obturation

A few patients, 1–2%, may suffer post-obturation flare-ups, inflammation, and pain. The primary cause is generally microbial; mechanical or chemical irritation of the apical tissues by instruments or obturating materials may also contribute (Siqueira, 2003). Attention to technical details, cleaning, and shaping, as described earlier, should prevent most flare-ups. Inflammatory pain should be addressed using nonsteroidal anti-inflammatory medications. Antibiotics should not be prescribed, except for rare diagnoses of acute apical abscess with systemic effects or with spread. Most flare-ups resolve within a couple of weeks. Reassurance is

key. Rarely, if symptoms do not resolve, nonsurgical retreatment may be indicated.

Restoration

The amount of remaining tooth structure after root canal treatment is directly related to long-term tooth survival. Access cavities must be conservative. Excessive tooth structure should not be removed when searching for canals, a common error. Instead, knowledge of normal canal anatomy and its variations along with careful preoperative case assessment should provide a precise plan and a conservative 3-D access preparation design. Additionally, supplementary lighting, magnification, and small instruments should be used. Excessive coronal, or even midroot, flaring beyond that needed for adequate cleaning and shaping should also be avoided. Dentin and enamel must be preserved whenever possible (Gluskin, Peters, and Peters, 2014).

Posts should only be used when there is no other way of providing retention or resistance form for the definitive coronal restoration. Posts entail removal of additional tooth structure, weakening teeth. Posts also direct occlusal forces apically, increasing the risk of root fractures. Post preparation also adds the risk of root perforation.

Coronal leakage is a major cause of endodontic failure. Bacteria must be excluded from the root canal system permanently through well-sealed durable restoration for decades. The quality of the restoration may be as important as the quality of the root canal treatment in achieving endodontic success.

Tooth fracture in anterior teeth

Anterior root canal-treated teeth should only rarely receive crowns, because crown preparation removes excessive tooth structure (Sorensen and Martinoff, 1984). Instead, anterior teeth should generally be restored using composite restorations, even if multiple restorations are needed in a single tooth. If the tooth is too dark, an opaque white-colored resin composite can be placed deep within the access cavity; this can be covered with a layer of tooth-colored resin composite.

Internal bleaching should use sodium perborate alone, without heat or superoxyl so as to avoid the complication of external resorption. Internal bleaching is highly effective in lightening teeth that have been stained by necrotic tissue or blood breakdown products. A glass ionomer or resin-modified glass ionomer barrier should be placed to just above the level of the periodontal attachment, usually a millimeter or so below the level of the cementoenamel junction so as to avoid external resorption.

Management of anterior tooth fracture

Porcelain veneers can be used to achieve excellent esthetic results. Again, conservative tooth preparation is important; most of the veneer should be kept within enamel.

Root fracture, especially vertical or oblique, may not be treatable, so prevention through conservation of tooth structure is the key.

Tooth fracture in posterior teeth

In contrast to anterior teeth, posterior teeth will benefit from receiving coronal coverage; they will be less likely to fracture (Zadik et al., 2008). Onlays are preferred to full crowns because more tooth structure is preserved. Almost all endodontically treated molars can be restored using an amalgam corono-radicular buildup instead of a post. Retention and resistance can be gained from the walls of the pulp chamber. Upon initiating root canal treatment in posterior teeth, occlusion should be reduced to eliminate both centric and eccentric contacts; this has little downside, because these teeth will be restored using onlays or crowns.

Complications with posts

Only if absolutely needed, and there is absolutely no other way to gain resistance and retention form, should posts be used (Sorensen and Martinoff, 1984). If used, they should maximize conservation of tooth structure. Posts should be passive, parallel sided, serrated, and vented (e.g., ParaPost, Coltene Whaledent, Altstatten, Switzerland). These features minimize the removal of precious tooth structure, minimize the wedge effect, and maximize retention.

Management of post complications

Post spaces are best made at the time of obturation under rubber dam isolation when the root anatomy is best understood. To avoid perforation, the post should be much narrower than the root, maybe one-fourth of the root width or less. Remember that many posterior roots have pronounced concavities that are not clearly seen on radiographs, for example, upper first premolars. Remember that canals may curve in or out of the plane of a radiograph, for example, the palatal root of an upper molar. First, a heated instrument should be used to remove gutta-percha to provide a pathway. Second, a Gates Glidden drill, one size smaller than the final post drill, is used to make an initial preparation; its rounded flutes try to follow the canal. Finally, the definitive post drill is used to finalize the shape and depth.

Once a post space has been made, it is critical that it not be contaminated by bacteria or saliva. Prefabricated posts are best placed at the time of obturation.

Should a post perforation occur, it must be recognized immediately; vigilance is important (Figure 3.14) (AAE, 2008). A rubber dam should be placed, if not already present. The wide end of a paper point can be used to check for clear tissue exudate or blood from a minor perforation. The post space is gently irrigated and rinsed and a nonsetting calcium hydroxide paste placed. The patient must be informed and referral to an endodontist for internal perforation repair made, likely using an endodontic microscope to place mineral trioxide aggregate.

Coronal microleakage

Reentry of bacteria to the root canal system is a key cause of endodontic failure. Bacteria must be excluded at all stages of root canal treatment and thereafter. Effective rubber dam isolation and durable leak-proof temporary restoration are critical, but the definitive restoration must be performed for decades. Ideally, a permanent restoration is placed at the time of obturation to avoid the risks of leakage that are inherent with temporary materials. Teeth that receive a permanent buildup or foundation restoration have a better prognosis than those that receive temporary restorations (Landys Borén, Jonasson, and Kvist, 2015).

Prevention and management of coronal microleakage

Definitive restorations are best placed at the time of obturation, before the rubber dam is removed. Glass ionomers seal well but are not strong enough to form an entire core or buildup. Glass ionomers may be used as liners or bases, sealing the pulpal floor. One technique is to remove gutta-percha to 1–2mm below the floor of the pulp chamber and replace it with a glass ionomer intra-orifice barrier. Amalgam or composite can be used for the bulk restoration.

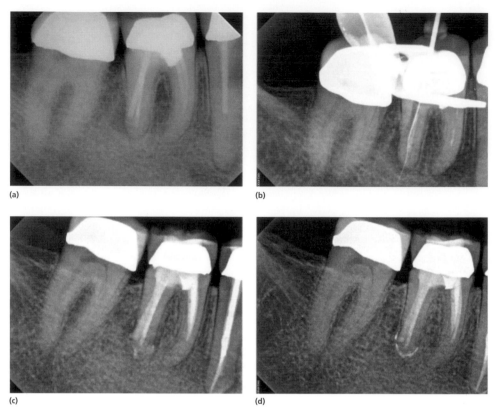

(a)   (b)

(c)   (d)

Figure 3.14 Management of a post perforation. (a) Patient presented for endodontic retreatment with symptomatic apical periodontitis due to a perforation that occurred many years previously; the lesion is centered on the end of the post. (b) The post was removed using ultrasonic vibration and the canal path was located. Calcium hydroxide paste was placed in the canals for 4 months. (c) After initial healing was confirmed, MTA was used to seal the perforation and obturate the distal canal. (d) Complete healing at 1.5-year recall; despite the short fills on the mesial roots, the periapical tissues are healthy and the patient is asymptomatic.

If there is to be even a minor delay between obturation and definitive restoration, a durable temporary restoration must be placed. Popular materials, zinc oxide eugenol based or soft and moldable, do not maintain a long-term seal, and soft moldable materials are particularly susceptible to being worn away in larger cavities. Instead, a glass ionomer or resin-modified glass ionomer is recommended. An opaque white temporary material can be used so as to facilitate its identification and removal for definitive restoration (e.g., white Fuji TRIAGE, GC; or blue Vitremer Core Buildup). Often a small cotton pellet is placed underneath a temporary restoration to facilitate restoration removal. But, damp cotton is a magnet for bacteria and a great culture medium. If a cotton pellet is to be used, it should be small so as to maximize the thickness of the temporary restoration. A little nonsetting calcium hydroxide paste can be added to the pellet to prevent bacterial growth. Alternatively, a small piece of a synthetic sponge can be used instead of cotton.

Should a gutta-percha obturation be exposed to the oral environment for more than a few days, retreatment is recommended. Obturation is just that filling rather than sealing. In the future, sealers that really seal against dentin will be developed. But, at this time, we must rely on a durable leak-proof restoration to exclude bacteria.

Systemic issues causing complications

Very few systemic issues are thought to adversely affect endodontic prognosis. Diabetes, particularly insulin-dependent diabetes, is associated with a reduced likelihood of successful healing after root canal treatment, increased symptoms, and an increased incidence of flare-ups (Fouad, 2003). However, other medical conditions, even HIV status, do not appear to influence the outcomes of root canal treatment (Quesnell *et al.*, 2005).

In fact, root canal treatment may be provided, even in the case of useless teeth so as to avoid extraction or surgery, in patients who have bleeding disorders, who have received high-dosage bisphosphonate therapy, or who are undergoing head and neck radiation. In these situations, great care must be taken to avoid traumatizing the gingiva during rubber dam clamp placement, etc. Increased age does not influence endodontic outcomes; however, increased calcification can increase the level of technical difficulty (Hamedy *et al.*, 2014).

Failure to heal after root canal treatment

Most root canal treatment results in healing. Root canal-treated teeth have extremely high survival rates, as measured by systematic review, the highest level of clinical evidence (Iqbal and Kim, 2007; Torabinejad *et al.*, 2007). Follow-up is needed to monitor the healing process. Usually positive signs, a decrease in the size of a periapical radiolucency and bony healing, become evident in 6 months to 1 year.

For teeth that had preoperative periapical radiolucencies, it is expected that the radiolucencies will resolve over time. A periapical lesion is an immunological response to bacteria and their breakdown products. After the root canal system has been properly cleaned, disinfected, and obturated, the periapical tissues can begin to heal and return to their normal architecture. If root canal treatment was not thorough, then remaining bacteria will prevent healing.

The healing and remodeling process takes time, sometimes years (Molven *et al.*, 2002). If a tooth has had NSRCT and a periradicular radiolucency is still present, it does not necessarily mean that the treatment is failing. It is irrational to extract, retreat, or surgically treat such a tooth based solely on radiographic findings. If the tooth is in the process of healing, soft tissue findings quickly return to normal; sinus tracts, edema, and deep periodontal probing defects usually resolve within a few weeks. An absence of tenderness to chewing, percussion,

and palpation is expected on an RCT-treated tooth that is healed or healing within normal limits.

Unhealed cases

In making the determination of whether the RCT is failing and further treatment is needed, it can be helpful to assess the quality of the existing treatment clinically and radiographically, but "radiographic esthetics" aren't necessarily an indicator of prognosis. We have all seen "radiographically beautiful" cases fail, and less than optimal cases succeed. The question is, have the biologic goals of removing bacteria and sealing the tooth been met? Unfortunately, the intraradicular bacterial status cannot be determined by looking at a radiograph. Nevertheless, cases with clear deficiencies, such as incomplete treatment or missed canals, may be retreated. The patient and treating dentist can provide useful information such as the date of the original treatment and treatment protocol, for example, whether a rubber dam was used.

Management of unhealed cases

If a periapical radiolucency does not decrease in size, or if a tooth remains symptomatic, nonsurgical retreatment is generally indicated (Figure 3.15) (Torabinejad *et al.*, 2009). Only if retreatment has not been successful, or if retreatment is not possible, should root end microsurgery be performed provided (Torabinejad *et al.*, 2015). A single tooth implant may be a viable alternative to apical surgery in a severely compromised tooth.

If a tooth requires endodontic retreatment, in the absence of irreparable iatrogenic damage, and is restorable, the chance of saving the tooth with endodontic retreatment or indeed even with retreatment followed by surgery is excellent.

Conclusion

Root canal treatment is a predictable and viable way to eliminate pain, inflammation, and infection of endodontic origin while saving precious natural teeth, but it is not easy. Thoughtful treatment planning and technical care are required to avoid all potential complications. Should complications be anticipated, or should they occur, endodontic specialists can be called upon. Patients prefer to save their natural teeth and appreciate the meticulous work that is endodontics.

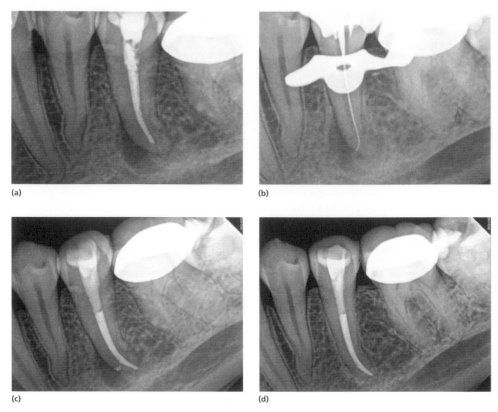

(a)

(b)

(c)

(d)

Figure 3.15 Nonsurgical endodontic retreatment. If the biological objectives can be met, cleaning and shaping the entire root canal system, the prognosis is excellent. (a) The original fill points toward the root apex and a small lesion, but it is over 1 mm short; interestingly, the larger lesion is centered to the mesial of the root apex. (b) A small precurved file is used to explore the entire apex, as well as the main canal; another portal of exit was located in the center of the larger lesion, mesial to the apex. (c) The main canal and mesial branch have been obturated and a definitive restoration has been placed. (d) A 1-year recall PA shows complete healing.

References

Ahmed, H.M., Cohen, S., Lévy, G., Steier, L. and Bukiet, F. (2014) Rubber dam application in endodontic practice: an update on critical educational and ethical dilemmas. *Australian Dental Journal*, **59**, 457–463.

American Academy of Pediatric Dentistry (AAPD) Council on Clinical Affairs. (2010) Clinical guideline on management of acute dental trauma. *AAPD Reference Manual* **32**: 202–212.

American Association of Endodontists (AAE). (2004) *Recommended Guidelines of the American Association of Endodontists for the Treatment of Traumatic Dental Injuries.* Chicago 2004. http://www.aae.org/uploadedFiles/Publications_and_ Research/Guidelines_and_Position_Statements/2004 TraumaGuidelines.pdf (accessed December 21, 2015).

AAE (2008) Procedural accidents: an online study guide. *Journal of Endodontics*, **34** (5 Suppl), e65–e70.

Baumgartner, J.C. and Xia, T. (2003) Antibiotic susceptibility of bacteria associated with endodontic abscesses. *Journal of Endodontics*, **29**, 44–47.

Cope, A., Francis, N., Wood, F., Mann, M.K. and Chestnutt, I.G. (2014) Systemic antibiotics for symptomatic apical periodontitis and acute apical abscess in adults. *Cochrane Database of Systematic Reviews*, **6**, CD010136.

Crump, M.C. and Natkin, E. (1970) Relationship of broken root canal instruments to endodontic case prognosis: a clinical investigation. *The Journal of the American Dental Association*, **80**, 1341–1347.

DiAngelis, A.J., Andreasen, J.O., Ebeleseder, K.A., Kenny, D.J., Trope, M., Sigurdsson, A., Andersson, L., Bourguignon, C., Flores, M.T., Hicks, M.L., Lenzi, A.R., Malmgren, B., Moule, A.J., Pohl, Y. and Tsukiboshi, M. (2012) International Association of Dental Traumatology guidelines for the management of traumatic dental injuries: 1. Fractures and luxations of permanent teeth. *Dental Traumatology*, **28**, 2–12.

Fedorowicz, Z., van Zuuren, E.J., Farman, A.G., Agnihotry, A. and Al Langawi, J.H. (2013) Antibiotic use for irreversible pulpitis. *Cochrane Database of Systematic Reviews*, **12**, CD004969.

Fouad, A.F. (2003) Diabetes mellitus as a modulating factor of endodontic infections. *Journal of Dental Education*, **67**, 459–467.

Gillen, B.M., Looney, S.W., Gu, L., Loushine, B.A., Weller, R.N., Loushine, R.J., Pashley, D.H. and Tay, F.R. (2011) Impact of the quality of coronal restoration versus the quality of root canal fillings on success of root canal treatment: a systematic review and meta-analysis. *Journal of Endodontics*, **37**, 895–902.

Gluskin, A.H., Peters, C.I. and Peters, O.A. (2014) Minimally invasive endodontics: challenging prevailing paradigms. *British Dental Journal*, **216**, 347–353.

Hamedy, R., Shakiba, B., Pak, J.G., Barbizam, J.V., Ogawa, R.S. and White, S.N. (2014) Prevalence of root canal treatment and periapical radiolucency in elders: a systematic review. *Gerodontology*, **33**, 116–127.

Hansen, J.R., Beeson, T.J. and Ibarrola, J.L. (2013) Case series: tooth retention 5 years after irretrievable separation of LightSpeed LSX instruments. *Journal of Endodontics*, **39**, 1467–1470.

Hülsmann, M. and Hahn, W. (2000) Complications during root canal irrigation: literature review and case reports. *International Endodontic Journal*, **33**, 186–193.

Iqbal, M.K. and Kim, S. (2007) For teeth requiring endodontic treatment, what are the differences in outcomes of restored endodontically treated teeth compared to implant-supported restorations? *The International Journal of Oral & Maxillofacial Implants*, **22** (Suppl), 96–116.

Kakehashi, S., Stanley, H.R. and Fitzgerald, R.J. (1965) The effects of surgical exposures of dental pulps in germ-free and conventional laboratory rats. *Oral Surgery, Oral Medicine, and Oral Pathology*, **20**, 340–349.

Krastl, G., Filippi, A., Zitzmann, N.U., Walter, C. and Weiger, R. (2011) Current aspects of restoring traumatically fractured teeth. *The European Journal of Esthetic Dentistry*, **6**, 124–141.

Kuttler, Y. (1955) Microscopic investigation of root apexes. *The Journal of the American Dental Association*, **50**, 544–552.

Landys Borén, D., Jonasson, P. and Kvist, T. (2015) Long-term survival of endodontically treated teeth at a public dental specialist clinic. *Journal of Endodontics*, **41**, 176–181.

Lubisich, E.B., Hilton, T.J. and Ferracane, J. (2010) Cracked teeth: a review of the literature. *Journal of Esthetic and Restorative Dentistry*, **22**, 158–167.

Madarati, A.A., Watts, D.C. and Qualtrough, A.J. (2008) Factors contributing to the separation of endodontic files. *British Dental Journal*, **204**, 241–245.

Maltz, M., Garcia, R., Jardim, J.J., de Paula, L.M., Yamaguti, P.M., Moura, M.S., Garcia, F., Nascimento, C., Oliveira, A. and Mestrinho, H.D. (2012) Randomized trial of partial vs. stepwise caries removal: 3-year follow-up. *Journal of Dental Research*, **91**, 1026–1031.

Mertz-Fairhurst, E.J., Curtis, J.W., Ergle, J.W., Rueggeberg, F.A. and Adair, S.M. (1988) Ultraconservative and cariostatic sealed restorations: results at year 10. *The Journal of the American Dental Association*, **129**, 55–66.

Mohammadi, Z. and Dummer, P.M. (2011) Properties and applications of calcium hydroxide in endodontics and dental traumatology. *International Endodontic Journal*, **44**, 697–730.

Molven, O., Halse, A., Fristad, I. and MacDonald Jankowski, D. (2002) Periapical changes following root-canal treatment observed 20–27 years postoperatively. *International Endodontic Journal*, **35**, 784–790.

Pak, J.G. and White, S.N. (2011) Pain prevalence and severity before, during, and after root canal treatment: a systematic review. *Journal of Endodontics*, **37**, 429–438.

Paqué, F., Balmer, M., Attin, T. and Peters, O.A. (2010) Preparation of oval-shaped root canals in mandibular molars using nickel-titanium rotary instruments: a micro-computed tomography study. *Journal of Endodontics*, **36**, 703–707.

Quesnell, B.T., Alves, M., Hawkinson, R.W., Johnson, B.R., Wenckus, C.S. and BeGole, E.A. (2005) The effect of human immunodeficiency virus on endodontic treatment outcome. *Journal of Endodontics*, **31**, 633–636.

Siqueira, J.F. (2001) Strategies to treat infected root canals. *Journal of the California Dental Association*, **29**, 825–837.

Siqueira, J.F. (2003) Microbial causes of endodontic flare-ups. *International Endodontic Journal*, **36**, 453–463.

Sjogren, U., Hagglund, B., Sundqvist, G. and Wing, K. (1990) Factors affecting the long-term results of endodontic treatment. *Journal of Endodontics*, **16**, 498–504.

Sjögren, U., Figdor, D., Spångberg, L. and Sundqvist, G. (1991) The antimicrobial effect of calcium hydroxide as a short-term intracanal dressing. *International Endodontic Journal*, **24**, 119–125.

Stojicic, S., Zivkovic, S., Qian, W., Zhang, H. and Haapasalo, M. (2010) Tissue dissolution by sodium hypochlorite: effect of concentration, temperature, agitation, and surfactant. *Journal of Endodontics*, **36**, 1558–1562.

Sorensen, J.A. and Martinoff, J.T. (1984) Intracoronal reinforcement and coronal coverage: a study of endodontically treated teeth. *The Journal of Prosthetic Dentistry*, **51**, 780–784.

Sundqvist, G.K., Eckerbom, M.I., Larsson, A.P. and Sjögren, U.T. (1979) Capacity of anaerobic bacteria from necrotic dental pulps to induce purulent infections. *Infection and Immunity*, **25**, 685–693.

Swanson, K. and Madison, S. (1987) An evaluation of coronal microleakage in endodontically treated teeth. Part I. Time periods. *Journal of Endodontics*, **13**, 56–59.

Torabinejad, M., Anderson, P., Bader, J., Brown, L.J., Chen, L.H., Goodacre, C.J., Kattadiyil, M.T., Kutsenko, D., Lozada, J., Patel, R., Petersen, F., Puterman, I. and White, S.N. (2007) Outcomes of root canal treatment and restoration, implant-supported single crowns, fixed partial dentures, and extraction without replacement: a systematic review. *The Journal of Prosthetic Dentistry*, **98**, 285–311.

Torabinejad, M., Corr, R., Handysides, R. and Shabahang, S. (2009) Outcomes of nonsurgical retreatment and endodontic surgery: a systematic review. *Journal of Endodontics*, **35**, 930–937.

Torabinejad, M., Landaez, M., Milan, M., Sun, C.X., Henkin, J., Al Ardah, A., Kattadiyil, M., Bahjri, K., Dehom, S., Cortez, E. and White, S.N. (2015) Tooth retention through endodontic microsurgery or tooth replacement using single implants: a systematic review of treatment outcomes. *Journal of Endodontics*, **41**, 1–10.

Witherspoon, D.E., Small, J.C. and Regan, J.D. (2013) Missed canal systems are the most likely basis for endodontic retreatment of molars. *Texas Dental Journal*, **130**, 127–139.

Zadik, Y., Sandler, V., Bechor, R. and Salehrabi, R. (2008) Analysis of factors related to extraction of endodontically treated teeth. *Oral Surgery, Oral Medicine, Oral Pathology, Oral Radiology, and Endodontics*, **106**, e31–e35.

Zehnder, M. (2006) Root canal irrigants. *Journal of Endodontics*, **32**, 389–398.

CHAPTER 4

Prosthodontics complications

Thomas S. Giugliano

Department of Prosthodontics, New York University College of Dentistry, New York, USA

Fixed prosthodontics

Common complications
Fractured porcelain

The porcelain fused to metal (PFM) restoration is still widely used in dentistry today for single crowns and fixed dental prostheses (FDPs). One of the most common complications with this type of restoration is fractured porcelain (Figure 4.1a–d). Studies have shown the incidence of porcelain fracture (Table 4.1) to be between 2 and 5% over a 10-year period (Coonaert, Adriaens, and de Boever, 1984, Ozcan, 2003a).

The most frequent reason for porcelain fracture is related to cracks within the ceramic material. Other reasons for fractured porcelain can be seen in Table 4.2 (Ozcan, 2003b).

Prevention

Adequate preparation of the tooth (teeth) is of vital importance to the successful fabrication of any single crown or FDP. Insufficient occlusal and/or axial reduction can lead to technical failures such as the metal or porcelain being too thin and increasing the chance of fracture. If a tooth is overreduced, inadequate height and surface area will result in decreased retention of the crown. Overreduction also increases the chance of pulpal exposure, requiring endodontic treatment and additional buildup to restore the tooth. When a clinical crown is short, grooves can be placed in the axial walls of the preparation to increase retention or crown lengthening may be indicated if there is adequate bone and root length.

Management

Fractured porcelain can be repaired most commonly in three ways:

1 Rebonding the fractured chip to the remaining fractured porcelain.
2 Bonding a porcelain veneer to the fractured porcelain.
3 Using a composite resin to restore the fractured porcelain (Figure 4.2a–f) (Yanikoglu, 2004). Porcelain repair kits are commercially available for this purpose.

The prognosis of a porcelain repair is highly dependent on the integrity of the bond between the ceramic and the composite resin (Yanikoglu, 2004) and the conditioning methods used (Kimmich and Stappert, 2013). If fractured porcelain remains unrepaired, sharp edges have the potential to cause ulceration of the surrounding soft tissue. If a fracture occurs along an incisal edge (Figure 4.1a, b), esthetics, speech, and occlusal function may be compromised.

Fractured metal frames

Any material, including metal, will fracture if the load applied exceeds that material's fracture strength (Baran, Boberick, and McCool, 2001). In the case of FDPs, one of the most important considerations to avoid metal frame fracture is the height and width of the connector. The connector is the weakest component of an FDP since it displays the highest concentration of stress (Wright, 1986). When an FDP metal framework is subject to loading, it will flex, causing deformation. The metal framework must be sufficiently rigid to withstand this deformation (Selby, 1994). If the forces consistently exceed two thirds of the stress limit value of the metal,

Avoiding and Treating Dental Complications: Best Practices in Dentistry, First Edition. Edited by Deborah A. Termeie.
© 2016 John Wiley & Sons, Inc. Published 2016 by John Wiley & Sons, Inc.

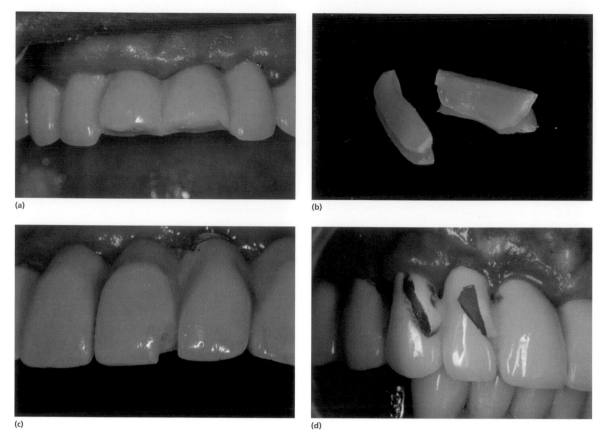

(a)

(b)

(c)

(d)

Figure 4.1 Examples of fractured porcelain. Reproduced with permission from T. Suzuki.

Table 4.1 Fracture rate of porcelain fused to metal restorations.

Author	Year	Fracture rate (%)	Time period (year)
Strub, Stiffler, and Scharer	1988	2.7	7
Karlsson	1986	4.2	10
Sailer et al.	2007	2.9	5

Table 4.2 Reasons for fractured porcelain.

- Cracks within the ceramic material
- Improperly designed metal substructure
- Different coefficients of expansion between metal and porcelain
- Excessive porcelain thickness
- Technical flaws in application of porcelain
- Occlusal forces
- Trauma

Data from Ozcan (2003b).

the continuous loading of occlusal forces will cause metal to fracture due to fatigue (Lundgren and Laurell, 1994).

Prevention

Imperfections in the casting, poor solder joints, and small connectors may increase the possibility of framework fracture (Selby, 1994) even if there is a passive, accurate fit of the framework (Sones, 1989). Case selection in providing FDPs is of critical importance to reduce the likelihood of fractured frameworks. Short clinical crowns and long spans should be avoided. One study found the recommended minimum dimensions for metal FDP connectors to be 4.1 mm in height and 4.0 mm in width for a single posterior tooth replacement and 2.9 mm in height and 3.0 mm in width for a maxillary anterior tooth replacement (Erhardson, Carlsson, and Wictorin, 1980). Since solder joints are common sites for fractures, FDPs should be cast in one piece if possible (Glantz and Nyman, 1982). If a framework must be cut and soldered,

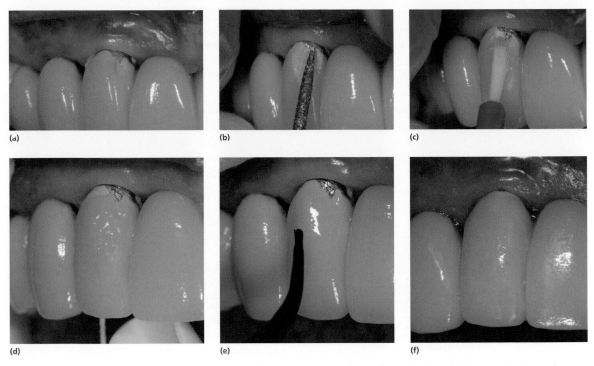

Figure 4.2 Procedure to repair porcelain with composite resin. (a) Fractured porcelain, (b) diamond bur roughening surface of porcelain and metal, (c) application of hydrofluoric acid, (d) allow acid adequate time to etch (according to manufacturer's instructions), (e) application of bonding agent, (f) finished repair with composite resin. Reproduced with permission from T. Suzuki.

midpontic solder joints (vertical and diagonal) have been shown to be stronger than a solder joint at the interproximal connector area (Ferencz, 1987).

Management

Fractured frameworks can be repaired, but the cause of the fracture should be determined in order to prevent the fracture from recurring. Possible causes to consider could be metal miscast, the span of the FDP being too long, or insufficient occlusal clearance for an adequate connector. The most predictable way to manage a fractured framework is to identify the cause of the fracture, modify the design of the framework as needed, then remake the FDP.

Crown/FDP loose

Occasionally a crown or FDP will begin to exhibit mobility. Sometimes the patient will notice movement and inform the dentist, other times the patient is unaware, and it is discovered during a routine recall examination. When a crown or FDP is perceived to have

mobility, it is important to determine exactly what is loose. It is possible that only the crown or FDP is loose and may simply require removal, cleaning, and recementation. However, it may also be possible that the tooth or one or more abutments of the FDP may be loose and the prosthesis is intact and stable. This can be due to bone loss, root fracture, or occlusal trauma.

Management

A thorough clinical examination with careful visual inspection is necessary to determine if the supporting abutments are mobile. Clinical judgment will determine how to proceed in these instances. If the crown or FDP is intact, and the mobility is due to bone loss, a referral to a periodontist is recommended to determine if any surgical intervention is indicated. Occlusion should be checked to rule out occlusal trauma. If the mobility is determined to be caused by occlusal trauma, an occlusal adjustment may be all that is necessary. If a radiographic examination reveals the mobility to be caused by a root fracture, a new appropriate treatment plan will be needed. Since root fractures often render a tooth unrestorable, extraction may become necessary. Clinical options such as fixed, removable, or implant prosthodontics must then be discussed with the patient to determine the method of tooth replacement.

If a crown is loose, it can almost always be removed intact. If an FDP is loose, it may not always be removed. At times, only one of several abutment crowns may have a defective cement seal on an FDP. If this is the case, the FDP may have to be cut off and replaced with a new one, if the supporting abutments are still restorable.

Crown/FDP fallen out

Sometimes a crown or FDP can fall out. Saliva contamination during the cementation process may wash out some cement before the cement has had a chance to fully set. If the occlusion was not properly adjusted, lateral forces on a crown can, over time, break the cement seal and cause looseness of a crown or FDP.

Prevention

Periodic recall examinations are critical for the long-term success of any prosthesis. A careful check of the occlusion in centric occlusion, protrusive, and lateral excursions is critical to discover if any occlusal interferences exist. These interferences must be eliminated prior to dismissing the patient after a crown or FDP cementation to prevent lateral forces from acting detrimentally on the crown or FDP. Periodontal health must also be monitored to detect active periodontal disease, which when left untreated can lead to prosthetic complications. Periodic radiographic examinations are indicated to detect recurrent decay, bone loss, or other pathology.

Management

Reexamine the crown (or FDP) for fractures, perforations, excessive wear, or any other complication that may prevent the recementation of the prosthesis. Reevaluate the tooth (or abutments) for recurrent decay and reassess the periodontal health. Confirm if the internal and interproximal fit of the crown is acceptable. Some studies (Levers and Darling, 1983) have shown that supraeruption is a continual process. So it is very important to check the occlusion, especially if the patient has had the crown out of his/her mouth for an extended period of time. It is perfectly acceptable to recement a crown or FDP if it is intact, it fits well, and the occlusal and interproximal contacts have been properly adjusted.

Removable prosthodontics

According to the American College of Prosthodontists, over 35 million Americans are completely edentulous, and 178 million Americans are partially edentulous. The US adult population in need of complete denture treatment will increase from 35.4 million in 2000 to nearly 37.9 million in 2020 (Douglass, Shih, and Ostry, 2002).

Common complications in complete dentures
Pain, difficulty eating, and loose dentures

Several studies have reported that when denture patients were surveyed, their most common complaints were pain, difficulty eating, and loose dentures (Kotkin, 1985; Smith and Hughes, 1988; Brunello and Mandikos, 1998). No significant relationship was found between the patients' gender, age, or overall health and the nature of the complaints (Brunello and Mandikos, 1998; Dervis, 2002). Clearly, if a patient has pain, he/she will have difficulty chewing and eating and may not wear the denture. Pain can be severe enough so that the patient cannot wear the denture. One of the most common causes of pain is denture-induced ulceration, most often in the frena and regions of muscular attachments (Bergman and Carlsson, 1972). Denture-induced lesions are the most common symptom among patients after delivery of complete dentures (Kivovics et al., 2007). Ulcerations can also be caused by thin, sharp, or overextended denture borders, resulting in discomfort and a poor fit.

Management

Poorly fitting dentures can be managed by detecting the cause of the poor fit. Prostheses with poor fit can be caused by distorted impressions, improper blockout and waxing, processing errors, or improper metal or acrylic finishing and polishing (Shetty and Shenoy, 2011). Overcompression of the tissue during impression making will result in a pressure area in the denture base that impinges on the soft tissue. It is important to check the internal adaptation of any denture prior to delivery. Disclosing agents (disclosing wax, pressure indicating paste, indelible applicators, sprays, etc.) can be used to determine the accuracy of fit. Proper adjustment of dentures prior to delivery will reduce the chances of complications.

Loss of retention

One of the most common complications among complete denture wearers is loss of retention (Brunello and Mandikos, 1998; Bilhan et al., 2013). One study (Brunello and Mandikos, 1998) found 88% of the patients examined had dentures with poor retention. This can be caused by improperly extended denture borders, poor tissue contact, or an inadequate posterior palatal seal resulting in an imperfect peripheral seal of the denture. Also, as the residual ridge resorbs, the fit of the denture base declines (Jorge et al., 2012). Although residual ridge resorption is a chronic and continuous process of bone remodeling (Kovačić et al., 2010), the rate at which it occurs varies significantly among individuals (Nishimura and Garrett, 2004).

Prevention

Prevention of complications in removable prosthodontics begins with a thorough and complete intraoral examination and proper diagnostic procedures. Accurate, distortion-free impressions are of utmost importance in the fabrication of all types of dentures. Diagnostic (preliminary) impressions are very important in order to fabricate accurate custom trays. Without properly extended custom trays, accurate border molding becomes very difficult, increasing the chances of an inaccurate impression and an inaccurately fitting prosthesis. The fabrication process in the dental laboratory is also critical to ensure properly fitting dentures. Occlusion should always be thoroughly checked upon delivery of any prosthesis. Denture teeth will often move during the final processing, resulting in occlusal contacts different from the final esthetic wax try-in. Premature occlusal contacts will cause unwanted movement in a denture and may lead to uncomfortable ulcerations. When dentures are fabricated, balanced occlusion should be used to achieve an even distribution of occlusal forces (Feng, Liao, and Chen, 2012). Patients with moderately or severely resorbed ridges may be candidates for implant-supported overdentures to provide more stability to the denture base.

Management

One of the most effective ways to manage a denture that has lost retention is to perform a chairside or laboratory reline. This can be done if the denture is intact and the existing denture teeth retain adequate anatomical detail to remain functional. One study showed that, on average, complete dentures needed to be relined after 5.9–7.4 years of use (Dorner et al., 2010).

Denture stomatitis

Oral mucosal lesions include denture stomatitis, angular cheilitis, traumatic ulcers, tissue hyperplasia, and fibrous or "flabby" ridges (Budtz-Jorgensen, 1981). Of these lesions, denture stomatitis, often referred to as candidiasis, is among the most common, affecting anywhere from 17% (Kovav-Kavcic and Skaleric, 2000) to over 70% (Budtz-Jorgensen, Holmstrup, and Krogh, 1996) of denture wearers. It is characterized by inflammation and erythema of the portion of the oral mucosa covered by a denture (Arendorf and Walker, 1987) and may have a "cottage cheese-like" appearance (Negm, 2013). Although most patients are asymptomatic, some complain of a burning sensation, discomfort, or bad taste (Chen and Zirwas, 2007). Candidiasis has been associated with numerous conditions (Table 4.3).

Numerous studies have reported a significant association between yeast colonization, especially *Candida albicans*, and denture stomatitis (Budtz-Jorgensen and Bertram, 1970; Webb et al., 1998; Baena-Monroy et al., 2005; Bilhan et al., 2009).

Prevention

Denture patients must be given very specific postdelivery oral hygiene instructions. Since poor denture hygiene has been associated with denture stomatitis (Kulac-Ozkan, Kazazoglu, and Arikan, 2002), patients

Table 4.3 Denture stomatitis has been associated with:

- Poor oral hygiene
- Poor denture hygiene
- Continual and nighttime wearing of dentures
- Accumulation of denture plaque
- Bacterial and yeast contamination of denture surface
- Trauma due to poor denture fit
- Increased age of the denture user
- Increased age of the denture

Data from Gendreau and Loewy (2011).

must be instructed to thoroughly brush their dentures every day. Use of an ultrasonic cleaning device has also been shown to be an effective cleansing alternative (Shay, 2000), especially for patients with limited manual dexterity. Soaking dentures overnight in a 1:50 dilution (0.02%) of sodium hypochlorite solution for several weeks (Webb *et al.*, 1998), as well as removing dentures at night while sleeping, will also help to reduce the incidence of denture stomatitis (Gendreau and Loewy, 2011).

Management

Several treatments have been shown to be effective in the treatment of denture stomatitis (Table 4.4).

Fractured dentures

Complete and partial dentures can fracture in a variety of ways. The causes of denture fracture include inaccurate fit of the denture base, poor occlusal balance, accidental dropping, and presence of a maxillary torus (Beyli and von Fraunhofer, 1981;

Table 4.4 Treatment of denture stomatitis.

Nystatin powder	Bergendal and Isacsson (1980)
Topical miconazole gel	Watson *et al.* (1982)
Nystatin oral rinse	DePaola *et al.* (1986)
Oral fluconazole	Budtz-Jorgensen, Holmstrup, and Krogh (1988)

Uzun and Herseck, 2002). Also, ongoing crestal resorption results in a lever effect atop the hard palatal midline (Cilingir *et al.*, 2013). Maxillary dentures were found to fracture twice as often as mandibular dentures (Beyli and von Fraunhofer, 1981). Of all types of denture repairs, 33% were due to debonded or detached teeth, 29% were due to midline fractures, and the remaining 38% were other types of fractures, including detachment of acrylic from metal in cast metal removable dental prostheses (RDPs) (Darbar, Huggett, and Harrison, 1994).

Prevention

Periodic recall examinations for completely and partially edentulous patients are critical in discovering the potential for future fractures. The oral hygiene of the individual patient will determine recall frequency. Every recall examination should include a thorough evaluation of the stability and retention of the prostheses. One technique used to improve the fracture resistance of complete dentures is the incorporation of metal into the denture base at the time of fabrication (Balch *et al.*, 2013). This can be achieved with a cast metal framework (Figure 4.3a, b) using chromium–cobalt or a variety of other metal strengtheners such as wires, plates, and mesh (Vallittu, 1995). Chrome–cobalt is chosen for casting because it has strength and rigidity with minimum bulk (Morrow *et al.*, 1968).

Other materials such as glass or nylon fibers embedded in the denture have been shown to increase its flexural strength (John, Gangadhar, and Shah, 2001). With the

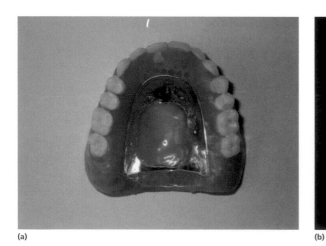
(a)

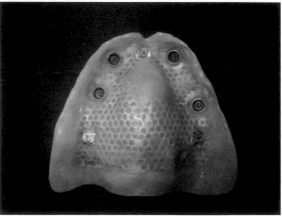
(b)

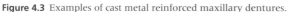

Figure 4.3 Examples of cast metal reinforced maxillary dentures.

advent of computer-aided design/computer-aided manufacturing (CAD–CAM), the days of denture repairs of this nature may shortly be behind us. Two manufacturers in the United States are fabricating dentures using CAD–CAM technology and are storing the fabrication data in their computer databases. In the not too distant future, a new, replacement denture may only be a phone call away.

Management

Some fractures require complete refabrication of the prosthesis, while some fractures can be repaired (Figure 4.4a, b). Fractures that can be managed by repair of the prosthesis have become very common, especially if they can be done chairside (Figure 4.5a–n). Although laboratory refabrication or repair has a better prognosis than a chairside repair, involving a lab can be costly and time consuming. Newer materials, such as light- or dual-cured bis-acryl composites, may offer some advantages (less shrinkage, lower setting temperatures, no odor) but also tend to be more brittle than traditional acrylic resins (polymethyl methacrylate).

Lost/missing/broken denture teeth

When a patient presents with a broken (Figure 4.6a–h) or lost (Figure 4.7a–j) denture tooth, sending the prosthesis to a commercial dental laboratory for a repair is costly and time consuming. Using composite resin for an in-office replacement of the broken or lost tooth eliminates the need for a laboratory repair

and can produce an esthetic result (Stameisen and Ruffino, 1987).

Prevention

Contamination with wax at the time of laboratory processing appears to be the main reason for detached teeth (Cunningham and Benington, 1997). Careful attention to detail in the laboratory is essential to avoid this contamination.

Management

A broken or missing tooth can also be replaced with another denture tooth of similar size and shade. The disadvantage of this technique is that it requires either a large inventory of denture teeth or the time consuming and costly delay of ordering new teeth. With mechanical retention, this can be a very predictable repair.

Similar to the repair of a complete denture, several materials (Figure 4.5j) can be used to reinforce and strengthen the replacement of a missing tooth.

Common complications in removable dental prostheses (RDPs)

RDPs have similar complications to that of complete dentures (Table 4.5). However, the one component an RDP has that a complete denture does not is a clasp. The most commonly seen complication found in RDPs is loss of retention (Bilhan *et al.*, 2012; Rehmann *et al.*, 2013).

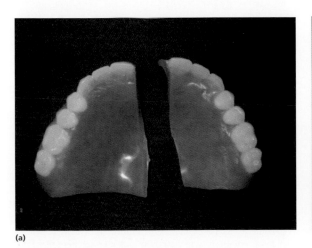

(a)

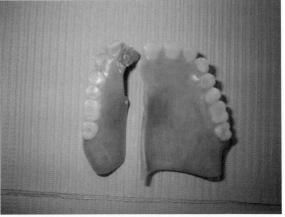

(b)

Figure 4.4 Examples of fractured maxillary dentures.

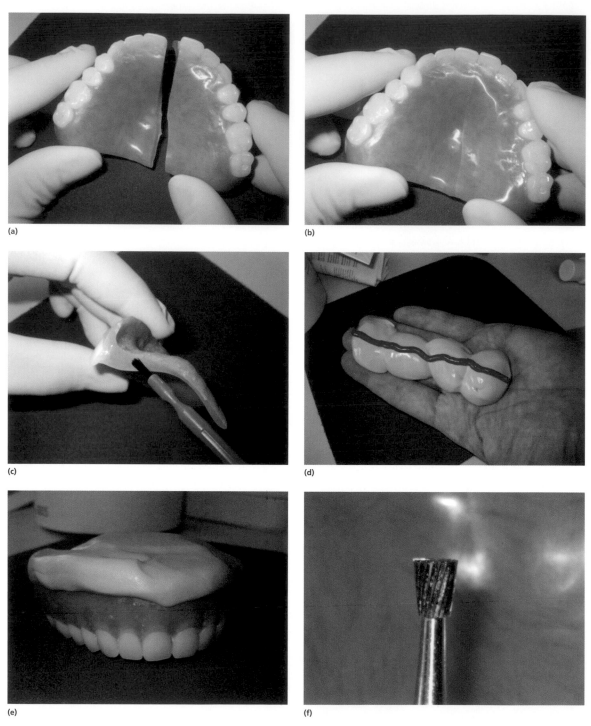

Figure 4.5 Repair procedure for a broken denture. (a) Fractured denture, (b) determine if denture can be reassembled cleanly, (c) small amount of cyanoacrylate to reassemble denture, (d) lab putty-polyvinyl siloxane (PVS), (e) PVS index of denture, (f) inverted cone acrylic bur used to make undercut notches, (g) undercut notches for mechanical retention (side view), (h) undercut notches for mechanical retention (occlusal view), (i) denture placed back on PVS index, (j) several different materials can be used to reinforce a repaired denture. Left to right: nylon mesh, orthodontic wire, perforated metal mesh, metal bar, (k) reinforcement material placed in notches, (l) reinforcement material shown below surface of denture, (m) application of powder and liquid repair acrylic to fill in voids, (n) allow repair acrylic to set, polish before delivery.

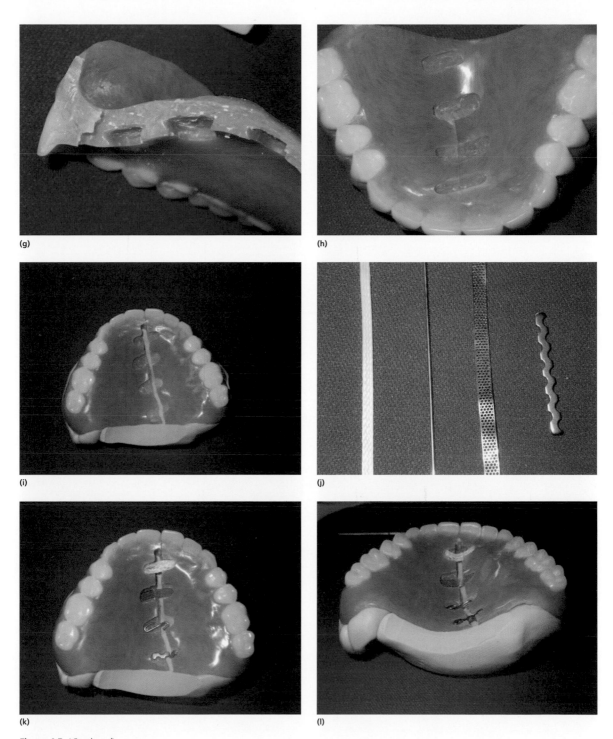

(g)

(h)

(i)

(j)

(k)

(l)

Figure 4.5 (*Continued*)

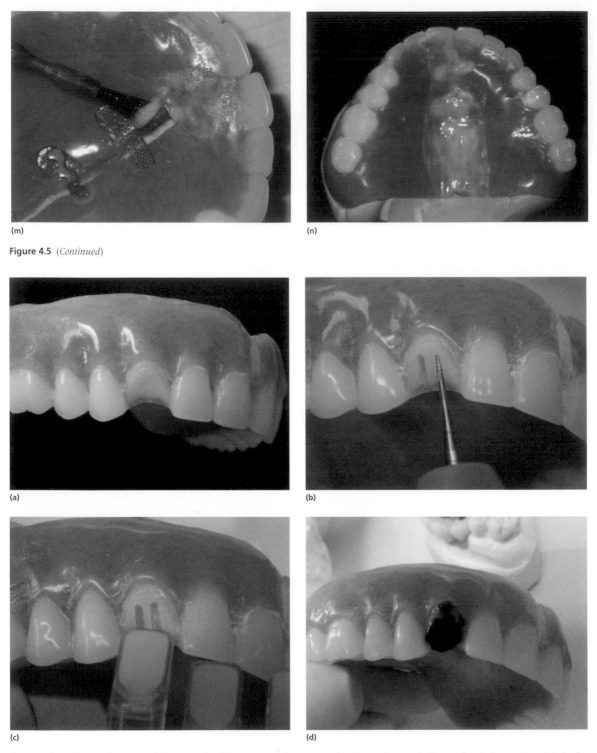

(m)

(n)

Figure 4.5 (*Continued*)

(a)

(b)

(c)

(d)

Figure 4.6 Broken tooth repair with composite. (a) Fractured denture tooth, (b) notches made for mechanical retention, (c) shade selection, (d) etchant applied, (e) bonding agent applied, (f) composite buildup, (g) light cure, (h) finished repair.

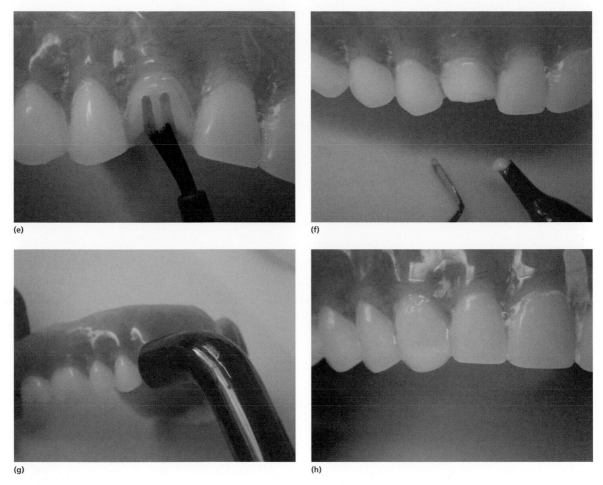

(e)

(f)

(g)

(h)

Figure 4.6 (*Continued*)

Loss of retention

Loss of retention in an RDP can be caused by residual ridge resorption, loosening of abutment teeth, loosening of clasps, or broken clasps. As in a complete denture, relining may become necessary to reestablish intimate tissue contact between the RDP and the soft tissue.

Loose clasps

An RDP can lose retention over time due to one or more retentive clasps no longer engaging the undercut it was intended to engage.

Prevention

To reduce the frequency of loose clasps, instruct the patient on proper removal and insertion of the RDP. Every time an RDP is inserted and removed, the retentive clasp flexes to engage and disengage the undercut. Excessive removal and insertion will accelerate fatigue of the metal. The patient should also be instructed to insert and remove the RDP along the proper path of insertion to avoid distorting or placing excess torque on the clasps.

Management

Clasps can be adjusted with the use of clasp-bending pliers, but it is important to keep in mind that only the terminal third of the clasp arm has enough flexibility to engage an undercut (Renner and Boucher, 1987). When bending a clasp to restore retention, there is always the possibility that the clasp will break or become more deformed (Sato, 1999).

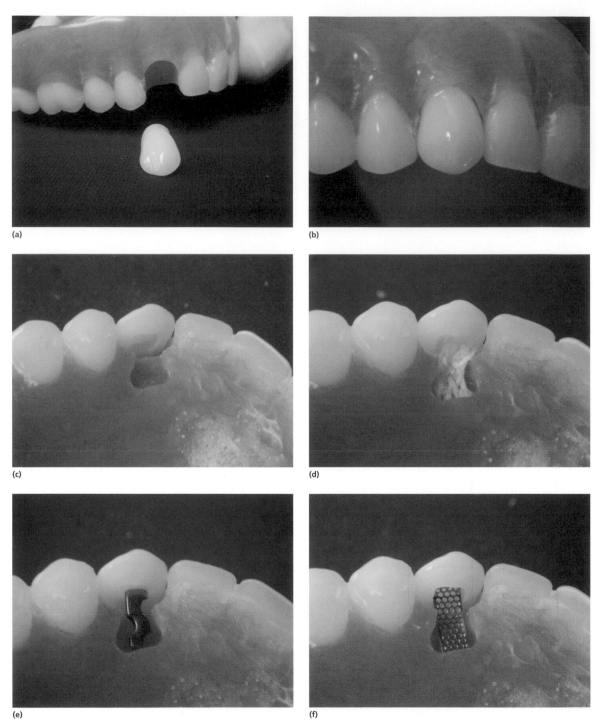

Figure 4.7 Broken tooth replacement with new denture tooth. (a) Tooth selection, (b) assess proper fit, size, and shade, (c) notches for mechanical retention, (d) nylon strip, (e) metal bar, (f) perforated metal mesh, (g) orthodontic wire, (h) powder and liquid repair acrylic, (i) finished repair, lingual view, (j) finished repair, facial view.

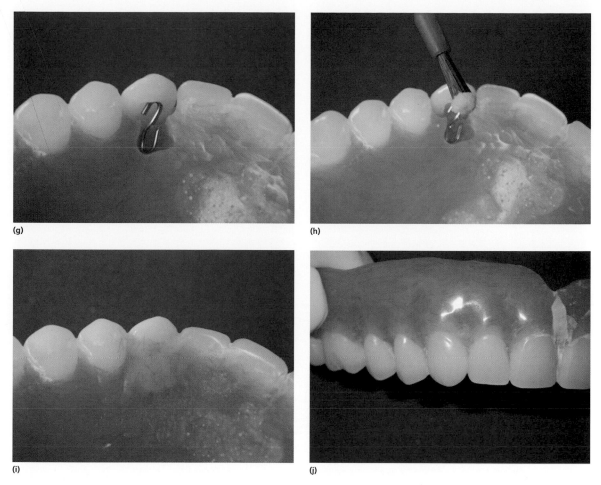

(g)
(h)
(i)
(j)

Figure 4.7 (*Continued*)

Table 4.5 The incidence and types of RDP complications.

		n	%
Complications	Loss of retention	64	64.6
	Irritation or ulceration	47	47.5
	Loss of artificial teeth	35	35.4
	Fracture of denture base	26	26.3
	Stomatitis	9	9.1
	Epulis fissuratum	5	5.1
	Fractured remaining clasps	4	4
	Existence of inflammatory papillary hyperplasia	2	2

Data from Bilhan *et al.* (2012). Reproduced with permission from The Korean Academy of Prosthodontics.

Broken clasps/frame/rest seats

Flexible clasps that engage undercuts on teeth are susceptible to fracture over time due to metal fatigue. Internal voids in the metal due to improper casting technique can predispose clasps and even major connectors to fracture (Lewis, 1978). Occlusal rest seats and embrasure clasps through the areas of the rest seat can also break (Figure 4.8a–c).

Prevention

Following proper design principles is crucial to minimize complications in RDP fabrication. The type and material of the clasp to be used will depend on the amount of undercut available on the tooth, soft tissue undercuts, and the periodontal health of the abutment tooth. The undercuts can be evaluated using a surveyor (McCord *et al.*,

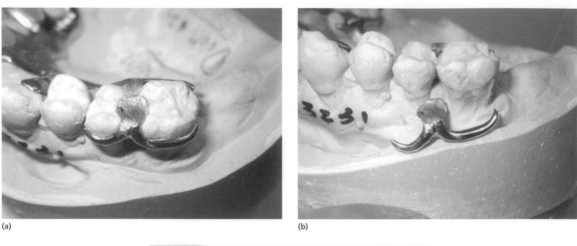

(a)　　　　　　　　　　　　　　　　　　　　　(b)

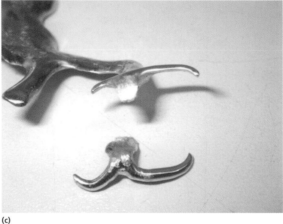

(c)

Figure 4.8 Fractured RDP clasp. (a) Embrasure clasp needs occlusal adjustment, (b, c) fractured clasp due to inadequate tooth reduction and inadequate occlusal clearance.

Table 4.6 Undercut needed for certain clasps.

Type of clasp	Amount of retentive undercut needed (in.)
Cast metal half-round circumferential clasps	0.01
Wrought wire or cast metal round clasps	0.02
Infrabulge clasp	0.01

Data from Bohnenkamp (2014).

2002). The selection of the type, placement, and number of clasps, major connector, and other components of the RDP must follow accepted design principles (Table 4.6) to ensure success (Bohnenkamp, 2014).

When preparing rest seats it is critical to ensure adequate reduction of tooth structure to accommodate the planned rest seat. This will provide adequate occlusal clearance for a rest seat. Similar to a crown preparation, insufficient tooth reduction or insufficient occlusal clearance will increase the number of complications. Occlusal rests should be of sufficient thickness and size to prevent fracture of the rest from the framework (Rice *et al.*, 2010). Different sources in the literature have recommended different suggestions as to just what size an adequate rest seat should be (Table 4.7).

Also important is to have accurately mounted and articulated casts to send to the laboratory technician. Be sure there is adequate occlusal clearance for the designed clasp before sending the casts to the laboratory.

Table 4.7 Recommendations for rest seats.

Author	Year	Width Buccolingually	Length Mesiodistally	Depth (mm)
Rudd *et al.*	1999	1/3 the crown width	1/3 to 1/2 crown length	1–2
Sato *et al.*	2003	2–2.5 mm	1/3 to 1/2 crown length	1–1.5
Luk *et al.*	2007	1 mm	2 mm	1.46

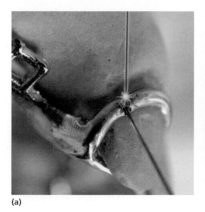
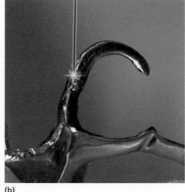
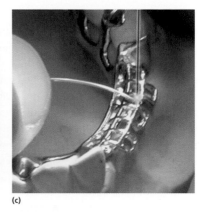

(a) (b) (c)

Figure 4.9 Examples of laser welding clasp and framework repair. Reproduced with permission from LaserStar Technologies.

Management

Broken claps are most commonly replaced with an added wrought wire clasp (Parr and Gardner, 1993). This can be done in the office if there is an adequate acrylic base to retain the clasp or sent to the lab to have a new clasp soldered into place. Broken clasps and broken RDP frames can also be repaired by welding. One of the oldest and most versatile welding processes is oxyfuel welding (conventional gas welding) which burns acetylene in oxygen (Kumar *et al.*, 2012). During the past decade, the use of laser welding (Figure 4.9a–c) had become more popular because of its ease of use and pinpoint area of heat, resulting in less damage to other parts of the RDP (Suzuki *et al.*, 2004).

Replacing a missing tooth in an RDP

If an RDP has lost a denture tooth due to fracture, it can be repaired in the same manner as a lost denture tooth in a complete denture. Although not the most common complication to occur in RDPs, occasionally a clasped natural abutment tooth is lost to periodontal disease or root fracture. One study showed it had an incidence of 8.6% of RDP complications (Behr *et al.*, 2012).

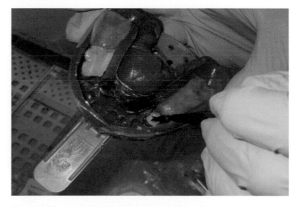

Figure 4.10 Applying acrylic into a pickup impression to replace a missing tooth in an RDP.

Management

A natural tooth can be replaced in an RDP in several ways. Prior to the extraction, a pickup impression is made using irreversible hydrocolloid (alginate) or polyvinyl siloxane (PVS) impression material. The clasps can then be bent inward to retain the powder and liquid acrylic placed in the impression of the tooth to be extracted (Figure 4.10). In this way an exact duplicate of the shape of the tooth that was extracted can be attached to the existing RDP.

In a similar manner, the clinical crown of the extracted natural tooth itself can be used, after disinfection, to attach to the RDP (Satapathy *et al.*, 2013). This can be especially effective for patients with high esthetic needs or when a shade is difficult to match. Whichever technique is used, it is important to check the repaired RDP intraorally, to determine if any adjustments are necessary.

Combination syndrome

Combination syndrome (CS) is commonly seen in patients with a complete maxillary denture opposed by mandibular natural anterior teeth and a bilateral distal extension partial denture (Langer, Laufer, and Cardash, 1995). The incidence of patients with CS has been found to be 24% among patients who wore maxillary complete dentures opposing mandibular natural anterior teeth, five times greater than completely edentulous denture wearers (Shen and Gongloff, 1989). It was first described by Kelly (1972) to include the following symptoms (Table 4.8).

The following destructive changes also occur (Table 4.9).

There is some controversy as to why these changes take place. Kelly (1972) suggests that bone loss in the anterior maxilla starts first, followed by the enlargement of the maxillary tuberosities. It is only after both dentures migrate downward posteriorly that

Table 4.8 Combination syndrome.

- Bone loss from the anterior maxilla
- Hypertrophy of the maxillary tuberosities
- Papillary hyperplasia in the hard palate
- Supraeruption of the mandibular anterior teeth
- Bone loss under the partial denture base

Data from Kelly (1972).

Table 4.9 Combination syndrome.

- Loss of vertical dimension of occlusion
- Occlusal plane discrepancy
- Anterior repositioning of the mandible
- Poor adaptation of the prostheses
- Epulis fissuratum
- Periodontal changes

Data from Saunders, Gllis, and Desjardins (1979).

supraeruption of the mandibular anterior teeth occurs (Langer, Laufer, and Cardash, 1995). Saunders, Gllis, and Desjardins (1979) believe that mandibular posterior support is lost first, leading to increased occlusal load in the anterior region.

Prevention

In a patient with a bilateral distal extension RDP, careful attention must be given to the proper design of the RDP. Since soft tissues contribute to the support of an RDP also, it is important that the denture base has properly extended borders, covering the retromolar pads and buccal shelves. Early replacement of lost teeth with implants has been suggested as a way to avoid the development of CS (Tolstunov, 2007).

Management

Preserving the health and function of remaining natural teeth can prevent progression of CS. Early detection of the symptoms of CS will enable the dentist to initiate corrective measures (Tolstunov, 2007). Prosthodontic treatment of CS should be designed to restore posterior occlusal support and reduce the occlusal pressure on the anterior maxilla as much as possible (Langer, Laufer, and Cardash, 1995). Proper occlusal records at the correct vertical dimension of occlusion are critical to determine if there has in fact been supraeruption of the mandibular anterior teeth.

Implant prosthodontics

Implant-supported restorations are designed in a variety of ways: fixed/removable combinations using fixed bars and a removable prosthesis, screw retained, cement retained, single unit, or multiple units.

Common complications

The incidence of individual implant prosthetic mechanical complications has been reported (Table 4.10), and four of the most commonly occurring implant prosthetic complications involved overdentures (Goodacre *et al.*, 2003).

For the edentulous patient, the disadvantages of complete dentures are well known (Table 4.11).

The implant-supported overdenture has become a viable and popular alternative to the complete denture, especially for the treatment of the edentulous mandible (Table 4.12).

Table 4.10 Most common implant prosthetic complications.

Complication	Mean incidence (%)
Overdenture clip/attachment loosening	30
Resin veneer fracture/fixed partial dentures	22
Overdenture relines needed	19
Overdenture clip/attachment fracture	17
Porcelain veneer fracture/fixed partial dentures	14
Overdenture fracture	12
Opposing prosthesis fracture	12
Esthetic complication with prosthesis	10
Acrylic resin base fracture	7
Prosthesis screw loosening	7
Phonetic complications	7
Abutment screw loosening	6
Prosthesis screw fractures	3
Metal framework fractures	3
Abutment screw fractures	2

Data from Goodacre *et al*. (2003). Reproduced with permission from Elsevier.

Table 4.11 Disadvantages of complete dentures.

- Fabrication requires attention to detail
- Lack of stability and retention
- Ongoing alveolar bone loss
- Compromised function when ill fitting
- Social concerns (slippage, unnatural appearance)

Data from Doundoulakis *et al*. (2003). Reproduced with permission from Elsevier.

Table 4.12 Advantages of the implant-supported overdenture.

- As few as two implants may be used for support
- Good stability and retention
- Improved esthetics and function
- Reduced residual ridge resorption
- Possible incorporation of existing denture into the new prosthesis

Data from Doundoulakis *et al*. (2003). Reproduced with permission from Elsevier.

An implant-supported overdenture can receive retention and stability from several types of inserts and attachments. These include bars, clips, balls, rubber rings, nylon inserts, and even magnets. One study (Berglundh, Persson, and Klinge, 2002) found the incidence of superstructure complications in overdentures to be 4–10 times greater than in fixed restorations. Even with the incidence of complications, patients still strongly preferred implant-supported overdentures over conventional complete dentures (Karabuda, Yaltink, and Bayraktar, 2008).

Loose clip/attachment

All types of overdenture attachments, clips, and inserts will exhibit wear over time during normal function, due to fatigue (Rutkunas, Mizutani, and Takahashi, 2005).

Prevention

It has been shown that the type of attachment used has a negligible effect on the prosthetic outcome (Cehreli *et al*., 2010). Proper fit and occlusion of the overdenture will reduce denture movement, extending the lifetime of overdenture attachments. Examination of the overdenture at periodic recall appointments will help identify worn attachments.

Management

It will become necessary to replace overdenture inserts periodically as they wear. If the overdenture is intact, most simple replacements of overdenture attachments can be performed chairside. Careful attention to the manufacturer's instructions will ensure success.

Overdenture fracture

The acrylic resin used to fabricate implant-supported overdentures becomes thinner and weaker after attachments are inserted into the denture (Domingo *et al*., 2013). Typically, the fracture of an overdenture, especially one with no metal reinforcement, will occur right in line with where the inserts are placed (Figure 4.11a–d). This is because the acrylic denture base is thinnest in this location.

Even metal frameworks imbedded in implant-supported overdentures will fracture if the metal is too thin to tolerate occlusal forces (Figure 4.12).

Prevention

Upon initial diagnosis and examination, it is important to have properly mounted and articulated diagnostic casts. This will reveal if there is adequate interocclusal space for the placement of overdenture attachments.

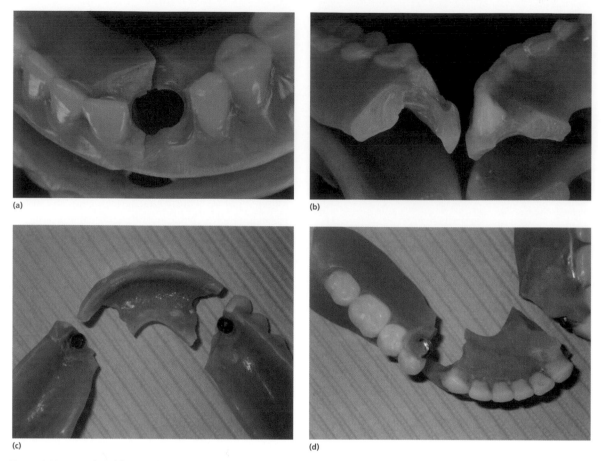

(a)

(b)

(c)

(d)

Figure 4.11 Examples of fractured overdentures. Reproduced with permission from T. Suzuki.

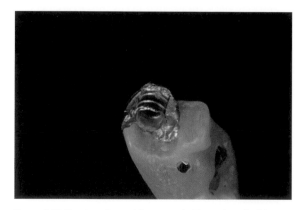

Figure 4.12 Fractured metal framework. Reproduced with permission from T. Suzuki.

Various types of overdenture attachments require different amounts of occlusal clearance. A thorough and complete clinical examination must be performed to establish if the patient is a candidate for preprosthetic surgery such as ridge reduction, alveoplasty, tuberosity reduction, etc. Metal reinforcement of the overdenture will reduce the incidence of fracture.

Regular recall maintenance is critical to monitor the wear of overdenture components. Patients with overdentures should be instructed to monitor the retention and stability of their denture. All patients, but especially patients with superstructures, need to understand the importance of good oral hygiene.

Management

Fractured overdentures can be repaired, but often they will fracture again if there is inadequate acrylic thickness to support normal function. Be sure to check intraorally that the height of each overdenture abutment is correct. If an abutment is too high (supragingivally), it may need to be removed and replaced with a new abutment with the proper height. Studies have shown no difference in patient satisfaction and function between conventional complete dentures and implant-supported overdentures *in the maxilla* (Cune, De Putter, and Hoogstraten, 1994; De Albuquerque Junior *et al.*, 2000). It has also been reported (Goodacre *et al.*, 2003) that maxillary implant-supported overdentures had the highest incidence of implant loss when compared to all other types of implant prostheses with survival rates as low as 71% at 5 years (Dudley, 2013). As a result, maxillary implant-supported overdentures should not be considered as a general treatment of choice in patients with good bony support for maxillary conventional prostheses (De Albuquerque Junior *et al.*, 2000).

Loose screws/loose crown/loose prosthesis

Screws loosen and break for several reasons (Table 4.13). Multiple factors should be considered before, during, and after prosthetic treatment. The

Table 4.13 Factors for screw loosening/breaking.

Factor	Author
Operator error	Brunski, Puleo, and Nanci (2000)
Torsion relaxation	
Thermal changes	
Amount of ridge resorption	Sones (1989)
Length and number of implants	
Opposing dentition	
Implant angulation	
Parafunctional habits	
Off-axis centric contacts	Binon (2000)
Excursive contacts	
Cantilevered loading	
Internal stresses created by misfits	
Settling	Al-Turki *et al.* (2002)
Misfit of the prosthesis	
Insufficient tightening force	
Biomechanical overload	
Differences in screw material	

incidence of screw loosening was found to be 6% (Goodacre *et al.*, 2003).

In the case of angulated implants requiring screw-retained custom abutments, occlusal forces are not directed along the long axis of the screw. This may generate more strain than the screw can tolerate, resulting in a fractured screw (Binon, 2000). The misfit of the superstructure has been shown to significantly contribute to screw instability (Al-Turki *et al.*, 2002). Radiographic examination can be helpful to determine if a metal framework fits accurately (Figure 4.13). If possible, it is important to determine the cause of the loose screw. Retightening the screw may alter its metallic properties causing progressive loss of torque retention and fracture (Weiss, Kozak, and Gross, 2000; Fauvell, Gialanella, and Penna, 2006).

Broken screws

The most common reason for screw fractures (Figure 4.14a–d) is undetected loosening (Fauvell, Gialanella, and Penna, 2006) which can be caused by bruxism, ill-fitting superstructure, overloading, or malfunction (Nergiz, Schmage, and Shahin, 2004). The mean incidence of occurrence is 4% (Goodacre *et al.*, 2003).

Prevention

Proper, thorough diagnosis and presurgical prosthetic treatment planning are the keys to reducing the number of complications in implant prosthetics. This includes close communication with the surgeon placing the

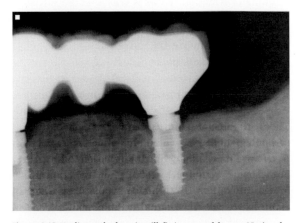

Figure 4.13 Radiograph showing ill-fitting metal frame. Notice the space between the implant platform and the metal framework.

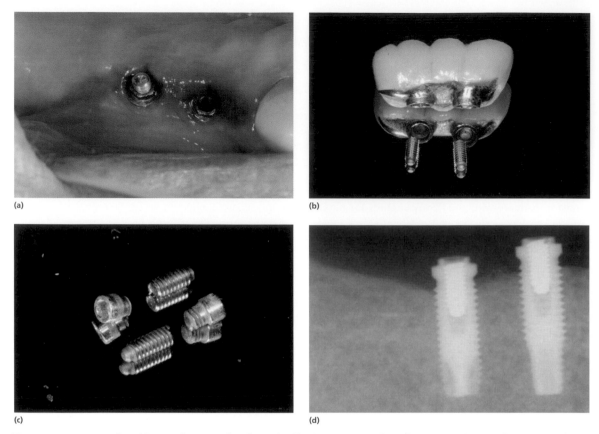

(a)

(b)

(c)

(d)

Figure 4.14 (a–c) Examples of fractured screws, (d) radiograph of broken screws inside implants. Reproduced with permission from T. Suzuki.

implants along with an accurate surgical template. Proper torquing of retention screws is critical to the success of any implant-supported prosthesis. It has been reported that the average torque placed on a screw by hand tightening with a screwdriver is only 10 N cm (Dellinges and Tebrock, 1993). A specific torque is recommended for each screw for different implant systems from different manufacturers (Burguete et al., 1994). Too small a torque may result in screw fatigue, failure, or loosening; too large a torque may break a screw or strip the threads of the screw (Siamos, Winkler, and Boberick, 2002).

Management
If an abutment screw fractures above the platform of the implant (Figure 4.14a), a hemostat or college pliers can be used to remove the broken screw. When the

screw fractures below the implant platform, in some instances an explorer can be used to engage the top of the broken screw. If that does not succeed, several other techniques have been described for screw retrieval:

- Placing a groove in the broken screw, use a self-made screwdriver (Williamson and Robinson, 2001)
- Creating a trough between the broken screw and the internal aspect of the implant, use a fine forceps (Maalhagh-Fard and Jacobs, 2010)
- Using one of several commercially available repair kits (Nergiz, Schmage, and Shahin, 2004)
- Using a piezoelectric ultrasonic scaler (Bhandari, Aggarwal, and Bakshi, 2013; Gooty et al., 2014)

Implant screw retrieval kits are available from different manufacturers.

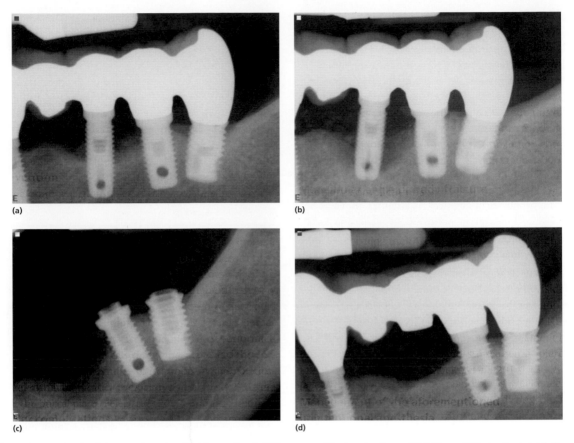

(a)

(b)

(c)

(d)

Figure 4.15 Example of "overengineering." (a) Intact 5 unit FDP supported by four implants, (b) failing middle implant, (c) failing implant removed, (d) same 5 unit FDP reinserted.

CASE: JUDY G.

- This case was saved by overengineering. A 5 unit FDP was supported by four implants (Figure 4.15a). One of the middle implants failed (Figure 4.15b), the screw-retained FDP was removed, the failed implant was removed (Figure 4.15c), and the FDP was given back to the patient (Figure 4.15d). This saved the patient from having to remake the FDP. Even in implant-supported overdentures, it has been suggested that more than two implants be used in the event one of the implants fails in the future (Doundoulakis *et al.*, 2003). If all the additional implants are not used in the prosthesis design, they are held in reserve if needed later.

Occasionally one implant will fail out of several implants that support a multiple unit FDP. One way to prevent costly remakes of FDPs is to think ahead—this is called "overengineering" (Figure 4.15). If adequate bone exists and there are no contraindications, place three implants if three teeth are to be replaced. The alternative of two implants and a three unit FDP leaves the patient vulnerable if one of the two implants fails.

Occlusal complications in implant prosthodontics

A successful implant-supported prosthesis requires careful attention to occlusion. Implants do not have a periodontal ligament (PDL) like a natural tooth. As a result, implants lack the mechanoreceptors and the shock-absorbing function that the PDL provides (Schulte, 1995). A natural tooth with a PDL has the reversible, adaptive ability to increase mobility when loaded (Gross, 2008). An osseointegrated implant does not have this ability. Hence, occlusal overload on an implant prosthesis tends to lead to mechanical complications such as screw loosening or fracture of the components (prosthesis, screw, or implant) (Schwarz, 2000; Pjetursson *et al.*, 2012). Although many concepts and theories on implant occlusion have been proposed, there is currently no evidence supporting a particular occlusal scheme (Kim *et al.*, 2005; Carlsson, 2009; Koyano and Esaki, 2015). Occlusal schemes in use appear to be based on clinical experience and expert opinion rather than evidence-based studies (Ben-Gal *et al.*, 2013).

Prevention

Although no firm clinical guidelines have been established for implant occlusion (Koyano and Esaki, 2015), some recommendations have been proposed to help prevent mechanical complications. Partial or full arch splinting and the avoidance of excursive contacts using shallow cuspal inclinations will reduce lateral forces on the prosthesis (Misch and Bidez, 2005; Klineberg, Trulsson, and Murray, 2013; Bergmann, 2014). Modification of the occlusal table and contacts to guide occlusal forces in an apical direction has also been suggested to reduce complications (Kim *et al.*, 2005).

Management

In order to service or repair an implant restoration after a complication, retrievability should be considered in the initial design. A screw-retained restoration is easily retrieved, while a cement-retained restoration may not always be retrievable, depending on the type of cement used (Chee and Jivraj, 2006). When natural teeth are adjacent to or in occlusion with an implant prosthesis, it cannot be assumed the occlusal relationship will stay the same over time. Natural teeth may move due to skeletal growth and supraeruption. Frequent monitoring of the occlusal contacts should be performed at regular hygiene maintenance visits (Bergmann, 2014).

Complications related to prosthodontics

Xerostomia

Xerostomia, more commonly known as "dry mouth," is defined as the subjective impression of oral dryness (Fox, Busch, and Baum, 1987; Ikebe *et al.*, 2002). It occurs more often in the elderly due to their increased

Table 4.14 Systemic diseases in patients with objective xerostomia.

Systemic diseases	*n* (%)
Diabetes	25 (36.7)
Sjögren syndrome	3 (4.4)
Oral cancer	5 (7.4)
Neck cancer	7 (10.3)
Depression	8 (11.8)
Hypertension	15 (22.0)
Gastrointestinal disorders	5 (7.4)

Data from Nikolopoulou, Tasopoulos, and Jagger (2013). Reproduced with permission from Quintessence Publishing Group Inc., Chicago, IL. *n* = 68.

use of drugs and susceptibility to disease (Sreenby and Schwartz, 1997). It has been estimated that approximately 20% of the population exhibits xerostomia, although prevalence in some studies has been as low as 10% (Matear *et al.*, 2006) and as high as 46% (Narhi, 1994).

Xerostomia is usually associated with hyposalivation and is caused most commonly by dehydration, medications, head and neck radiotherapy, diabetes mellitus, and other specific diseases (Arslan *et al.*, 2009). Nikolopoulou, Tasopoulos, and Jagger reported the following associations between xerostomia and systemic diseases in 2013 (Table 4.14).

Also, certain classes of drugs have been shown to be associated with xerostomia, especially antidepressants, anticholinergics, antihistamines, and diuretics (Table 4.15).

Prevention

Adhesive force developed between saliva and the denture base functions to retain a denture (Massad and Cagna, 2002). Cast metal denture bases can be used as an alternative to acrylic, since the increased wettability of metal over acrylic improves the surface coverage with saliva (Lloyd, 1996). It has also been reported that cast metal denture bases enable patients to feel temperature changes more than acrylic denture bases, resulting in enhanced flavor and enjoyment of food (Hummel *et al.*, 1999).

Table 4.15 Drugs associated with xerostomia.

Author	Year	Drugs associated
Osterberg, Landahl, and Hedegard	1984	Anticholinergics, antihistamines
Rindal *et al.*	2005	Antidepressants
Thomson *et al.*	2006	Antidepressants, diuretics

Table 4.16 CFDP success rates.

Author	Year	Success rate (%)	Tooth or implant supported	Time period (year)
Pjetursson *et al.*	2004	81.8	Tooth	10
Tan *et al.*	2004	89.1	Tooth	10
Pjetursson *et al.*	2004	86.7	Implant	10
Aglietta *et al.*	2009	88.9	Implant	10

Management

A thorough and complete medical history, including medications being taken, is critical to the management of xerostomia. If one or more medications are shown to have xerostomia as a side effect, perhaps the patient's physician can prescribe an alternate drug. Since patients with xerostomia develop significantly more carious lesions, especially cervical or root surface caries, appropriate use of topical fluorides has been suggested (Hopcraft and Tan, 2010; Plemons, Al-Hashimi, and Marek, 2014). Several over-the-counter saliva substitutes are available for the relief of xerostomia. More frequent recalls are indicated for patients with xerostomia to enable more careful monitoring of their dental health.

Cantilevers

The cantilever fixed dental prosthesis (CFDP) is a restoration with one or more abutments at one end and unsupported at the other end (Wright, 1986). It has been recommended that a cantilevered pontic have at least two abutments (Schweitzer, Schweitzer, and Schweitzer, 1968; Wright and Yettram 1979). Research has shown similar success rates over time for implant-supported CFDPs and natural tooth-supported CFDPs (Table 4.16).

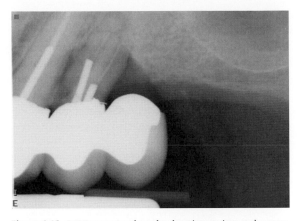

Figure 4.16 CFDP on natural teeth, showing caries, and severe bone loss.

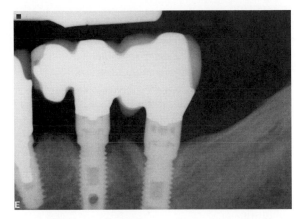

Figure 4.17 Nineteen year postoperative still functioning CFDP.

Among tooth-supported CFDPs, one study found after 10 years, the most common complications were loss of pulp vitality (32.6%) and caries (Figure 4.16) at the abutment teeth (9.1%) (Pjetursson *et al.*, 2004).

Among implant-supported CFDPs, two additional studies concurred that after 5 years the most common complications were porcelain veneer fractures (10.2%) and screw loosening (8.1%) (Aglietta *et al.*, 2009; Romeo and Storelli, 2012). Even with some complications, the tooth-supported (Wright, 1986; Hochman, Ginio, and Ehrlich, 1987; Himmel *et al.*, 1992) and the implant-supported CFDP (Aglietta *et al.*, 2009; Greenstein and Cavallaro, 2010; Romeo and Storelli, 2012) both remain a valid treatment modality (Figure 4.17), especially in areas with anatomical limitations (Figure 4.18).

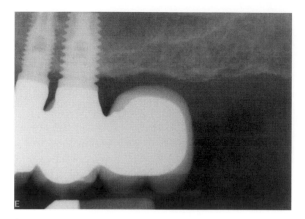

Figure 4.18 Maxillary sinus lift avoided.

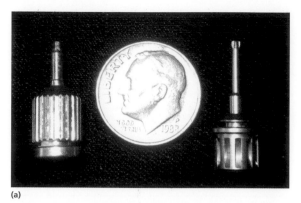

(a)

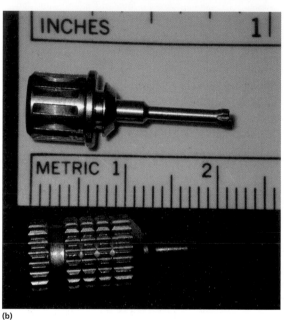

(b)

Figure 4.19 Relative size of some implant drivers (a, b).

Prevention

Since implants are at risk for peri-implantitis and natural teeth are at risk for periodontitis, proper oral hygiene and regular recall maintenance are critical in maintaining healthy abutments. A CFDP is a class 1 lever and the abutment adjacent to the cantilever acts as a fulcrum (Greenstein and Cavallaro, 2010). Like a seesaw, a class 1 lever places a fulcrum between the effort and the load. This means a downward force on one side of the fulcrum will result in an upward force on the other side of the fulcrum. As a result, occlusal force directly on the cantilever will exert a vertical dislodging force on the abutment farthest away from the cantilever.

Management

Some of the suggestions that have been made in the literature to reduce potential complications in CFDPs include:

- The abutment tooth farthest from the cantilever should be extremely retentive to resist vertical dislodgement (Himmel *et al.*, 1992).
- Narrow the occlusal table on the cantilever to reduce the loads transferred to the abutments (Wright, 1986).
- Increase the thickness in height and width of the metal substructure to increase resistance to deformation (Greenstein and Cavallaro, 2010).
- Avoid off-axis loading (English, 1993).
- Place cantilever in infraocclusion (Carlsson, 2009).
- Minimize cantilever length (Rodriguez *et al.*, 1993).
- Eliminate cantilevers when possible in bruxers (Misch, 2002).

Ingestion (swallowing) or aspiration

Many components used in dentistry are very small (Figure 4.19a, b) and have the possibility of being dropped into the back of a patient's mouth during a dental procedure.

This can result in accidental swallowing or aspiration. Although ingestion is more common than aspiration (Venkataraghavan *et al.*, 2011; Obinata *et al.*, 2011; Santos *et al.*, 2012), both situations should be treated as a medical emergency (Cosellu *et al.*, 2013).

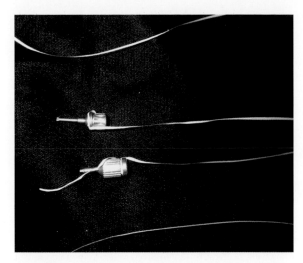

Figure 4.20 Dental floss tied around implant drivers.

Prevention

Incidents of aspiration or ingestion can be reduced by following some simple precautionary techniques. A rubber dam should always be used whenever practical. A ligated throat pack (pharyngeal drape) of gauze can be used to protect the airway (Wandera and Conry, 1993). Dental floss should be tied to any prosthetic component that has the possibility of being dropped (Figure 4.20).

Management

If a patient feels any item falling into the back of the mouth, coughing should be encouraged to try to eject the item (Cossellu *et al.*, 2013). The patient must be seen at a hospital emergency room immediately to determine if the item has been aspirated or swallowed. Consultation with the appropriate specialist(s) should be done to determine the most appropriate course of treatment (endoscopy, bronchoscopy, surgery, etc.). While waiting for emergency help to arrive, it is imperative to maintain the patient's airway. The Heimlich maneuver or cricothyroidotomy may be necessary if appropriate and indicated (Obinata *et al.*, 2011; Cossellu *et al.*, 2013).

Conclusion

To reduce the incidence of all prosthodontic complications requires the following:

- Proper diagnosis and careful treatment planning
- Cooperation and communication with other specialists, if necessary

- Accurate, detailed, and distortion-free impressions
- Proper design and fit of all aspects of the prosthesis
- Talented laboratory technicians with whom there is good communication
- Careful attention to occlusion
- Carefully following manufacturer's instructions when indicated
- Educating the patient to understand the importance of hygiene maintenance
- Meticulous postoperative care and recall

Acknowledgments

The author would like to thank Takanori Suzuki, DDS, Ph.D., for the photographs in Figures 4.1a–d, 4.2a–f, 4.11a, b, 4.12, and 4.14a–c; LaserStar Technologies for the photographs in Figure 14.9a–c; and Dr. Roger Warren for his inspiration and encouragement.

References

Aglietta, M., Siciliano, V.I., Zwahlen, M., Bragger, U., Pjetursson, B.E., Lang, N. and Salvi, G. (2009) A systematic review of the survival and complication rates of implant-supported fixed dental prostheses with cantilever extensions after an observation period of at least 5 years. *Clin Oral Impl Res*, **20**, 441–451.

Al-Turki, L.E.E., Chai, J., Lautenschlager, E.P. and Hutten, M.C. (2002) Changes in prosthetic screw stability because of misfit of implant-supported prostheses. *Int J Prosthodont*, **15**, 38–42.

Arendorf, T.M. and Walker, D.M. (1987) Denture stomatitis: a review. *J Oral Rehabil*, **14**, 217–227.

Arslan, A., Orhan, K., Canpolat, C., Delilbasi, C. and Dural, S. (2009) Impact of xerostomia on oral complaints in a group of elderly Turkish removable denture wearers. *Arch Gerontol Geriatr*, **49**, 263–267.

Baena-Monroy, T., Moreno-Maldonado, V., Franco-Martinez, F., Aldape-Barrios, B., Quindos, G. and Sanchez-Vargas, L.O. (2005) *Candida albicans*, *Staphylococcus aureus* and *Streptococcus mutans* colonization in patients wearing dental prosthesis. *Med Oral Pathol Oral Cir Bucal*, **10** (Suppl 1), E27–E39.

Balch, J.H., Smith, P.D., Marin, M.A. and Cagna, D.R. (2013) Reinforcement of a mandibular complete denture with internal metal framework. *J Prosthet Dent*, **109**, 202–205.

Baran, G., Boberick, K. and McCool, J. (2001) Fatigue of restorative materials. *Crit Rev Oral Biol Med*, **12**, 350–360.

Behr, M., Zeman, F., Passauer, T., Koller, M., Hahnel, S., Buergers, R., Lang, R., Handel, G. and Kolbeck, C. (2012)

Clinical performance of cast clasp-retained removable partial dentures: a retrospective study. *Int J Prosthodont*, **25**, 138–144.

Ben-Gal, G., Lipovetsky-Adler, M., Haramaty, O., Sharon, E. and Smidt, A. (2013) Existing concepts and a search for evidence: a review on implant occlusion. *Compend Contin Educ Dent*, **34**, 26–31.

Bergendal, T. and Isacsson, G. (1980) Effect of nystatin in the treatment of denture stomatitis. *Scand J Dent Res*, **88**, 446–454.

Berglundh, T., Persson, L. and Klinge, B. (2002) A systematic review of the incidence of biological and technical complications in implant dentistry reported in prospective longitudinal studies of at least 5 years. *J Clin Periodontol*, **29**, 197–212.

Bergman, B. and Carlsson, G.E. (1972) Review of 54 complete denture wearers. Patient's opinions 1 year after treatment. *Acta Odontol Scand*, **30**, 399–414.

Bergmann, R.H. (2014) Occlusal considerations for dental implant restorations. *Compend Contin Educ Dent*, **35**, 455–458.

Beyli, M.S. and vonFraunhofer, J.A. (1981) An analysis of causes of fracture of acrylic resin dentures. *J Prosthet Dent*, **46**, 238–241.

Bhandari, S., Aggarwal, N. and Bakshi, S. (2013) Ultrasonic oscillations for conservative retrieval of a rare fracture of implant healing abutment. *J Oral Implantol*, **39**, 475–478.

Bilhan, H., Sulun, T., Erkose, G., Kurt, H., Erturan, Z., Kutay, O. and Bilgin, T. (2009) The role of *Candida albicans* hyphae and *Lactobacillus* in denture-related stomatitis. *Clin Oral Investig*, **13**, 363–368.

Bilhan, H., Erdogan, O., Ergin, S., Celik, M., Ates, G. and Geckili, O. (2012) Complication rates and patient satisfaction with removable dentures. *J Adv Prosthodont*, **4**, 109–115.

Bilhan, H., Geckili, O., Ergin, S., Erdogan, O. and Ates, G. (2013) Evaluation of satisfaction and complications in patients with existing complete dentures. *J Oral Sci*, **55**, 29–37.

Binon, P.P. (2000) Implants and components: entering the new millennium. *Int J Oral Maxillofac Implants*, **15**, 76–94.

Bohnenkamp, D.M. (2014) Removable partial dentures clinical concepts. *Dent Clin N Am*, **58**, 69–89.

Brunello, D. and Mandikos, M. (1998) Construction faults, age, gender, and relative medical health: factors associated with complaints in complete denture patients. *J Prosthet Dent*, **79**, 545–554.

Brunski, J.B., Puleo, D.A. and Nanci, A. (2000) Biomaterials and biomechanics of oral and maxillofacial implants: current status and future developments. *J Oral Maxillofac Implants*, **15**, 15–46.

Budtz-Jorgensen, E. (1981) Oral mucosal lesions associated with the wearing of removable dentures. *J Oral Pathol*, **10**, 65–80.

Budtz-Jorgensen, E. and Bertram, U. (1970) Denture stomatitis. I. The etiology in relation to trauma and infection. *Acta Odontol Scand*, **28**, 71–92.

Budtz-Jorgensen, E., Holmstrup, P. and Krogh, P. (1988) Fluconazole in the treatment of *Candida*-associated denture stomatitis. *Antimicrob Agents Chemother*, **32**, 1859–1863.

Budtz-Jorgensen, E., Mojon, P., Banon-Clement, J.M. and Baehni, P. (1996) Oral candidosis in long-term hospital care: comparison of edentulous and dentate subjects. *Oral Dis*, **2**, 285–290.

Burguete, R.L., Johns, R.B., King, T. and Patterson, E.A. (1994) Tightening characteristics for screwed joints in osseointegrated dental implants. *J Prosthet Dent*, **71**, 592–599.

Carlsson, G.E. (2009) Dental occlusion: modern concepts and their application in implant prosthodontics. *Odontology*, **97**, 8–17.

Cehreli, M.C., Karasoy, D., Kokat, A.M., Akca, K. and Eckert, S.E. (2010) Systematic review of prosthetic maintenance requirements for implant-supported overdentures. *Int J Oral Maxillofac Implants*, **25**, 163–180.

Chee, W. and Jivraj, S. (2006) Screw versus cemented implant supported restorations. *Br Dent J*, **201**, 501–507.

Chen, A. and Zirwas, M. (2007) Denture stomatitis. *Skinmed*, **6**, 92–94.

Cilingir, A., Bilhan, H., Baysal, G., Sunbuloglu, E. and Bozdag, E. (2013) The impact of frenulum height on strains in maxillary denture bases. *J Adv Prosthodont*, **5**, 409–415.

Coonaert, J., Adriaens, P. and de Boever, J. (1984) Long-term clinical study of porcelain-fused-to-gold restorations. *J Prosthet Dent*, **51**, 338–342.

Cosellu, G., Farronato, G., Carrassi, A. and Angiero, F. (2013) Accidental aspiration of foreign bodies in dental practice: clinical management and prevention. *Gerodontology*, **32**, 229–233.

Cune, M.S., De Putter, C. and Hoogstraten, J. (1994) Treatment outcome with implant-retained overdentures: Part II Patient satisfaction and predictability of subjective treatment outcome. *J Prosthet Dent*, **72**, 152–158.

Cunningham, J.L. and Benington, I.C. (1997) A survey of the pre-bonding preparation of denture teeth and the efficiency of dewaxing methods. *J Dent*, **25**, 125–128.

Darbar, U.R., Huggett, R. and Harrison, A. (1994) Denture fracture – a survey. *Br Dent J*, **176**, 342–345.

De Albuquerque Junior, R.F., Lund, J.P., Tang, L., Larivee, J., de Grandmont, P., Gauthier, G. and Feine, J.S. (2000) Within-subject comparison of maxillary long-bar implant-retained prostheses with and without palatal coverage: patient-based outcomes. *Clin Oral Implants Res*, **11**, 555–565.

Dellinges, M.A. and Tebrock, O.C. (1993) A measurement of torque values obtained with hand-held drivers in a simulated clinical setting. *Int J Prosthodont*, **2**, 212–214.

DePaola, L.G., Minah, G.E., Leupold, R.J., Faraone, K.L. and Elias, S.A. (1986) The effect of antiseptic mouth rinses on oral microbial flora and denture stomatitis. *Clin Prev Dent*, **8**, 3–8.

Dervis, E. (2002) Clinical assessment of common patient complaints with complete dentures. *Eur J Prosthodont Restor Dent*, **10** (3), 113–7.

De Santana Santos, T., Antunes, A.A., Vajgel, A., Cavalcanti, T.B.B., Nogueira, L.R. and Filho, J.R. (2012) Foreign body ingestion during dental implant procedures. *J Craniofac Surg*, **23**, 119–123.

Domingo, K.B., Burgess, J.O., Litaker, M.S. and McCracken, M.S. (2013) Strength comparison of four techniques to secure implant attachment housings to complete dentures. *J Prosthet Dent*, **110**, 8–13.

Dorner, S., Zeman, F., Koller, M., Lang, R., Handel, G. and Behr, M. (2010) Clinical performance of complete dentures: a retrospective study. *Int J Prosthodont*, **23**, 410–417.

Douglass, C.W., Shih, A. and Ostry, L. (2002) Will there be a need for complete dentures in the United States in 2020? *J Prosthet Dent*, **87**, 5–8.

Doundoulakis, J.H., Eckert, S.E., Lindquist, C.C. and Jeffcoat, M.K. (2003) The implant-supported overdenture as an alternative to the complete mandibular denture. *J Am Dent Assoc*, **134**, 1455–1458.

Dudley, J. (2013) Maxillary implant overdentures: current controversies. *Aust Dent J*, **58**, 420–423.

English, C.E. (1993) Biomechanical concerns with fixed partial dentures involving implants. *Implant Dent*, **2**, 221–242.

Erhardson, S., Carlsson, J. and Wictorin, L. (1980) Fracture mechanics of dental gold soldered joints. *Swed Dent J Suppl*, **5**, 1–62.

Fauvell, S.A., Gialanella, G. and Penna, K.J. (2006) The lumen technique. *N Y State Dent J*, **72**, 43.

Feng, S., Liao, P. and Chen, M. (2012) Prosthodontic treatment of a patient with combination syndrome: a clinical case report. *J Prosthodont Implant Dentistry*, **1**, 22–25.

Ferencz, J.L. (1987) Tensile strength analysis of midpontic soldering. *J Prosthet Dent*, **57**, 696–703.

Fox, P.C., Busch, K.A. and Baum, B.J. (1987) Subjective reports of xerostomia and objective measures of salivary gland performance. *J Am Dent Assoc*, **115**, 581–584.

Gendreau, L. and Loewy, Z.G. (2011) Epidemiology and etiology of denture stomatitis. *J Prosthod*, **20**, 251–260.

Glantz, P.-O. and Nyman, S. (1982) Technical and biophysical aspects of fixed partial dentures for patients with reduced periodontal support. *J Prosthet Dent*, **47**, 47–51.

Goodacre, C.J., Bernal, G., Rungcharassaeng, K. and Kan, J.Y.K. (2003) Clinical complications with implants and implant prostheses. *J Prosthet Dent*, **90**, 121–132.

Gooty, J.R., Palakuru, S.K., GuntaKalla, V.R. and Nera, M. (2014) Noninvasive method for retrieval of broken dental implant abutment screw. *Contemp Clin Dent*, **5**, 264–267.

Greenstein, G. and Cavallaro, J. (2010) Cantilevers extending from unilateral implant-supported fixed prostheses. A review of the literature and presentation of practical guidelines. *J Am Dent Assoc*, **141**, 1221–1230.

Gross, M.D. (2008) Occlusion in implant dentistry. A review of the literature of prosthetic determinants and current concepts. *Australian Dent J*, **53** (Suppl), S60–S68.

Himmel, R., Pilo, R., Assif, D. and Aviv, I. (1992) The cantilever fixed partial denture – a literature review. *J Prosthet Dent*, **67**, 484–487.

Hochman, N., Ginio, I. and Ehrlich, J. (1987) The cantilever fixed partial denture: a 10-year follow-up. *J Prosthet Dent*, **58**, 542–545.

Hummel, S.K., Marker, V.A., Buschang, P. and DeVengencie, J. (1999) A pilot study to evaluate different palate materials for maxillary complete dentures with xerostomic patients. *J Prosthod*, **8**, 10–17.

Hopcraft, M.S. and Tan, C. (2010) Xerostomia: an update for clinicians. *Aust Dent J*, **35**, 238–244.

Ikebe, K., Sajima, H., Kobayashi, S., Hata, K., Morii, K., Nokubi, T. and Ettinger, R.L. (2002) Association of salivary flow rate with oral function in a sample of community-dwelling older adults in Japan. *Oral Surg Oral Med Oral Pathol Oral Radiol Endod*, **99**, 704–710.

John, J., Gangadhar, S.A. and Shah, I. (2001) Flexural strength of heat polymerized polymethyl methacrylate denture resin reinforced with glass, aramid or nylon fibers. *J Prosthet Dent*, **86**, 424–427.

Jorge, J.H., Quishida, C.C.C., Vergani, C.E., Machado, A.L., Pavarina, A.C. and Giampolo, E.T. (2012) Clinical evaluation of failures in removable partial dentures. *J Oral Sci*, **54**, 337–342.

Karabuda, C., Yaltink, M. and Bayraktar, M. (2008) A clinical comparison of prosthetic complications of implant-supported overdentures with different attachment systems. *Implant Dent*, **17**, 74–81.

Karlsson, S. (1986) A clinical evaluation of fixed bridges, 10 years following insertion. *J Oral Rehabil*, **13**, 423–432.

Kelly, E. (1972) Changes caused by a mandibular removable partial denture opposing a maxillary complete denture. *J Prosthet Dent*, **27**, 140–150.

Kim, Y., Oh, T., Misch, C.E. and Wang, H. (2005) Occlusal considerations in implant therapy: clinical guidelines with biomechanical rationale. *Clin Oral Impl Res*, **16**, 26–35.

Kimmich, M. and Stappert, C. (2013) Intraoral treatment of veneering porcelain chipping of fixed dental restorations. *J Am Dent Assoc*, **144**, 31–44.

Kivovics, P., Jahn, M., Borbely, J. and Marton, K. (2007) Frequency and location of traumatic ulcerations following placement of complete dentures. *Int J Prosthodont*, **20**, 397–401.

Klineberg, I.J., Trulsson, M. and Murray, G.M. (2013) Occlusion on implants – is there a problem? *J Oral Rehabil*, **39**, 522–537.

Kotkin, H. (1985) Diagnostic significance of denture complaints. *J Prosthet Dent*, **53**, 73–77.

Kovac-Kavcic, M. and Skaleric, U. (2000) The prevalence of oral mucosal lesions in a population in Ljubljana, Slovenia. *J Oral Pathol Med*, **28**, 331–335.

Kovacić, I., Celebić, A., Zlatarić, D.K., Petricević, N., Buković, D., Bitanga, P., Mikelić, B., Tadin, A., Mehulić, K. and Ognjenović, M. (2010) Decreasing of residual alveolar ridge height in complete denture wearers. A five year follow up study. *Coll Antropol*, **34**, 1051–1056.

Koyano, K. and Esaki, D. (2015) Occlusion on oral implants: current clinical guidelines. *J Oral Rehabil*, **42**, 153–161.

Kulac-Ozkan, Y., Kazazoglu, E. and Arikan, A. (2002) Oral hygiene habits, denture cleanliness, presence of yeasts, and stomatitis in elderly people. *J Oral Rehabil*, **29**, 300–304.

Kumar, S.M., Sethumadhava, J.R., Kumar, V.A. and Manita, G. (2012) Effects of conventional welding and laser welding on the tensile strength, ultimate tensile strength and surface characteristics of two cobalt-chromium alloys: a comparative study. *J Indian Prosthodont Soc*, **12**, 87–93.

Langer, Y., Laufer, B. and Cardash, H.S. (1995) Modalities of treatment for the combination syndrome. *J Prosthod*, **4**, 76–81.

Levers, B.G.H. and Darling, A. (1983) Continuous eruption of some human adult teeth of ancient populations. *Arch Oral Biol*, **28**, 401–408.

Lewis, A.J. (1978) Failure of removable partial denture castings during service. *J Prosthet Dent*, **39**, 147–149.

Lloyd, P.M. (1996) Complete denture therapy for the geriatric patient. *Dent Clin North Am*, **40**, 239–254.

Luk, N.K., Wu, V.H., Liang, B.M., Chen, Y.M., Yip, K.H. and Smales, R.J. (2007) Mathematical analysis of occlusal rest design for cast removable partial dentures. *Eur J Prosthodont Restor Dent*, **15**, 29–32.

Lundgren, D. and Laurell, L. (1994) Biomechanical aspects of fixed bridgework supported by natural teeth and endosseous implants. *J Periodontol 2000*, **4**, 23–40.

Maalhagh-Fard, A. and Jacobs, L.C. (2010) Retrieval of a stripped abutment screw: a clinical report. *J Prosthet Dent*, **104**, 212–215.

Massad, J.J. and Cagna, D.R. (2002) Removable prosthodontic therapy and xerostomia. Treatment considerations. *Dent Today*, **21**, 80–87.

Matear, D.W., Locker, D., Stephens, M. and Lawrence, H.P. (2006) Associations between xerostomia and health status indicators in the elderly. *J R Soc Health*, **126**, 79–85.

McCord, J.F., Grey, N.J.A., Winstanley, R.B. and Johnson, A. (2002) A clinical overview of removable prostheses: 3. Principles of design for removable partial dentures. *Dent Update*, **29**, 474–481.

Misch, C.E. (2002) The effect of bruxism on treatment planning for dental implants. *Dent Today*, **21**, 76–81.

Misch, C.E. and Bidez, M.W. (2005) Occlusal consideration for implant-supported prostheses: implant protected occlusion, in *Dental Implant Prosthetics*, 1st edn (ed C.E. English), Mosby, St. Louis, MO, pp. 472–510.

Morrow, R.M., Reiner, P.R., Feldmann, E.E. and Rudd, K.D. (1968) Metal reinforced silicone-lined dentures. *J Prosthet Dent*, **19**, 219–229.

Narhi, T.O. (1994) Prevalence of subjective feelings of dry mouth in the elderly. *J Dent Res*, **73**, 20–25.

Negm, S. (2013) *Candida albicans* on tongue. *Int J Dent Clinics*, **5**, 31–32.

Nergiz, I., Schmage, P. and Shahin, R. (2004) Removal of a fractured implant abutment screw: a clinical report. *J Prosthet Dent*, **91**, 513–517.

Nikolopoulou, F., Tasopoulos, T. and Jagger, R. (2013) The prevalence of xerostomia in patients with removable prostheses. *Int J Prosthodont*, **26**, 525–526.

Nishimura, I. and Garrett, N. (2004) Impact of human genome project on treatment of frail and edentulous patients. *Gerodontology*, **21**, 3–9.

Obinata, K., Satoh, T., Towfik, A.M. and Nakamura, M. (2011) An investigation of accidental ingestion during dental procedures. *J Oral Sci*, **53**, 495–500.

Osterberg, T., Landahl, S. and Hedegard, B. (1984) Salivary flow, saliva, pH and buffering capacity in 70-year-old men and women. Correlation to dental health, dryness in the mouth, disease and drug treatment. *J Oral Rehabil*, **11**, 157–170.

Ozcan, M. (2003a) Evaluation of alternative intra-oral repair techniques for fractured ceramic-fused-to-metal restorations. *J Oral Rehabil*, **30**, 194–203.

Ozcan, M. (2003b) Fracture reasons in ceramic-fused-to-metal restorations. *J Oral Rehabil*, **30**, 265–269.

Parr, G.R. and Gardner, L.K. (1993) Removable partial denture repairs. *Compend Contin Educ Dent*, **14**, 846–853.

Pjetursson, B.E., Tan, K., Lang, N.P., Bragger, U., Egger, M. and Zwahlen, M. (2004) A systematic review of the survival and complication rates of fixed partial dentures (FPD's) after an observation period of at least 5 years. *Clin Oral Impl Res*, **15**, 667–676.

Pjetursson, B.E., Thoma, D., Jung, R., Zwahlen, M. and Zembic, A. (2012) A systematic review of the survival and complication rates of implant supported fixed dental prostheses (FPDs) after a mean observation period of at least 5 years. *Clin Oral Implants Res*, **23** (Suppl), 22–38.

Plemons, J.M., Al-Hashimi, I. and Marek, C. (2014) Managing xerostomia and salivary gland hypofunction. *J Am Dent Assoc*, **145**, 867–873.

Rehmann, P., Orbach, K., Ferger, P. and Wostmann, B. (2013) Treatment outcomes with removable partial dentures: a retrospective analysis. *Int J Prosthodont*, **26**, 147–150.

Renner, R.P. and Boucher, L.J. (1987) *Removable Partial Dentures*, Quintessence Publishing, Chicago, IL.

Rice, J.A., Lynch, C.D., McAndrew, R. and Milward, P.J. (2010) Tooth preparation for rest seats for cobalt-chromium removable partial dentures completed by general dental practitioners. *J Oral Rehabil*, **38**, 72–78.

Rindal, D.B., Rush, W.A., Peters, D. and Maupome, G. (2005) Antidepressant xerogenic medications and restoration rates. *Community Dent Oral Epidemiol*, **33**, 74–80.

Rodriguez, A.M., Aquilino, S.A., Lund, P.S., Ryther, J.S. and Southard, T.E. (1993) Evaluation of strain at the terminal abutment site of a fixed mandibular implant prosthesis during cantilever loading. *J Prosthodont*, **2**, 93–102.

Romeo, E. and Storelli, S. (2012) Systematic review of the survival rate and the biological, technical, and esthetic complications of fixed partial prostheses with cantilevers on implants reported in longitudinal studies with a mean of 5 years follow up. *Clin Oral Implants Res*, **23**, 39–49.

Rudd, R.W., Bange, A.A., Rudd, K.W. and Montalvo, R. (1999) Preparing teeth to receive a removable partial denture. *J Prosthet Dent*, **82**, 536–549.

Rutkunas, V., Mizutani, H. and Takahashi, H. (2005) Evaluation of stable retentive properties of overdenture attachments. *Stomatologija*, **7**, 115–120.

Sailer, I., Pjetursson, B., Zwahlen, M. and Hammerle, C. (2007) A systematic review of the survival and complication rates of all-ceramic and metal-ceramic reconstructions after an observation period of at least 3 years. Part II: Fixed dental prostheses. *Clin Oral Impl Res*, **18**, 86–96.

Sato, Y. (1999) Clinical methods for adjusting retention force of cast clasps. *J Prosthet Dent*, **82**, 557–561.

Sato, Y., Shindoi, N., Koretake, K. and Hosokawa, R. (2003) The effect of occlusal rest size and shape on yield strength. *J Prosthet Dent*, **89**, 503–507.

Saunders, T.R., Gillis, R.E. and Desjardins, R.P. (1979) The maxillary complete denture opposing the mandibular bilateral distal-extension partial denture: treatment considerations. *J Prosthet Dent*, **41**, 124–128.

Satapathy, S.K., Pillai, A., Jyothi, R. and Annapurna, P.D. (2013) Natural teeth replacing artificial teeth in a partial denture: a case report. *J Clin Diagn Res*, **7**, 1818–1819.

Schulte, W. (1995) Implants and the periodontium. *Intl Dent J*, **45**, 16–26.

Schwarz, M.S. (2000) Mechanical complications of dental implants. *Clin Oral Implants Res*, **11** (Suppl), 156–158.

Schweitzer, J.M., Schweitzer, R.D. and Schweitzer, J. (1968) Free-end pontics used on fixed partial dentures. *J Prosthet Dent*, **20**, 120–138.

Selby, A. (1994) Fixed prosthodontic failure. A review and discussion of important aspects. *Aust Dent J*, **39**, 150–156.

Shay, K. (2000) Denture hygiene: a review and update. *J Contemp Dent Pract*, **1**, 1–8.

Shen, K. and Gongloff, R.K. (1989) Prevalence of the combination syndrome among denture patients. *J Prosthet Dent*, **62**, 642–644.

Shetty, M.S., and Shenoy, K.K. (2011) Techniques for evaluating the fit of removable and fixed prosthesis. *ISRN Dent*, epub 2011 Jul 14, doi: 10.5402/2011/348372. 1–4, article ID 348372.

Siamos, G., Winkler, S. and Boberick, K.G. (2002) The relationship between implant preload and screw loosening on implant-supported prostheses. *J Oral Implantol*, **28**, 67–73.

Smith, J.P. and Hughes, D. (1988) A survey of referred patients experiencing problems with complete dentures. *J Prosthet Dent*, **60**, 583–586.

Sones, A.D. (1989) Complications with osseointegrated implants. *J Prosthet Dent*, **62**, 581–585.

Sreenby, L.M. and Schwartz, S.S. (1997) A reference guide to drugs and dry mouth – 2nd ed. *Gerodontology*, **14**, 33–47.

Stameisen, A.E. and Ruffino, A. (1987) Replacement of lost or broken denture teeth with composites. *J Prosthet Dent*, **58**, 119–120.

Strub, J.R., Stiffler, S. and Scharer, P. (1988) Causes of failure following oral rehabilitation: biologic versus technical factors. *Quintessence Int*, **19**, 215–222.

Suzuki, Y., Ohkubo, C., Abe, M. and Hosoi, T. (2004) Titanium removable partial denture clasp repair using laser welding: a clinical report. *J Prosthet Dent*, **91**, 418–420.

Tan, K., Pjetursson, B.E., Lang, N.P. and Chan, E.S. (2004) A systematic review of the survival and complication rates of fixed partial dentures (FPDs) after an observation period of at least 5 years. *Clin Oral Implants Res*, **15**, 654–656.

Thomson, W.M., Chalmers, J.M., Spencer, A.J., Slade, G.D. and Carter, K.D. (2006) A longitudinal study of medication exposure and xerostomia among older people. *Gerodontology*, **23**, 205–213.

Tolstunov, L. (2007) Combination syndrome: classification and case report. *J Oral Implantol*, **33**, 139–151.

Uzun, G. and Hersek, N. (2002) Comparison of the fracture resistance of six denture base acrylic resins. *J Biomater Appl*, **17**, 19–29.

Vallittu, P.K. (1995) A review of methods used to reinforce polymethyl methacrylate resin. *J Prosthod*, **4**, 183–187.

Venkataraghavan, K., Anantharaj, A., Praveen, P., Prathibha Rani, S. and Krishnan, B. (2011) Accidental ingestion of foreign object: systemic review, recommendations and report of a case. *Saudi Dent J*, **23**, 177–181.

Wandera, A. and Conry, J.P. (1993) Aspiration and ingestion of a foreign body during dental examination by a patient with spastic quadriparesis: case report. *Pediatr Dent*, **15**, 362–363.

Watson, C.J., Walker, D.M., Bates, J.F. and Newcombe, R.G. (1982) The efficacy of topical miconazole in the treatment of denture stomatitis. *Br Dent J*, **152**, 403–406.

Webb, B.C., Thomas, C.J., Wilcox, M.D., Harty, D.W. and Knox, K.W. (1998) Candida-associated denture stomatitis. Aetiology and management: a review. Part 3. Treatment of oral candidosis. *Aust Dent J*, **43**, 244–249.

Weiss, E.I., Kozak, D. and Gross, M.D. (2000) Effect of repeated closures on opening torque values in seven abutment-implant systems. *J Prosthet Dent*, **84**, 194–199.

Williamson, R.T. and Robinson, F.G. (2001) Retrieval technique for fractured implant screws. *J Prosthet Dent*, **86**, 549–550.

Wright, W.E. (1986) Success with the cantilever fixed partial denture. *J Prosthet Dent*, **55**, 537–539.

Wright, W.E. and Yettram, A.L. (1979) Reactive force distributions for teeth when loaded singly and when used as fixed partial denture abutments. *J Prosthet Dent*, **42**, 411–416.

Yanikoglu, N. (2004) The repair method for fractured metal-porcelain restorations: a review of the literature. *Eur J Prosthodont Rest Dent*, **12**, 161–165.

CHAPTER 5

Oral surgery complications

Shahrokh C. Bagheri[1,2,3,4,5,6], Behnam Bohluli[7] and Roger A. Meyer[1,5,6,8,9]

[1]Chief, Department of Surgery, Division of Oral and Maxillofacial Surgery, Northside Hospital, Atlanta, GA, USA
[2]Private Practice, Georgia Oral and Facial Reconstructive Surgery, Atlanta, GA, USA
[3]Adjunct Assistant Professor of Oral and Maxillofacial Surgery, School of Medicine, University of Miami, Miami, FL, USA
[4]Adjunct Assistant Professor of Oral and Maxillofacial Surgery, Department of Surgery, School of Medicine, Emory University, Atlanta, GA, USA
[5]Adjunct Associate Professor of Oral and Maxillofacial Surgery, Augusta University, Augusta, GA, USA
[6]Diplomate, American Board of Oral and Maxillofacial Surgery, Chicago, IL, USA
[7]Oral and Maxillofacial Surgery, Azad University of Medical Sciences, Tehran, Iran
[8]Maxillofacial Consultations Ltd, Greensboro, GA, USA
[9]Georgia Oral and Facial Reconstructive Surgery, Marietta, GA, USA

A surgical complication is any event occurring during or after an operation that if unsuspected, undiagnosed, or ignored may have adverse effects on the patient (Meyer, 1987). A complication can be an unfortunate part of any surgical procedure in which risks are inherent components. Basic oral surgical procedures are commonly performed by clinicians who are not oral and maxillofacial surgeons. Every dental practitioner has an ethical and professional obligation to perform only those procedures, surgical or otherwise, in which he/she is adequately trained, not only in the operative techniques but also in the postoperative **management** of the patient. This obligation dictates the need for basic clinical and didactic training in the recognition and management of complications. The goal of this chapter is to present complications that may be encountered during basic oral surgery procedures and suggestions for their appropriate management. An in-depth presentation of complications related to major oral maxillofacial surgery (OMFS) procedures is beyond the scope of this textbook, and readers are referred to comprehensive surgical publications on this topic (see Kaban, Pogrel, and Perrott, 1997; Bagheri, Bell, and Khan, 2011; Miloro, 2015).

Complications related to any type of surgical operation can be arbitrarily divided into four categories:

1 Minor complications confined to the anatomic area of the surgical field (dry socket, localized infections, localized bleeding)
2 Major complications confined to the oral and maxillofacial regions (mandible fracture, nerve injury, osteomyelitis, infections of the fascial spaces, osteonecrosis)
3 Minor systemic complications, which require more specific localized or systemic treatments (allergic reaction, syncope, other minor, non-life-threatening cardiopulmonary events)
4 Major, potentially life-threatening systemic complications, which require other expert surgical or medical interventions (seizures, major cardiac or pulmonary events, sepsis, shock)

The focus of this chapter is on the first category: minor complications confined to the anatomic area of the surgical field.

All surgical procedures will trigger some type of soft tissue inflammatory response or other localized reactions (such as pain, edema, ecchymosis). The degree of invasiveness of the procedure can impact on the severity of the inflammatory manifestation. These manifestations are not necessarily complications but expected consequences of the surgical trauma. The inflammatory responses can be minimized with a gentle surgical technique and postoperative measures that reduce inflammation (steroids, non-steroidal anti-inflammatory drugs/NSAIDs, cold compresses, elevation of the patient's head, limitation of strenuous physical activity). Excessive swelling and/or bruising that is out of proportion to the procedure should be investigated for a possible secondary etiology that may need active intervention (infection, uncontrollable bleeding from a ruptured artery or vein). Other diagnoses, such as dry socket (pain secondary to alveolar osteitis), may require only supportive care (Noroozi and Philbert, 2009; Bowe, Rogers, and Stassen, 2010; Cardoso et al., 2010; Daly et al., 2012; Laraki, Chbicheb, and El Wady, 2012). Less common but more significant complications, such as mandibular fractures, nerve injuries, and fascial abscesses, should warrant immediate consultation with an experienced oral and maxillofacial surgeon (Meyer, 1987; Bagheri, Bell, and Khan, 2012; Ethunandan, Shanahan, and Patel, 2012; Marciani, 2012; Bagheri and Meyer, 2014).

Minor complications can be divided into intraoperative and postoperative complications.

Intraoperative complications

Intraoperative bleeding
Intraoperative bleeding obscures the surgical field, puts extra stress on the dentist, and, if the surgery is continued, may cause other complications, such as errors in surgical technique due to haste or poor visibility (McCormick, Moore, and Meechan, 2014a; McCormick et al., 2014b; Mingarro-de-León, Chaveli-López, and Gavaldá-Esteve, 2014).

Prevention
The following steps might decrease the incidence of intraoperative bleeding:
1 Adequate preoperative evaluation to determine if the patient has any type of bleeding disorder. Knowledge of the patient's medical conditions will alert the dentist, who can be prepared to handle any event that may arise.
2 The use of a local anesthetic agent with proper vasoconstrictor (e.g., epinephrine 1:100 000 or 1:200 000) and waiting several minutes for the full effect of the vasoconstrictor on surrounding tissues can considerably diminish soft tissue bleeding.

3 Precise radiographic evaluation to detect any possible proximity of the surgical site to the inferior alveolar canal (IAC) will inform the clinician and help reduce the risk of injury to the inferior alveolar artery and vein (Duda, 2002; Durmus et al., 2004; Bouloux, Steed, and Perciaccante, 2007; Huang, Wu, and Worthington, 2007; Brauer, 2008; Huang, Chen, and Chuang, 2011).

Treatment
To control intraoperative bleeding, one should attempt to find the origin of bleeding. A wet gauze is placed with gentle pressure over the surgical site for a short time. Then, using a small suction tip and adequate light (preferably a headlight), the surgical site is explored. After finding the origin of the bleeding, the following steps may be taken to control the bleeding:
1 Soft tissue bleeding may be controlled by placing gauze over the wound and maintaining firm pressure for 5 min. If slow oozing of blood continues, the injection of a small amount (1–2 ml) of local anesthetic solution containing a vasoconstrictor into the bleeding area may aid in obtaining hemostasis. As a definitive measure, clamping of a bleeding vessel and application of electrocautery may be required in an occasional patient. In most instances, barring other considerations (e.g., the overall status of the patient), the surgery may be continued once the bleeding has been controlled.
2 Some lesions (such as periapical granulomas, pyogenic granulomas, and giant cell granulomas) are usually highly vascular, and their excision is often accompanied by brisk (albeit a small total amount of) bleeding. The best action is to completely remove the lesion without delay; once the lesion is excised, the bleeding should stop spontaneously. However, in more problematic lesions (such as hemangiomas and arterial–venous malformations, recognized on preoperative imaging studies and often creating a palpable thrill or bruit on auscultation) massive, life-threatening bleeding may occur. For patients with these conditions, any proposed surgery should be postponed, and consultation should be requested with an experienced surgeon.
3 During excision of pathologic lesions (e.g., apical granuloma, cyst) or removal of mandibular molar teeth whose roots are in proximity to the IAC, the inferior alveolar artery and veins may be damaged,

which can cause brisk bleeding from the depth of the extraction socket or bone cavity. These bleeding episodes are easily controlled by placing a wet gauze or surgical hemostatic agents (gelfoam, Surgicel) into the extraction socket and exerting firm pressure for several minutes. Note: using heated applicators or electrocautery may damage the inferior alveolar nerve (IAN) and must be avoided.

Tooth displacement

Accidental displacement of a tooth is a relatively rare complication. Improper angle of application or exertion of excessive force on tooth elevators might displace the tooth or fragments thereof into adjacent soft tissues. Additional desperate or vain attempts to retrieve the displaced fragment in a poorly lit or poorly visualized surgical field often only result in further damage to surrounding tissues and/or even further displacement of the tooth. Maxillary and mandibular third molars are the teeth that are most commonly displaced, into the pterygopalatine (also, pterygomaxillary) fossa or maxillary sinus and sublingual space, respectively. However, other teeth and root fragments can be displaced into their adjacent tissues as well (Duda, 2002; Durmus *et al.*, 2004; Bouloux, Steed, and Perciaccante, 2007; Huang, Wu, and Worthington, 2007; Brauer, 2008; Huang, Chen, and Chuang, 2011).

Treatment

Several modalities can be used to retrieve a displaced tooth or tooth fragment. It is generally believed that a displaced tooth should be removed as soon as possible. That is true only if the operator is, by training and experience, technically capable of accessing the pterygopalatine fossa, the maxillary sinus, or the sublingual space; is familiar with the pertinent anatomy of these important areas; and has adequate lighting, instrumentation, and assistance to complete the procedure without undue risk to the patient. However, "discretion is often the better part of valor," and the prudent practitioner may elect to abort the procedure, obtain further imaging studies to document the exact location of the displaced object, and refer the patient to an oral and maxillofacial surgeon who will retrieve the object under more favorable conditions. A delay or postponement of the definitive surgery will allow fibrous tissue to form, surrounding the displaced tooth and preventing its further displacement by the manipulations of surgical intervention. In any case,

for this procedure the technology of three-dimensional (3-D) imaging, such as cone beam computed tomography (CBCT), should be part of a well-equipped operating room (Duda, 2002; Durmus *et al.*, 2004; Bouloux, Steed, and Perciaccante, 2007; Huang, Wu, and Worthington, 2007; Brauer, 2008; Huang, Chen, and Chuang, 2011).

The following are among the most common displacement sites, and each needs its own special considerations.

Tooth displaced into the maxillary sinuses. The root apices of most maxillary molars have a very close relationship to the floor of the maxillary sinuses. Sometimes with well-pneumatized sinuses or intrusive molar roots, only a delicate layer of bone or only a sinus epithelial membrane separates the roots from the sinus. Any careless pressure by a surgical instrument may destroy the bony barrier and dislodge the root fragment (Figure 5.1a, b) or, in rare occasions, the entire tooth into the maxillary sinuses. In such situations, treatment must be focused on removing the displaced tooth and managing the newly formed oroantral fistula (OAF) (Bouloux, Steed, and Perciaccante, 2007; Huang, Wu, and Worthington, 2007). Prompt referral to an oral and maxillofacial surgeon is always indicated.

Prevention

Gentle and meticulous surgical technique is the mainstay in avoiding displacement of tooth segments into the sinus and injury to the sinus itself. Radiographic assessment may help the surgeon detect susceptible cases. Conical roots, thin osseous separation between sinus floor and root apices, and the presence of pathologic lesions (e.g., apical cyst or granuloma) when detected on preoperative imaging should alert the practitioner to the added risks. Injudicious application of elevators and excessive force applied by extractions forceps are the forerunners of a complication in such patients.

Treatment

When a maxillary molar tooth fragment disappears in the surgical field, and tooth displacement is suspected, the following steps may help to retrieve the tooth fragment (Bouloux, Steed, and Perciaccante, 2007; Huang, Wu, and Worthington, 2007):

1 The patient is carefully examined under proper visualization (adequate light, strong high-power surgical suction, perhaps 2× power surgical loupes).

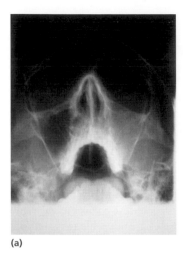
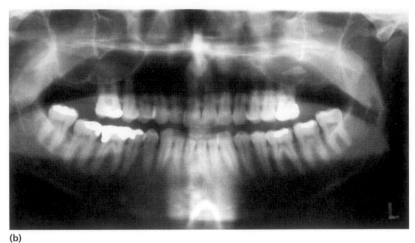

(a)   (b)

Figure 5.1 (a, b) Careless manipulation of maxillary posterior roots or tooth segments may dislodge the root to maxillary sinus.

Displaced root fragments may be observed and retrieved by a delicate suction cannula or a mosquito forceps. Irrigation and careful suctioning of the extraction socket may help to remove the displaced fragment or bring it back into the field of vision. If these maneuvers don't work, further manipulation or widening of the bony communication is not recommended, but standard sinus approaches might be considered.

2 The open sinus lift approach may provide the best access to the sinus. In some cases, the displaced tooth fragment lies beneath the Schneiderian (sinus) membrane in the sinus floor, and this relatively conservative approach may allow good visualization of the foreign body while the sinus membrane remains intact. In cases where the membrane is disrupted, conventional entry into the sinus is made (the Caldwell–Luc approach through a bony window in the canine fossa on the facial aspect of the maxilla superior to the apical region of the maxillary premolars, created with high-speed drill and rongeurs), and the foreign body is visualized, grasped, and removed. Alternatively, the patient may be placed in the supine position and then the sinus space is rinsed with normal saline and suctioned with a delicate cannula. The tooth fragment may float in the irrigating solution and can be grasped by a suction tip.

3 When a tooth or a fragment enters the maxillary sinus, an OAF (communication between mouth and sinus) is created through the tooth socket. Thus, after

removal of the foreign body, the OAF is located and documented and a treatment plan is made to manage it. This usually requires a soft tissue flap closure of the fistula (such as a buccal advancement flap or a pedicled buccal fat pad advancement flap) and creation of temporary drainage from the maxillary sinus, if necessary.

Tooth displacement into the pterygopalatine fossa

Inadvertent posterior/superior movement of a maxillary third molar tooth may cause it to be entrapped in the soft tissue between the maxillary process and the pterygoid process (Figure 5.2a–c). The tooth usually disappears from the surgical field when it slips from the extraction forceps, travels superoposterolaterally, and enters the soft tissue adjacent to the lateral or posterior aspect of the maxilla. Distal angulation, depth of impaction, and improper use of elevators may predispose the tooth and the operator to this situation (Bouloux, Steed, and Perciaccante, 2007; Huang, Wu, and Worthington, 2007).

Treatment

The first effort by an experienced surgeon may yield the displaced tooth, but if this effort fails, further manipulations may worsen the condition by forcing the tooth deeper into soft tissue. It is often advisable to postpone further surgery for 3 weeks to let the soft tissues around the tooth to heal and become fibrous. Before the second surgery, the exact position of the displaced tooth is

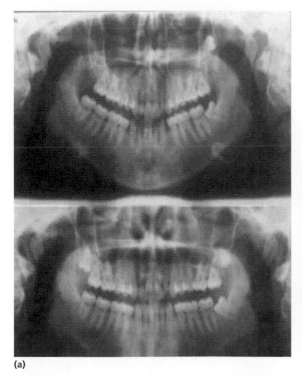

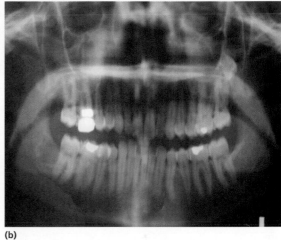

(a)   (b)

Figure 5.2 (a, b) Improper technique has forced maxillary third molar to pterygomaxillary space.

determined by 3-D imaging, such as CBCT. A 25-gauge long needle may be used to mark the tooth location on an imaging study prior flap reflection. The flap is then reflected and the fibrous tooth is easily grasped and extracted (Bouloux *et al.*, 2007; Huang, Wu, and Worthington, 2007).

Tooth displacement into the submandibular/sublingual spaces

The lingual cortex in the posterior mandible is relatively thin and may be easily fractured during surgical extraction of the mandibular third molars (Figure 5.3). As a result, root fragments (or, occasionally, the entire tooth) may be dislodged through the fractured lingual cortex and be entrapped in the soft tissue (of the sublingual space, which lies superior to the mylohyoid muscle in the floor of the mouth) (Figure 5.4b) (Durmus *et al.*, 2004; Bouloux, Steed, and Perciaccante, 2007; Huang, Wu, and Worthington, 2007). This may also render the lingual nerve at risk of injury since it usually courses within 1–2 mm of the lingual cortex.

Treatment

1 A finger-sweeping maneuver beneath the ipsilateral side of the tongue may help to redirect the tooth superiorly to its socket. Then, under proper visualization, the socket is carefully checked to find the root and grasp it.

2 If the first effort (aforementioned, #1) fails, further surgical intervention is avoided for 2–3 weeks to let the fibrous tissue surround the tooth.

3 After this interval, 3-D imaging should be obtained to locate the tooth fragment, and a 25-gauge needle might be used as a probe to find the tooth in soft tissue or as a marker on a CBCT image. The needle is inserted into the soft tissue until it touches the tooth, and then a gentle soft tissue dissection is done to reach the fibroid tooth fragment and remove it (Durmus *et al.*, 2004; Bouloux, Steed, and Perciaccante, 2007; Huang, Wu, and Worthington, 2007; Brauer, 2008). Alternatively, the use of intra-operative 3-D CT-guided imaging can be used to locate and retrieve the segment.

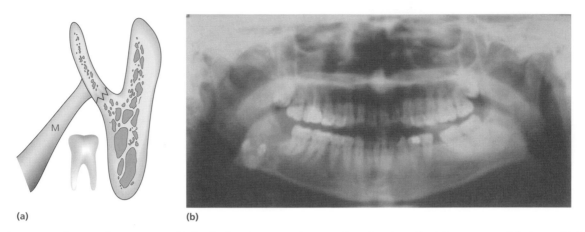

(a)   (b)

Figure 5.3 (a, b) Lingual cortex in mandibular third molar area is often very thin. There is a risk of displacement of the lower third molar into the adjacent sublingual or submandibular space.

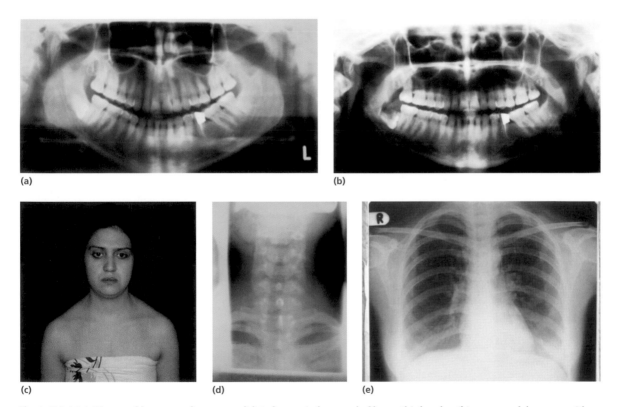

(a)   (b)

(c)   (d)   (e)

Figure 5.4 (a) A 30-year-old woman who was candidate for surgical removal of lower third molar, (b) unsuccessful surgery with high-speed handpiece, and (c) development of severe emphysema in the face, (d) neck, and (e) upper chest.

Alveolar bone and jaw fracture

Alveolar bone fracture is a relatively common complication of exodontia that ranges from a simple crack in the alveolar bone to a maxillary tuberosity fracture. Less common but more severe injuries include complete fractures of the mandibular symphysis, body, or angle (Peleg, *et al.*, 2009; Bodner, Brennan, and McLeod, 2011; Cankaya *et al.*, 2011; Chrcanovic and Freire-Maia, 2011;

Saksena *et al.*, 2014). Improper use of surgical instruments and uncontrolled forces are the main causes of bone injury. Additional risk is added if the patient's mandible is atrophic or osteoporotic. Depth of impaction, length of roots and their divergence, width of the PDL, age of the patient, and the skill of the surgeon may directly affect the incidence of bone fracture (Peleg *et al.*, 2009; Bodner, Brennan, and McLeod, 2011; Cankaya *et al.*, 2011; Chrcanovic and Freire-Maia, 2011; Saksena *et al.*, 2014).

Prevention
Proper case selection may be the first step in avoiding bone fracture.

It is generally recommended to leave deeply impacted teeth, which are not involved in a pathologic process (infection, cyst, tumor, root resorption of adjacent teeth) in situ. In special circumstances, where there is a need for its removal, an experienced surgeon, with the correct surgical plan, might elect to remove a deeply embedded tooth in a hazardous (proximity to IAC, inferior border of the mandible or adjacent tooth roots, associated pathology) position. Tooth sectioning may help the surgeon to remove long and divergent roots. A sharp periosteal elevator may easily pass through a narrow PDL and save the buccal plate (Peleg *et al.*, 2009; Bodner, Brennan, and McLeod, 2011; Cankaya *et al.*, 2011; Chrcanovic and Freire-Maia, 2011; Saksena *et al.*, 2014). In patients where there is a close relationship between the roots of a mandibular third molar tooth and the IAC and there is pathology associated with the tooth crown only, the surgeon may elect to do a "partial odontectomy" in which the tooth crown is removed and its roots (which lie in close proximity to the IAC) are left in situ, thus avoiding IAN injury (Freedman, 1997; Pogrel, Lee, and Muf, 2004).

Treatment
1 A separated bone fragment with no attachment to the periosteum has lost its blood supply and should be removed lest it become a foreign body and a nidus for infection. The bone that maintains its periosteal attachment is viable and may be carefully freed from the tooth by a periosteal elevator or other appropriate instruments and left in place with the hope that it will heal and assist in maintaining local alveolar bone.
2 The same principles may be applied to bigger segments, such as a maxillary tuberosity. A loose tuberosity without periosteal attachment is essentially a free bone graft and has a reduced chance of survival

and significant risk of infection. Therefore, it is usually removed before soft tissue closure is performed. In cases where a fractured tuberosity has periosteal and soft tissue connections, extraction is withheld and an effort is made to immobilize the fractured bone. Transdental wiring may fixate the fracture. After 4–6 weeks when the tuberosity is seen to have stabilized from osseous regeneration, careful surgical extraction of the tooth can be performed (Peleg *et al.*, 2009; Saksena *et al.*, 2014).

Mandibular angle or body fracture
Fracture of the mandible during exodontia is a major complication. A cracking or grinding sound, sharp pain with jaw movement or attempts at chewing food, mobility of the bone in the surgical site, and inability of the patient to bring the teeth together into normal occlusion are the main findings of a jaw fracture. This complication may happen intraoperatively if the mandible is atrophic, a large area of bone must be removed to expose the tooth in an otherwise diminutive mandible, or when the dentist applies instruments with unfavorable mechanical force on a deeply embedded tooth or, later, postoperatively because the mandible is weakened by excessive or unavoidable bone removal during the surgery and is now unable to withstand normal forces of mastication or minor physical contact (Bodner, Brennan, and McLeod 2011; Cankaya *et al.*, 2011; Chrcanovic and Freire-Maia, 2011; Saksena *et al.*, 2014).

Prevention
To minimize the likelihood of iatrogenic mandibular fracture, the following actions are generally recommended:
1 Precise evaluation (including appropriate preoperative imaging studies) of each case. Surgery may not be recommended for asymptomatic, deeply impacted third molar teeth.
2 When removal of a difficult tooth is indicated, proper surgical planning and instrumentation (such as tooth sectioning or bone removal with piezosurgery or lasers) have been reported to considerably reduce complications (Jing, Yang, Zheng *et al.*, 2014; Romero *et al.*, 2015).

Treatment
If an intraoperative or postoperative mandibular fracture is suspected, the best course of action is to refer the patient immediately to an oral and maxillofacial

surgeon. Further manipulation of a surgical site and any effort to complete the surgery may turn a greenstick fracture into a complex (displaced, compound, comminuted) fracture. The decision on whether to preserve the tooth in a fracture line or to extract the tooth should be made only after a complete assessment of the condition by the person who will be treating the fracture. Treatment varies (depending on the severity of the injury) from close observation and a liquid diet, to closed reduction with intermaxillary fixation, to open reduction and rigid internal fixation of the fracture (Bodner, Brennan, and McLeod, 2011; Cankaya *et al.*, 2011; Chrcanovic and Freire-Maia, 2011).

Extraction of the wrong tooth

This seemingly inexplicable complication is frequently reported in the literature as the main cause of legal actions against dentists (Lee, Curley, and Smith, 2007; Weiss, Stern, and Dym, 2011; Dym and Weiss, 2012). Several factors may increase the risk of this serious complication.

The following are predisposing factors (Lee, Curley, and Smith, 2007; Weiss, Stern, and Dym, 2011; Dym and Weiss, 2012):

1 "Add-on" emergency patients requiring dental extractions in an otherwise already overloaded, hectic clinic schedule

2 Miscommunication between clinicians (the dentist who sets the treatment plan and the clinician who performs the extraction)

3 Unclear identification of a tooth (discrepancy between the named tooth and its number)

4 Previously extracted teeth and/or a missing tooth with space closure that causes confusion in the correct designation of the remaining teeth (Lee, Curley, and Smith, 2007; Weiss, Stern, and Dym, 2011; Dym and Weiss, 2012)

Treatment

1 The extracted tooth can be managed as an "iatrogenic avulsed tooth." The operator is obliged to tell the patient about the complication and immediately replant and stabilize the tooth in its socket (or refer the patient to an oral and maxillofacial surgeon) as soon as possible. Further frequent follow-up is necessary until the ultimate status of the tooth can be determined. If the tooth fails to reattach and is lost, arrangements are made for permanent replacement (e.g., dental implant or fixed bridge).

2 In orthodontic patients, the orthodontist must also be informed about the event. Sometimes, with modifications in a treatment plan, orthodontic treatment can move adjacent teeth into position to close the space and achieve an occlusion as good as if the lost tooth had not been removed. Again, the responsible dentist continues follow-up and contact with the patient until the situation is resolved to the patient's and the orthodontist's satisfaction.

3 For partially edentulous patients that are due to receive dental implants, an immediate reevaluation should be made. Sometimes modification of the treatment plan may alleviate the need for replantation of the extracted tooth. The new treatment plan may include placement of a dental implant and restoration to substitute for the extracted tooth.

4 When reevaluation shows the tooth can be preserved, the replanted tooth should be securely splinted (arch bar or orthodontic appliance) for 4–6 weeks until stable. If the tooth is in an adult and the periapical opening is small and unlikely to facilitate revascularization of the dental pulp, an endodontic intervention may be indicated, as is often done with an avulsed tooth. In a child whose permanent tooth may still have a large periodical opening (so-called, "blunderbuss" pulp canal), revascularization is possible and endodontic treatment might be avoided.

Tooth and root fracture

Fracture of a tooth during extraction is a relatively common event. An extensively carious tooth, a tooth that has had previous endodontic treatment, and a tooth with a large restoration are common risk factors for tooth fracture.

Prevention

Careful attention to the basic principles of exodontia, including proper patient positioning for good visualization and access by the dentist, correct use of forceps and elevators, and sectioning of the tooth, where indicated, can considerably decrease the incidence of tooth fracture during extraction.

Treatment

In the past, before the availability of modern medications and improved surgical training and armamentarium, it was sometimes advocated to avoid surgical intervention and leave small, uninfected root fragments in situ ("leave sleeping dogs lie."). In modern dental practice, it is recommended that all the remaining roots or other tooth fragments be removed in order to provide an appropriate milieu for possible dental implant surgery.

When a tooth is broken during an attempted simple (i.e., forceps) extraction, an "open" (surgical flap) procedure will most likely be necessary to remove the remaining parts. The use of tooth sectioning, careful manipulation of the soft tissue, and preservation of crestal alveolar bone are helpful in maintaining the best conditions for possible dental implant surgery. Recontouring or rebuilding alveolar bone for implant surgery may require the use of autogenous bone (locally harvested from the mandibular symphysis or ramus or distantly harvested from the iliac crest or the tibia), processed bank bone, or bone substitutes.

Infection and abscess
Infections and abscesses are two well-known and related complications of oral surgery. It is estimated that 7–10% of extractions may result in an infection. Most of these infections are self-limiting and will regress or need only supportive care and routine oral health instructions. Some initially simple, localized infections may spread to the adjacent fascial spaces and need aggressive surgical intervention. Because of this, all infections and abscesses should be closely monitored (Yang *et al.*, 2006; Arai *et al.*, 2009; Moghimi *et al.*, 2013).

Prevention
Prophylactic antibiotic coverage when indicated in selected patients, use of properly sterilized instruments, preoperative mouth rinsing, and atraumatic surgery are the mainstays in preventing postoperative infections. Preoperative mouth rinse (e.g., chlorhexidine, sterile saline) has a positive effect on reducing the oral flora count immediately before the procedure and thus the rate of subsequent infection; daily mouth rinsing may be continued for 7–10 days until the sutures are removed. Whether there is an actual antibacterial effect or simply the mechanical effect of the rinsing is open to some debate. Simple infections (confined to the immediate surgical area) should be treated as soon as they are recognized. A localized periapical abscess is easily drained and brought under control, following which the tooth might be treated with an endodontic approach when it is possible to retain the tooth. A neglected or mismanaged periapical abscess may easily extend to adjacent

(or distant) fascial spaces and ultimately cause systemic, possible life-threatening illness (see later text). Pericoronitis, more likely to develop around a partially erupted mandibular third molar tooth, is easily managed in its initial presentation, but, if ignored, it can easily extend into the space of the body of the mandible and then into the masticator and other adjacent fascial spaces, which will produce fever, chills, trismus, and dysphagia and can progress to airway obstruction, systemic sepsis, and death (Yang *et al.*, 2006; Arai *et al.*, 2009; Moghimi *et al.*, 2013).

Treatment
1 The first step is to eradicate the source of infection, which is done by extirpation of the necrotic pulp using an endodontic approach, extraction of the tooth, or removal of a foreign body (necrotic tooth fragment). This step may be postponed only in special situations, such as a systemic disorder or severe trismus.
2 Surgical incision and drainage. In cases where the diagnosis of any fascial space abscess or cellulitis is made, incision and drainage must be planned and performed as soon as possible (Figure 5.6b, c). This step may be postponed in patients with unstable systemic conditions until the disorder is under control and permission for surgery has been issued by an appropriate medical consultant (e.g., infectious disease specialist). For a healthy patient with a localized, well-defined abscess (such as a vestibular abscess), incision and drainage would be adequate to resolve the problem and no additional intervention should be necessary.
3 Use of antibiotics. Antibiotics, used in conjunction with the two first steps, may help the patient's immune system to overcome the abscess. The decision to use an antibiotic is completely dependent on the patient's clinical condition and the experience and clinical judgment of the treating dentist (Yang *et al.*, 2006; Arai *et al.*, 2009; Moghimi *et al.*, 2013).

Emphysema during tooth extraction
The use of high-speed dental hand pieces with air coolant in surgical extraction may push air through the flap or fresh wounds, and this can result in a collection of air in adjacent soft tissues (subcutaneous emphysema). This condition may be immediately observed during the surgery or gradually appear after a few hours (Figure 5.4) (Yang *et al.*, 2006; Arai *et al.*, 2009).

Prevention

Standard surgical hand pieces (not the dental drills used for tooth cavity preparations for restorations) do not produce externalized air exhaust and are best to use in all types of surgical manipulations of soft and hard tissues.

Treatment

Subcutaneous emphysema that occurs following oral surgery is usually self-limiting and subsides in few days. On rare occasions, emphysema may progress and descend toward the trachea and mediastinum, which can result in a life-threatening encroachment on the patient's airway. Therefore, it is recommended to closely monitor the patient until the air is completely evacuated. The following steps are usually recommended (Yang *et al.*, 2006; Arai *et al.*, 2009):

1 The patient is asked to rest/sleep in a sitting or semi-sitting position to avoid downward movement of the air.
2 Antibiotics are prescribed to prevent any possible infection.
3 When downward movement of emphysema or difficulty in breathing is observed, an immediate medical consultation is necessary.
4 Prompt consultation with a physician (preferably a general surgeon) is highly recommended to assist in the evaluation and follow-up of the patient until the condition has resolved.

Postoperative complications

Dry socket

Alveolar osteitis (so-called, "dry socket") is a painfully debilitating complication that can occur after tooth extraction. Usually, the patient presents one to several days after the extraction complaining of severe, aching lower jaw pain, often radiating to the ipsilateral ear, inadequately relieved by pain medications, and a bad taste and foul odor to the breath. Etiology, prevalence, and treatment of this condition are extensively discussed in the literature (Pogrel, 1997). In dry socket, a blood clot that has a dominant role in socket healing is prematurely disintegrated, partially or totally, within one to four days after surgery, and free nerve endings and bone are exposed to the oral cavity. This condition may be observed in both maxillary and mandibular teeth, though it has been shown that it is much more prevalent in mandibular teeth (especially mandibular third molar teeth) (Noroozi and Philbert, 2009; Bowe, Rogers, and Stassen, 2010; Cardoso *et al.*, 2010; Daly *et al.*, 2012; Laraki, Chbicheb, and El Wady, 2012). Patients who seem to be most at risk of developing alveolar osteitis after tooth extractions are females who are taking estrogen-containing birth control medications and any patient who has had a localized dental infection (e.g., pericoronitis in the area of the tooth to be extracted) within the 3 months prior to the extraction.

Signs and symptoms

(Noroozi and Philbert, 2009; Bowe, Rogers, and Stassen, 2010; Daly *et al.*, 2012; Laraki, Chbicheb, and El Wady, 2012)

1 Throbbing pain that usually starts 2 or 3 days after extraction and radiates to the ipsilateral ear
2 Foul odor (bad breath)
3 Foul taste

Predisposing factors

1 Difficult extraction and traumatic surgery. Many studies have shown a direct correlation between this complication and the technical skills of the surgeon.
2 Improper postoperative care. Adequate postoperative care will help the tissues to heal properly. Biting on hard foods, vigorous spitting, overly forceful mouth rinsing, drinking warm liquids, and wound picking by the tongue or toothbrush may disrupt the clot and lead to dry socket.
3 Smoking imposes a negative pressure on the clot causing its possible dislodgment. In addition, the increased temperature changes and the chemical components of tobacco smoke are other factors that may adversely affect socket healing and result in a dry socket.
4 Previous history of dry socket.
5 Site of surgery. Mandibular molar teeth, especially wisdom teeth, are clearly more susceptible to dry socket.
6 The use of estrogen-containing birth control medications may cause early clot breakdown.
7 Infection in the area of the extraction within the three previous months.

Prevention

(Bowe, Rogers, and Stassen, 2010; Cardoso *et al.*, 2010; Daly *et al.*, 2012; Laraki, Chbicheb, and El Wady, 2012; Noroozi and Philbert, 2009)

1 Females can be advised to withhold birth control medications beginning several days before tooth extractions with resumption of medication 72 h afterward.
2 Patients who have had recent local tooth-related infections should be advised to wait for 3 months after the complete resolution of the infection before proceeding with extractions. The administration of preoperative antibiotics does not exert a protective influence against the development of alveolar osteitis in at-risk patients.
3 Meticulous surgical technique is critical in the prevention of dry socket.
4 Adequate attention to postoperative instructions will help clot formation and normal healing.
5 Both preoperative and postoperative chlorhexidine mouth rinses have been shown to effectively reduce the incidence of dry socket. Some researchers advocate the use of chlorhexidine gel to help preclude dry socket in susceptible patients. Overly vigorous postoperative mouth rinsing is not advisable.

Treatment

Many modalities are proposed to treat dry socket. The primary goal after diagnosis is the provision of adequate pain relief while the condition heals. The first step is to differentiate alveolar osteitis from other postextraction pain. This is easily done by first reviewing the history and symptoms (typically, onset of severe, throbbing pain one to several days after the extraction, radiation of pain to the ipsilateral ear, foul taste, bad breath). In some patients, the administration of a long-acting local anesthetic block provides good, rapid pain relief and allows the clinician to proceed to evaluate the patient. The socket is gently and thoroughly irrigated with tepid saline solution or chlorhexidine to remove all debris. Usually exposed alveolar bone is visible in the socket. Then, significant effort should be made to alleviate the pain and to redirect the socket healing to its normal process. A small cotton ball or gauze strip is soaked in eugenol (oil of clove) and gently but firmly placed into the involved socket. Pain relief (if a local anesthetic block has not been administered) usually occurs within one to several minutes. This effect is often dramatic, and the patient frequently remarks about its effectiveness. Antibiotics are not necessary, as this is not a true infectious process but merely surface exposure of bone to oral flora and debris. Curettage of the socket or osteoplasty is not indicated, as the simple supportive care of

socket irrigation and analgesic dressing usual solves the problem. The condition resolves when the exposed alveolar bone becomes covered with fresh granulation tissue. This takes about 7–14 days to occur; during that time, the patient could be seen every 2 or 3 days for removal and replacement of the socket dressing.

Trismus

Trismus is spasm of the muscles of mastication (masseter, temporalis, lateral and medial pterygoids) resulting in difficulty or restriction of the range of mouth opening. The normal maximal incisal opening (MIO) of an adult is 35–55 mm. Whenever the dentist is evaluating a patient for any type of procedure, a baseline measurement of MIO is an important piece of data that should be recorded in the patient's record; it can be used to assess postoperative recovery of mandibular range of motion. A MIO of less than 35 mm is almost always due to some type of restriction, most commonly due to an effect on the masticatory muscles. When it occurs after a surgical procedure in the mouth, it is generally caused by an irritation of the masticatory muscles during the surgical procedure. There are three general procedures, which are known to damage these muscles (Ogle and Mahjoubi, 2012; Coulthard et al., 2014).

1 Local anesthesia. During a mandibular nerve block placed into the pterygomandibular space, the needle may pass inadvertently through the medial pterygoid muscle. Sometimes, in an effort to find the best place of injection, several directional changes are made, which intensifies this damage. The other possible damaging factor is the needle tip. In both the IAN block and the Gow-Gates technique (routine mandibular anesthetic techniques), the needle bumps the medial surface of the mandibular ramus. Sometimes, this unintentional contact creates a small barb on needle tip. This barb can damage the soft tissue within its pathway when the needle is then redirected one or more times before injection and withdrawal, bringing it into contact with the medial pterygoid muscle. The needle should be checked after each injection in a given patient; if a barb has been created, the needle is discarded and replaced before giving subsequent injections to the same patient (Ogle and Mahjoubi, 2012).
2 Flap reflection. Anterior fibers of the temporal muscles are attached to the coronoid process and extend inferiorly to the distal aspect of mandibular third

molars. Distal extension of a buccal periosteal flap and wide dissection for exposure of a mandibular third molar may directly damage these fibers, which often results in mild to severe trismus (Ogle and Mahjoubi, 2012).

3 Extension of infection to the masticator fascial space. Bacterial infection of the masticatory space directly affects the masticatory muscles and may lead to severe trismus. This progressive condition may limit the surgical access to the mouth; thus, it is considered an urgent situation that should be managed by an oral and maxillofacial surgeon (Coulthard *et al.*, 2014).

Prevention

It is easy to avoid this debilitating complication if the etiology of trismus is understood.

1 *The needle may be changed after each block injection.* Alternatively, the needle can be passed through a piece of gauze, and if the gauze is torn, it should be changed for the next injection (Figure 5.5). Standard mandibular techniques do not require many direc-

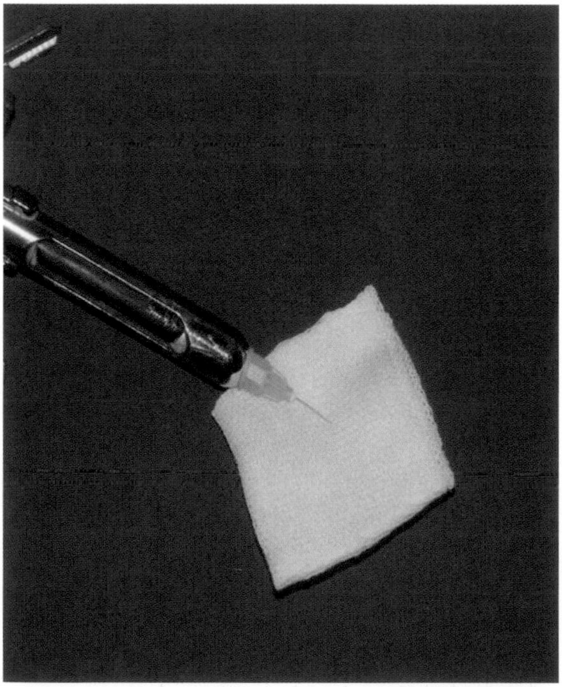

Figure 5.5 Needle may be passed through a surgical gauze to check possible barb formation in the second use of a needle for a patient.

tional changes and are performed with minimum soft tissue trauma (Coulthard *et al.*, 2014).

2 *Flap design.* The surgical flap technique for the removal of mandibular third molars may be extended anteriorly. Alternatively, a releasing incision may be performed in deep incisions, and posterior extension must be limited to only few millimeters posterior to the third molars. With this approach, temporalis muscle fibers are less likely to be at risk of injury (Coulthard *et al.*, 2014).

3 *Infection of masticatory spaces.* Infection from localized abscesses can spread along the path of least resistance to anatomically adjacent fascial spaces (space of body of the mandible, masticator space). It is recommended to treat all abscesses early before possible potential extension to other anatomic locations (Coulthard *et al.*, 2014).

Treatment

As the first step, it is necessary to differentiate trismus from other common causes of diminished mouth opening. After establishing the diagnosis, anti-inflammatory drugs are prescribed for traumatic injuries (such as local anesthesia or flap design). A soft diet is recommended, and the patient should be reassured that the situation will resolve in a few days. In infection cases, vigorous surgical intervention is necessary. Incision and drainage are performed, and the causative factor is eliminated as soon as possible. In some patients, severe, persistent trismus may require aggressive treatment, and referral to a physical therapist will be necessary in order to reestablish the preoperative level of mouth opening and other mandibular movements that the thorough clinician will have determined and recorded preoperatively (Ogle and Mahjoubi, 2012; Coulthard *et al.*, 2014).

Use of antibiotics to reduce complications of oral surgery

The role of antibiotics in the prevention of postoperative sequelae in oral surgery is extensively discussed in the literature (Jeske and Suchko, 2003; Schwartz and Larson, 2007; Susarla, Sharaf, and Dodson, 2011; Lodi *et al.*, 2012; Oomens and Forouzanfar, 2012). Lodi *et al.* performed a comprehensive meta-analysis on available clinical trials. The results of these studies show that the use of prophylactic antibiotics may slightly decrease the incidence of infection. Postoperative pain was also influenced where lowered incidence was observed in the cases receiving antibiotics. The evidence that antibiotics may reduce the risk of dry socket is questionable, at best. Prophylactic antibiotic coverage does not affect the degree of trismus and postoperative pain (Jeske and Suchko, 2003).

The decision to prescribe prophylactic antibiotics is best made by the surgeon on a case-by-case basis, tempered by accepted guidelines and clinical judgment. However, based on the current evidence, it is not recommended to use prophylactic antibiotics for an otherwise healthy patient who is without infection and is undergoing a simple (localized to the dento-alveolar region with minimal soft tissue dissection and without extensive bone exposure or removal) surgical procedure (Schwartz and Larson, 2007; Susarla, Sharaf, and Dodson, 2011; Lodi *et al.*, 2012; Oomens and Forouzanfar, 2012).

In patients with immune deficiency or systemic disease, as well as in difficult surgical cases, the risk of aforementioned complications is higher, and despite insufficient evidence, the use of prophylactic antibiotics is logically recommended (Schwartz and Larson, 2007; Susarla, Sharaf, and Dodson, 2011; Lodi *et al.*, 2012; Oomens and Forouzanfar, 2012).

Management of oral surgery complications in patients receiving hemostasis-altering drugs

Antiplatelet and antithrombotic drugs are commonly used to prevent myocardial infarction, stroke, pulmonary blood clots, and other thromboembolic dysfunctions. These medications are used to avoid platelet aggregation and clot formation. However, in tooth extractions and minor oral surgeries, it is prudent to be able to stop the bleeding (Wahl and Howell, 1996; Wahl, 2000; Jeske and Suchko, 2003; Pototski and Amenábar, 2007). The question is: What level of anticoagulation is acceptable in a patient about to undergo a tooth extraction? Current evidence for the commonly used drugs shows the following:

1 *Aspirin.* In minor oral surgery, the routine use of aspirin (>100 mg/day) may be continued, though local measures in bleeding control and postoperative instructions must be precisely considered.

2 *Dual antiplatelet therapy.* This includes patients who are on a combination of aspirin and other antiplatelet medications. Routine minor oral surgery and simple extractions are safely performed without any modifications in their daily drug use, though local hemostatic measures should be adequately provided (Wahl and Howell, 1996; Wahl, 2000; Jeske and Suchko, 2003; Pototski and Amenábar, 2007).

3 *Anticoagulant drugs.* A critical decision should be made whether to continue the medication and risk possible uncontrollable bleeding. Wahl conducted a systematic review in which he showed that the risk of a thromboembolic event is three times higher if the drug is interrupted when compared to bleeding (when the drug is continued). Therefore, this study (and several other similar studies) has recommended to not interrupt the anticoagulant in simple extractions, soft tissue biopsies, and minor oral surgeries. International normalized ratio (INR) will show the relative risk of hemorrhage after oral surgery. An INR of 2.5 is ideal for performing minor oral surgery, meaning that the risk of both bleeding and thrombocmbolic events is minimal. Nevertheless, minor surgeries might be safely done up to an INR of four. Some patients take both antiplatelet and anticoagulant medications. The same INR protocol may be applied safely. It is imperative that preoperative consultation with the physician managing the patient's medical condition be done and any decisions regarding medication/dose changes and/or interruption should be made by the responsible physician (Wahl and Howell, 1996; Wahl, 2000; Jeske and Suchko, 2003; Pototski and Amenábar, 2007).

Oroantral fistula

OAF is an iatrogenic opening between the maxillary sinus and the oral cavity. Extraction of a maxillary molar tooth is the most common cause, though eradication of benign and malignant lesions, implant surgery, and many other procedures in the posterior maxilla can result in this relatively common complication. An oroantral communication, pathway, or tract that is not obliterated by a stable blood clot and persists beyond 24 h is called an OAF. This communication, if it persists, is gradually covered by a layer of epithelium (Visscher, Van Minnen, and Bos, 2010; Dym and Wolf, 2012).

Predisposing factors

(Visscher, Van Minnen, and Bos, 2010; Dym and Wolf, 2012)

1 Long divergent maxillary molar roots
2 Large pneumatized sinus with a thin layer of bone between the sinus and roots
3 Thin, narrow periodontal ligament (PDL) and partial or total loss of PDL

Diagnosis

Inadvertent misdirection of a surgical instrument (such an elevator into the maxillary sinus), a large piece of bone attached to the tip of maxillary roots, and blood or air bubbling from the extraction socket indicate an OAF has occurred. When any doubt exists in the diagnosis, it may be assumed that a small OAF exists and further attempts at diagnosis, such as blowing the nose while the nostrils are kept closed by fingers or clinical examinations, may turn a simple or incomplete OAF to a complete or wider communication (Visscher, Van Minnen, and Bos, 2010; Dym and Wolf, 2012).

Treatment

1 Small defects, up to 3 mm. Small communications sometimes gradually close by themselves. The patients should be questioned about pressure differential or fluid movement between the oral cavity and maxillary sinus. The patient can be asked to swallow a small amount of water, while the practitioner observes for evidence of flow of fluid out of the ipsilateral nasal passage.

2 Medium defects, 3–5 mm. Many approaches are available to close a medium-sized OAF, though it is recommended to use the most effective techniques with the least possible morbidity:

o Buccal flap. In this technique, the soft tissue edges of the OAF are refreshed, and then a trapezoid flap is designed and reflected. This flap is advanced palatally to cover the defect (Figure 5.6a–c). When the flap does not freely cover the defect, a periosteal releasing incision may be done at the base of flap and closure is then performed. The potential drawback of this technique is missing keratinized gingiva. Therefore, for the critical levels of keratinized gingiva, this approach should be avoided.

o Pedicled buccal fat pad advancement flap. Buccal fat pads are two bulky fat tissues deeply located beneath the buccinator muscle on each side of the face. A pedicled fat flap may be prepared and advanced over the oroantral defect. This tissue has been predictably used to cover medium-sized fistulas. After 2 weeks, normal epithelial tissue covers the flap and the OAF is predominantly resolved (Figure 5.7a–c).

To prepare a fat flap, a buccal flap is widely reflected, a full periosteal incision is made, and the buccal fat pad is identified. The fat pad is gently advanced toward the defect. It is sutured to normal palatal tissue and the buccal flap is placed back without any advancement (Rapidis et al., 2000; Visscher, Van Minnen, and Bos, 2010; Dym and Wolf, 2012).

3 Defects wider than 5 mm and recurrent fistulas. Wide fistulas are challenging for the surgeon. Many flap techniques, such as the palatal rotational flap,

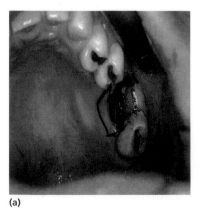
(a)

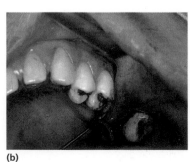
(b)

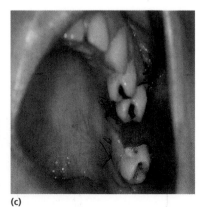
(c)

Figure 5.6 (a) Buccal flap is designed to restore a traumatic OAF, (b) trapezoid buccal flap is advanced to cover the defect, and (c) flap edges are passively sutured.

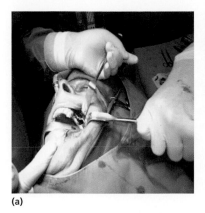
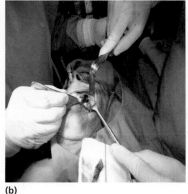
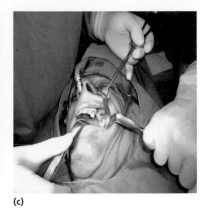

(a)   (b)   (c)

Figure 5.7 (a) Buccal fat flap is planned to cover a 1 cm OAF and (b) buccal fat is prepared and advanced to freely cover the defect, and (c) flap is precisely sutured in place.

palatal island flap, tongue flap, and a combination of all the aforementioned techniques, are frequently used. These complex reconstructions need to be performed by an experienced oral and maxillofacial surgeon (Rapidis *et al.*, 2000; Dym and Wolf, 2012; Visscher, Van Minnen, and Bos, 2010; Wahl and Howell, 1996).

4 When a patient has sustained a suspected opening into the maxillary sinus due to a dental procedure, it is mandatory that the dentist arrange a timely referral of the patient to an oral and maxillofacial surgeon for further evaluation, prompt treatment, and follow-up. When a previously sterile or clean maxillary sinus is opened to the fluids and debris of the oral cavity, it rapidly becomes contaminated and irritated. The resulting inflammatory response causes proliferation of polypoid tissue within the sinus, which can block the normal outflow from the sinus into the nasal cavity. Such obstruction rapidly leads to acute maxillary sinusitis, a condition that should be avoided if at all possible, as its treatment is much more extensive than that of a simple opening between the oral cavity and the sinus.

In this chapter, we have outlined some of the minor complications of oral surgery that are confined to the anatomic area of the surgical field. All clinicians performing oral surgical procedures should at minimum be trained in recognition of major complication (such as mandible fracture, nerve injuries, drug-induced osteonecrosis, osteomyelitis, sepsis, odontogenic facial space infections, or systemic complications), so that prompt referral to a trained oral and maxillofacial surgeon can be made.

References

Arai, I., Aoki, T., Yamazaki, H., Ota, Y. and Kaneko, A. (2009) Pneumomediastinum and subcutaneous emphysema after dental extraction detected incidentally by regular medical checkup: a case report. *Oral Surgery, Oral Medicine, Oral Pathology, Oral Radiology, and Endodontology*, **107**, e33–e38.

Bagheri, S.C. and Meyer, R.A. (2014) When to refer a patient with a nerve injury to a specialist. *Journal of the American Dental Association*, **145**, 859–861.

Bagheri, S.C., Bell, R.B. and Khan, H.A. (2012) Current Therapy in Oral and Maxillofacial Surgery.   Elsevier/Saunders, St. Louis.

Bagheri, S.C., Meyer, R.A., Cho, S.H., Thoppay, J., Khan, H.A. and Steed, M.B. (2012) Microsurgical repair of the inferior alveolar nerve: success rate and factors that adversely affect outcome. *Journal of Oral and Maxillofacial Surgery*, **70**, 1978–1990.

Bodner, L., Brennan, P.A. and McLeod, N.M. (2011) Characteristics of iatrogenic mandibular fractures associated with tooth removal: review and analysis of 189 cases. *British Journal of Oral and Maxillofacial Surgery*, **49**, 567–572.

Bouloux, G.F., Steed, M.B. and Perciaccante, V.J. (2007) Complications of third molar surgery. *Oral and Maxillofacial Surgery Clinics of North America*, **19**, 117–128.

Bowe, D.C., Rogers, S. and Stassen, L. (2010) The management of dry socket/alveolar osteitis. *Journal of the Irish Dental Association*, **57**, 305–310.

Brauer, H.U. (2008) Unusual complications associated with third molar surgery: a systematic review. *Quintessence International*, **40**, 565–572.

Cankaya, A.B., Erdem, M.A., Cakarer, S., Cifter, M. and Oral, C.K. (2011) Iatrogenic mandibular fracture associated with third molar removal. *International Journal of Medical Sciences*, **8**, 547.

Cardoso, C.L., Rodrigues, M.T.V., Júnior, O.F., Garlet, G.P. and De Carvalho, P.S.P. (2010) Clinical concepts of dry socket. *Journal of Oral and Maxillofacial Surgery*, **68**, 1922–1932.

Chrcanovic, B.R. and Freire-Maia, B. (2011) Considerations of maxillary tuberosity fractures during extraction of upper molars: a literature review. *Dental Traumatology*, **27**, 393–398.

Coulthard, P., Bailey, E., Esposito, M., Furness, S., Renton, T.F. and Worthington, H.V. (2014) Surgical techniques for the removal of mandibular wisdom teeth. *Database of Systematic Reviews* CD004345.

Daly, B., Sharif, M.O., Newton, T., Jones, K. and Worthington, H.V. (2012) Local interventions for the management of alveolar osteitis (dry socket). *Database of Systematic Reviews* CD006968.

Duda, M. (2002) Forcing of the root into the maxillary sinus during tooth extraction – and what next? *Annales Universitatis Mariae Curie-Sklodowska. Sectio D: Medicina*, **58**, 38–41.

Durmus, E., Dolanmaz, D., Kucukkolbsi, H. and Mutlu, N. (2004) Accidental displacement of impacted maxillary and mandibular third molars. *Quintessence International*, **35**, 375–377.

Dym, H. and Weiss, A. (2012) Exodontia: tips and techniques for better outcomes. *Dental Clinics of North America*, **56**, 245–266.

Dym, H. and Wolf, J.C. (2012) Oroantral communication. *Oral and Maxillofacial Surgery Clinics of North America*, **24**, 239–247.

Ethunandan, M., Shanahan, D. and Patel, M. (2012) Iatrogenic mandibular fractures following removal of impacted third molars: an analysis of 130 cases. *British Dental Journal*, **212**, 179–184.

Freedman, G.L. (1997) Intentional partial odontectomy: review of cases. *Journal of Oral and Maxillofacial Surgery*, **655**, 524.

Huang, I.-Y., Wu, C.-W. and Worthington, P. (2007) The displaced lower third molar: a literature review and suggestions for management. *Journal of oral and maxillofacial surgery*, **65**, 1186–1190.

Huang, I.-Y., Chen, C.-M. and Chuang, F.-H. (2011) Caldwell-Luc procedure for retrieval of displaced root in the maxillary sinus. *Oral Surgery, Oral Medicine, Oral Pathology, Oral Radiology, and Endodontology*, **112**, e59–e63.

Jeske, A.H. and Suchko, G.D. (2003) Lack of a scientific basis for routine discontinuation of oral anticoagulation therapy before dental treatment. *The Journal of the American Dental Association*, **134**, 1492–1497.

Jing, G., Yang, C., Zheng, J.-W., He, D.-M., Zheng, L.-Y. and Hu, Y.-H. (2014) Four osteotomy methods with piezosurgery to remove complicated mandibular third molars: a retrospective study. *Journal of Oral and Maxillofacial Surgery*, **72**, 2126–2133.

Kaban, L.B., Pogrel, M.A. and Perrott, D.H. (1997) *Complications in Oral and Maxillofacial Surgery*, WB Saunders Co., Philadelphia.

Laraki, M., Chbicheb, S. and El Wady, W. (2012) Alveolitis: review of the literature. *Odonto-stomatologie tropicale*, **35**, 19–25.

Lee, J.S., Curley, A.W. and Smith, R.A. (2007) Prevention of wrong-site tooth extraction: clinical guidelines. *Journal of Oral and Maxillofacial Surgery*, **65**, 1793–1799.

Lodi, G., Figini, L., Sardella, A., Carrassi, A., Del Fabbro, M. and Furness, S. (2012) Antibiotics to prevent complications following tooth extractions. *Database of Systematic Reviews* CD003811.

Marciani, R.D. (2012) Complications of third molar surgery and their management. *Atlas of the Oral and Maxillofacial Surgery Clinics*, **20**, 233–251.

McCormick, N., Moore, U., and Meechan, J. (2014a) Haemostasis. Part 1: The management of post-extraction haemorrhage. *Dental Update*, **41**, 290–292, 294–296.

McCormick, N., Moore, U., Meechan, J., and Norouzi, M. (2014b) Haemostasis. Part 2: Medications that affect haemostasis. *Dental Update*, **41**, 395–396, 399–402, 405.

Meyer, R.A. (1987) Complications of exodontia, in *Textbook of Practical Oral and Maxillofacial Surgery*, 3rd edn (ed D.E. Waite), Lea & Febiger, Philadelphia, pp. 145–167.

Miloro, M. (2015) *Complications in Oral and Maxillofacial Surgery*, Springer, New York.

Mingarro-de-León, A., Chaveli-López, B. and Gavaldá-Esteve, C. (2014) Dental management of patients receiving anticoagulant and/or antiplatelet treatment. *Journal of Clinical and Experimental Dentistry*, **6**, e155.

Moghimi, M., Baart, J.A., Karagozoglu, K.H. and Forouzanfar, T. (2013) Spread of odontogenic infections: a retrospective analysis and review of the literature. *Quintessence International*, **44**, 351–361.

Noroozi, A.-R. and Philbert, R.F. (2009) Modern concepts in understanding and management of the "dry socket" syndrome: comprehensive review of the literature. *Oral Surgery, Oral Medicine, Oral Pathology, Oral Radiology, and Endodontology*, **107**, 30–35.

Ogle, O.E. and Mahjoubi, G. (2012) Local anesthesia: agents, techniques, and complications. *Dental Clinics of North America*, **56**, 133–148.

Oomens, M.A. and Forouzanfar, T. (2012) Antibiotic prophylaxis in third molar surgery: a review. *Oral Surgery, Oral Medicine, Oral Pathology and Oral Radiology*, **114**, e5–e12.

Peleg, O., Givot, N., Halamish-Shani, T. and Taicher, S. (2009) Wrong tooth extraction: root cause analysis. *Quintessence International*, **41**, 869–872.

Pogrel, M.A. (1997) Complications of third molar surgery, in *Complications in Oral and Maxillofacial Surgery* (eds L.B. Kaban, M.A. Pogrel and D.H. Perrott), W.B. Saunders Co., Philadelphia, pp. 59–68.

Pogrel, M.A., Lee, J.D. and Muf, D.F. (2004) Coronectomy: a technique to protect the inferior alveolar nerve. *Journal of Oral and Maxillofacial Surgery*, **62**, 1447–1453.

Pototski, M. and Amenábar, J.M. (2007) Dental management of patients receiving anticoagulation or antiplatelet treatment. *Journal of Oral Science*, **49**, 253–258.

Rapidis, A.D., Alexandridis, C.A., Eleftheriadis, E. and Angelopoulos, A.P. (2000) The use of the buccal fat pad for reconstruction of oral defects: review of the literature and report of 15 cases. *Journal of Oral and Maxillofacial Surgery*, **58**, 158–163.

Romero, U., Libotte, F., Palaia, G., Tenore, G., Dalanakis, A. and Annibali, S. (2015) Is erbium:yttrium-aluminum-garnet laser versus conventional rotary osteotomy better in the postoperative period for lower third molar surgery? Randomized split-mouth clinical study. *Journal of Oral and Maxillofacial Surgery*, **73**, 211–218.

Saksena, A., Pemberton, M., Shaw, A., Dickson, S. and Ashley, M. (2014) Preventing wrong tooth extraction: experience in development and implementation of an outpatient safety checklist. *British Dental Journal*, **217**, 357–362.

Schwartz, A.B. and Larson, E.L. (2007) Antibiotic prophylaxis and postoperative complications after tooth extraction and implant placement: a review of the literature. *Journal of Dentistry*, **35**, 881–888.

Susarla, S.M., Sharaf, B. and Dodson, T.B. (2011) Do antibiotics reduce the frequency of surgical site infections after impacted mandibular third molar surgery. *Oral and Maxillofacial Surgery Clinics of North America*, **23**, 541–546.

Visscher, S.H., Van Minnen, B. and Bos, R.R. (2010) Closure of oroantral communications: a review of the literature. *Journal of Oral and Maxillofacial Surgery*, **68**, 1384–1391.

Wahl, M.J. (2000) Myths of dental surgery in patients: receiving anticoagulant therapy. *The Journal of the American Dental Association*, **131**, 77–81.

Wahl, M.J. and Howell, J. (1996) Altering anticoagulation therapy: a survey of physicians. *The Journal of the American Dental Association*, **127**, 625–638.

Weiss, A., Stern, A. and Dym, H. (2011) Technological advances in extraction techniques and outpatient oral surgery. *Dental Clinics of North America*, **55**, 501–513.

Yang, S.-C., Chiu, T.-H., Lin, T.-J. and Chan, H.-M. (2006) Subcutaneous emphysema and pneumomediastinum secondary to dental extraction: a case report and literature review. *The Kaohsiung Journal of Medical Sciences*, **22**, 641–645.

CHAPTER 6

Complications of local anesthesia, sedation, and general anesthesia

James W. Tom[1,2]

[1] Division of Endodontics, General Practice Dentistry, Herman Ostrow School of Dentistry of USC, Los Angeles, CA, USA
[2] Division of Public Health and Pediatric Dentistry, Herman Ostrow School of Dentistry of USC, Los Angeles, CA, USA

Complications of local anesthesia

Dental needle breakage or separation

Although the incidence of dental needle breakage in clinical use has long remained low since the introduction of nonreusable stainless steel needles, the risk of needle breakage still remains a possible complication despite a scarcity of published reports. The most common site of needle breakage during dental procedures occurs during the performance of the inferior alveolar nerve block (IANB), with reports as high as 79% of reported complications. Among these, the overwhelming majority of broken needles involved a 30-gauge needle and separation almost exclusively occurred at the hub of the needle (Malamed, Reed, and Poorsattar, 2010).

Prevention

Based on the common characteristics of reported broken dental needles, prevention of this occurrence should be focused on (i) avoiding bending the dental needle at the hub for soft tissue injections, (ii) minimizing needle insertion completely to the needle hub, (iii) minimizing the use of short needles for the IANB, (iv) minimizing the use of 30-gauge needles for the IANB, (v) minimizing patient movement during injection, and (vi) avoiding forceful contact with bony structures such as the medial aspect of the ramus.

Management

If a portion of the needle is readily visible and easily identified, the clinician may attempt to remove using a hemostat or other grasping instrument. However, in the majority of cases, the fragment will be submerged within tissue and requires immediate referral to a surgical specialist. Depending on the location of the needle fragment, migration can occur into fascial planes and, in the case of IANB broken needle situations, the pterygomandibular space (Gerbino et al., 2013). Three-dimensional imaging, fluoroscopic guided surgery, and stereotactic exploration to remove the needle fragments are all considerations in the management of such a complication, and surgery itself can potentiate further tissue damage (Altay et al., 2014).

Postinjection pain and trismus

It is not uncommon for a patient to experience significant orofacial pain and associated limited mouth opening, termed "trismus," after local anesthesia injections. Multiple factors contribute to this complication, yet the incidence can be reduced using preventative measures during local anesthesia administration. The more common etiologies include trauma during injection, multiple injections in close proximity, dull needles, needle tract infection, and development of hematomas. Less common factors include edema, chemical injury or irritation, recurrent aphthous stomatitis (RAS) lesions (Preeti et al., 2011) of varying presentation, and sloughing of tissues.

Trismus, classically defined as the prolonged, tetanic spasm of the jaw muscles by which the normal opening of the mouth is restricted, may accompany the pain after local anesthesia administration—particularly mandibular anesthesia. The aforementioned factors, including a single needle penetration, can all contribute

Avoiding and Treating Dental Complications: Best Practices in Dentistry, First Edition. Edited by Deborah A. Termeie.
© 2016 John Wiley & Sons, Inc. Published 2016 by John Wiley & Sons, Inc.

to limited, and often painful, mouth opening. Common techniques of anesthetizing the inferior alveolar nerve involve needle penetration of the medial pterygoid muscle of mastication and can result in hemorrhage, swelling, infection, and inflammation of this muscle and surrounding tissues. Symptoms can present up to a week after injection and persist indefinitely depending on etiology.

Prevention

Prevention of postinjection pain involves the following:
1 Using a new, sterile, and sharp local anesthesia needle
2 Limiting prolonged exposure to topical anesthetics
3 Slow anesthetic deposition (recommended 1 ml/min)
4 Limiting multiple injections in close proximity
5 Avoidance of dental treatment during bouts of RAS
Prevention of trismus involves the following:
1 Using a new, sterile, and sharp local anesthesia needle
2 Limiting the amount of anesthetic solution to only what is recommended and necessary
3 Limiting multiple injections in close proximity
4 Using alternate techniques to avoid penetration into the medial pterygoid or limiting injections into the medial pterygoid muscle

Management

Management of postinjection pain includes the use of systemic anti-inflammatories such as oral NSAIDs and corticosteroids. Injection pain can also be associated with, and must be differentiated from, dental treatment or surgery rendered concurrently with the anesthetic injections. While most pains originating from anesthetic injections are generally self-limiting and persist for a period of 4–6 days postinjection as the result of an inflammatory process, active management helps to limit its course. Mucosal irritation and RAS should be managed with topical and systemic corticosteroids, anti-inflammatories, antiseptics, and analgesics. Oral rinses such as 0.2% chlorhexidine and triclosan can be considered, as well as the use of topical diclofenac with hyaluronic acid to decrease discomfort (Belenguer-Guallar, Jimenez-Soriano, and Claramunt-Lozano, 2014).

Management of trismus generally follows a similar initial therapeutic plan. Since the complication often involves injury and inflammation to the medial pterygoid muscle, therapies involving active stretching of the affected muscle are indicated. Initial management must include preventing hypomobility by having the

patient stretch and progressively open the mouth to prevent muscle splinting and eventual fibrosis (myofibrotic contracture). Soft bite sticks, stacked tongue blades, commercially available mandibular range of movement rehabilitation devices (TheraBite™), warm liquid rinses, and consideration of mandibular manipulation under general anesthesia are all effective therapies in injection-induced trismus. Consideration of advanced imaging to rule out needle tract infection of the medial pterygoid or associated structures should be considered if traditional therapies prove futile. Consequently, antibiotics will be indicated once a needle tract infection is identified. The progression of therapy should be meticulously recorded, such as documenting incisal opening, to monitor incremental improvement in opening or lack thereof. Finally, the clinician should always consider referral to an appropriate specialist in any phase of the management of this complication (Beddis *et al.*, 2014).

Allergy

Allergy has been reported anecdotally by patients to encompass a wide variety of symptoms ranging from lightheadedness and heart palpitations to near death experiences. Reports of allergy by patients may be mistaken for the effects of beta-adrenergic stimulation by vasoconstrictors used in many dental local anesthesia preparations. Yet the reports of true, immunoglobulin E (IgE)-mediated allergy to local anesthesia are still exceptionally uncommon in dentistry given the number of injections delivered to patients on a daily basis (Berkun *et al.*, 2003). Urticaria, hives, rash, itching, edema, wheezing, or other symptoms related to histamine release are classic signs of true allergy. Ester-type anesthetics (benzocaine used in topical anesthesia, tetracaine, procaine) are derived from para-aminobenzoic acid (PABA) and elicit more reported allergic responses than any of the amide-type local anesthetics (articaine, bupivacaine, lidocaine, etc.) used commonly in dentistry. Methylparaben, a bacteriostatic agent, has been excluded from *dental* local anesthesia cartridges in all commercially prepared solutions. Methylparaben, however, is included in multidose vials (MDVs) used more commonly in healthcare settings other than dentistry and should be excluded from allergy testing specific to dental local anesthesia. Another potential allergen, sodium metabisulfite, an antioxidant commonly used to preserve fruits and vegetables, is included in all local anesthesia agents containing a vasoconstrictor such as epinephrine. Yet, to date, there is no documented case of a true allergic reaction to bisulfite-containing local anesthetic in dentistry.

Psychogenic manifestations of local anesthetic sensitivity are perhaps the most common complications that are often mistaken by the patient and sometimes by the clinician as allergy. Some of these reactions may convince the patient that powerful reactions to local anesthesia preclude their use, and therefore, treatment must be rendered under general anesthesia. The most common psychogenic reaction reported is vasovagal syncope followed by acute stress reactions that may include a rapid heart rate, diaphoresis, and nausea and vomiting.

Diagnosis of true allergic response involves ruling out psychogenic reactions to needle phobias and other stressors. Typically, once the psychogenic reactions have been ruled out, a differential diagnosis of allergic response to local anesthetics will fall into either an immediate (5–30 min onset), type I, IgE-mediated or delayed (8–12 h onset), type IV, cell-mediated reaction. Consultation with an allergist familiar with dental local anesthesia solutions is advisable if true allergy is suspected.

Prevention

Patient report and history to local anesthesia allergy must be investigated thoroughly, and if needed, appropriate referral to an appropriate allergy specialist should be considered. Despite the extremely limited occurrence of amide local anesthesia allergy in dentistry, the additional medicolegal concerns of administering an unwanted agent to a patient warrant extensive patient education and clinical evidence.

The clinician should be aware that local anesthesia allergy testing must involve local anesthesia preparations used exclusively in dental local anesthesia cartridges and not in MDVs used commonly in medicine. As stated earlier, dental preparations of local anesthesia are manufactured without a methylparaben bacteriostatic agent used in MDVs (Macy, 2003).

Patients reporting allergy to sulfites (not "sulfa" drugs, which refer to the sulfonamide class of drugs) should not receive local anesthetics containing epinephrine. Epinephrine-containing local anesthetics contain an antioxidant—metabisulfite, sodium bisulfite, or potassium bisulfite—to prolong shelf life. This antigen elicits a non-IgE hypersensitivity response that often manifests in rhinitis, rash, headache, dyspnea, and cramping (Simon, 1996).

Patients reporting allergy and sensitivity to PABA derivatives should not be exposed to ester local anesthetics found in many topical anesthetic preparations and ester-type local anesthetics. Other newer intranasal formulations of local anesthetics may employ an ester-type local anesthetic such as tetracaine (Ciancio *et al.*, 2013). These formulations should also be avoided.

Patients reporting allergy to latex should not be exposed to latex that may be contained in the diaphragms and stoppers of dental local anesthesia cartridges. Although there have been no reports of latex allergic reactions to dental local anesthesia cartridges in the literature, caution is urged for those patients who report severe latex allergic (anaphylactic) reactions and appropriate precautions should be implemented to avoid the use of latex-containing armamentarium and local anesthesia cartridges (Shojaei and Haas, 2002).

Finally, increases in heart rate and the patient being alarmed by such should be explained as a normal consequence of epinephrine administration. Empirically, some authors have cautioned practitioners to avoid using more than 0.040 mg (40 μg) of epinephrine in patients with significant cardiovascular disease (Malamed, 2013). Patients, however, should be counseled in respect to not mistaking increases in heart rate and sympathetic nervous system activation with true allergic response.

Management

Allergy and anaphylaxis are medical emergencies that need to be addressed promptly with antihistamines and, in the case of anaphylaxis, epinephrine. Delayed hypersensitivity reactions are typically treated with oral or parenteral H1 and H2 antihistamines such as diphenhydramine and ranitidine, respectively. Nebulized or metered-dose inhaled (MDI) albuterol can also be an effective bronchodilator when administered continuously. Corticosteroids can also be considered for late-effect allergic symptoms and should be continued for 2–3 days after initial presentation of allergic symptoms. Finally, for anaphylaxis, epinephrine (0.3 mg IM for adults, 0.15 mg for children) and glucagon are proven effective agents when used as directed (Liberman and Teach, 2008).

Psychogenic reactions such as syncope and hyperventilation should be treated in accordance with accepted medical emergency management in a dental-based setting. This also includes consideration of transporting the patient to an emergency medical care facility.

Failure to achieve anesthesia

The common complications of not achieving satisfactory local anesthesia to perform various dental procedures stem from a variety of etiologies. It is important to consider that the patient's perception of pain, or inadequate local anesthesia, may involve an overwhelming psychological component. The International Association for the Study of Pain (IASP) defines "pain" as "an unpleasant sensory and emotional experience associated with actual or potential tissue damage, or described in terms of such damage" (IASP, 2015). Simply, local anesthesia may not be sufficient to control or obviate the surgical trauma of dentistry or dental surgery, and one must consider alternate means once local anesthesia avenues have been exhausted.

Numerous hypotheses have been investigated regarding the failure of local anesthesia that included needle deflection, missing of landmarks or accessory nerve branches, the presence of infection, tetrodotoxin resistant sodium channels, or inadequate volume of local anesthetic solution. However, investigations have failed to isolate a singular etiology of oral local anesthesia failures (Brau et al., 2000). Maxillary anesthesia has classically not had a failure rate approaching that of the mandible. Moreover, the incidence of failed local anesthesia occurs primarily in attempting to achieve pulpal anesthesia in the mandible with the IANB and has been reported to be as high as 32% in the lateral incisors, particularly in dentition diagnosed with irreversible pulpitis.

When anesthetizing dentition near to the midline of both maxillary and mandibular arches, cross innervation of dentition, hard tissue and soft tissue from contralateral innervation can also result in a failure to achieve adequate local anesthesia (Clark et al., 2002).

Prevention and management

Adequate and reliable local anesthesia hinges upon proper administration and accurate deposition. The clinician must ensure that appropriate extraoral and intraoral landmarks are identified prior to injection and that an understanding of the areas anesthetized by a particular injection technique will provide appropriate coverage. Of particular note, the posterior

superior alveolar (PSA) and the greater palatine nerve block do leave the mesial buccal root of the maxillary first molar and the maxillary first premolar, respectively, unanesthetized in roughly 30% of the population (Malamed, 2013). Supplemental injections, namely, the supraperiosteal (infiltration) injection, will give the patient full anesthesia of these often overlooked anatomical variations. For the anterior dentition, additional anesthesia from the contralateral side may provide anesthetic coverage for those teeth that are cross-innervated (Clark et al., 2002).

A second injection of a different anesthetic solution from the commonly used 2% lidocaine with 1:100000 epinephrine concentration has not been shown to be effective in the IANB (Kanaa, Whitworth, and Meechan, 2012). Increasing the concentration of epinephrine in local anesthetic formulations has demonstrated no increased efficacy in randomized, double-blind comparisons (Mason et al., 2009).

In the treatment of dentition with irreversible pulpitis, several strategies are available to provide anesthesia. After ruling out a missed injection, alternate injections are advised that provide anesthesia to the proximal nerve trunk: Gow-Gates or Vazirani-Akinosi (closed mouth mandibular nerve injection technique with the needle introduced from the ipsilateral and anterior aspect, at the level of the maxillary marginal gingiva parallel to the maxillary occlusal plane) nerve blocks in the mandible and PSA, greater palatine, or Division 2 nerve blocks in the maxilla.

Additionally, the clinician should consider alternate injection techniques such as a buccal infiltration in the mandible with 4% articaine, intraosseous injections, or intrapulpal injections. Deposition of local anesthesia solution near or at the mental foramen (mental incisive nerve block) can improve the outcome of IANB in the premolar and mandibular first molar. Anesthetizing the mylohyoid nerve has not been shown to improve anesthetic efficacy of the IANB (Nusstein, Reader, and Drum, 2010).

Lastly, when taking into consideration the IASP definition of pain, the clinician must consider deferring treatment under a central nervous system (CNS) depressant used in moderate sedation to general anesthesia.

Paresthesia

Mechanical, chemical, or surgical trauma can lead to both temporary and permanent nerve damage that can alter sensation and motor control. Any alteration or abnormal sensation from normal is encompassed by the broad definition of paresthesia. Subdivisions of paresthesia include anesthesia, a total loss of sensation; dysesthesia, burning or tingling; allodynia, pain in response to normal stimuli; and hyperesthesia, increased pain response to all stimuli. Of the most commonly studied paresthesias related to dental local anesthesia, the IANB technique with resultant paresthesia to the lingual nerve accounts for as high as 70% of published reports with local anesthesia solutions in the 4% concentration (40 mg/ml). Several mechanisms of local anesthesia-mediated paresthesias have been proposed ranging from neural apoptosis to mechanical needle injury to a unifascicular lingual nerve (Malamed, 2006).

Inferior alveolar nerve paresthesia from surgery or other dental-related treatment may be difficult to distinguish from local anesthesia-related nerve injury upon initial presentation. Third molar removal (Kim *et al.*, 2012), extrusion of endodontic sealer into the mandibular canal (Gambarini *et al.*, 2011), mandibular implant placement (Alhassani and AlGhamdi, 2010), and other surgical procedures have all been implicated in paresthesias that affect the inferior alveolar nerve. Several diagnostic and preventative measures exist to assist the clinician in establishing a differential diagnosis of iatrogenic paresthesia (see section on "Paresthesia Management" following this section).

Prevention

According to Garisto *et al.*, in a series of continuing studies published reporting the occurrence of lingual nerve paresthesia involving prolonged anesthetic effects of the lower lip, clinicians should carefully weigh the risks versus the benefits of using 4% anesthetic solutions, namely, 4% articaine and 4% prilocaine, in the IANB (Garisto *et al.*, 2010). This recommendation, however, has been somewhat controversial, and others have argued that the damage to the lingual nerve may involve a mechanical component. Malamed (2006) explains that factual and causal relationship between 4% anesthetic solutions and lingual nerve paresthesia is yet to be established and postulates a reporting bias and that the traditional Halstead approach to the IANB results in overstretching and mechanical needle trauma to the lingual nerve (Moore and Haas, 2010). Moreover, the seemingly disparate incidence of mechanical injury to the use of any local anesthetic solution for IANB overall still remains unexplored.

Heller and Shankland (2001) have described a method using mandibular local anesthesia infiltration techniques, rather than traditional block techniques, to preserve sensory function of the inferior alveolar nerve during implant placement. The technique maintains the ability of the patient to "alert" the surgeon or dentist to possible compromise of the integrity of the mandibular canal and nerve contained within (Heller and Shankland, 2001). While not specifically anesthesia-related injury, choice of local anesthesia technique can aid in preventing surgical-related paresthesias.

Management

Most paresthesias will resolve without therapeutic intervention within 8 weeks of local anesthesia administration (Garisto *et al.*, 2010). Particular attention must be made by the clinician to document the initial finding, reassure the patient that most paresthesias are self-limiting, and document the patient's report with high fidelity. For example, if the patient reports a numbness that evolves into a "tingling" or "fuzzy" sensation, these descriptors should be documented verbatim in the patient's chart to provide a scale of improvement, if any, over a regular time interval until resolution. If the paresthesia does not begin to exhibit improvement over time, or if the patient reports a profound loss of normal sensation at the outset, it may be appropriate to promptly refer to an appropriate specialist.

The increasing use of the cone-beam computerized tomography (CBCT) or other diagnostic imaging can be of utility when identifying compromise of the mandibular canal due to implant placement, mandibular surgery, endodontic instrumentation, flap retraction, or other dental or maxillofacial procedures (Park, Kim, and Moon, 2012). Appropriate surgical management or other therapies are indicated if the surgical etiology of the paresthesia is evident, and anesthesia-related nerve injury may be ruled out.

Unintended anesthesia

Anesthesia of areas not intended to be anesthetized can be quite unsettling for many patients and, in some cases, can lead to discomfort, temporary loss of function, and possible injury. The most commonly reported case of unintended anesthesia related to dental local anesthesia is facial nerve paralysis, but other areas of the head and neck region can be affected. Ophthalmologic involvement, while rare, has been reported and is often attributed to local anesthesia solutions migrating toward the orbit and affecting the oculomotor cranial nerves II, IV, and VI (Von Arx, Lozanoff, and Zinkernagel, 2014). The disruption of sympathetic innervation to the eye is often referred to as Horner syndrome. Horner syndrome is described to consist of a triad of symptoms—ptosis, miosis, and anhydrosis—and results from anesthetic solution migrating into the area of the cavernous sinus (Huang et al., 2013; Faix, 2001).

The unintended anesthesia of the facial nerve can be a disconcerting and alarming complication of local anesthesia administration when attempting to deliver mandibular block anesthesia. In careful examination of the surrounding anatomy and innervation of the inferior alveolar nerve, the parotid gland and the course of the seventh cranial nerve (CN VII) lie in close proximity to the target local anesthesia landmarks. Coursing from the posterior border of the ramus of the mandible, the trunk of the facial nerve is commonly anesthetized during IANB if the deposition of local anesthesia is too far posterior or overinsertion of the needle is performed. Often referred to as Bell's palsy, the acute facial nerve paralysis can mimic symptoms of stroke and also be confused with idiopathic nerve paralysis.

Ocular complications

Various mechanisms have been proposed in the loss of vision or other ocular complications related to intraoral local anesthesia administration. In Von Arx, Lozanoff, and Zinkernagel's (2014) review of the current literature, four mechanisms have been postulated: (i) intravascular injection of local anesthetic, (ii) reflex vasospasm, (iii) cervical sympathetic block, and (iv) diffusion of local anesthetic into ocular structures. Commonly, the IANB and the PSA nerve block were attributed to ocular complications. Diplopia (double vision) was reported as the most frequent ocular disturbance at almost 40% of reported complications, and of that percentage, roughly 87% involved anesthesia of the lateral rectus and the abducens nerve (Von Arx, Lozanoff, and Zinkernagel, 2014). One report by Chisci, Chisci, and Chisci (2013) outlined a case of vertical and lateral diplopia arising from retrograde venous flow or an arterial flow path resulting in anesthesia to the IV cranial nerve, specifically the superior oblique muscle, from a PSA injection of 4% articaine with 1 : 200 000 epinephrine. When anesthesia affects the sympathetic innervation of the eye, as in Horner syndrome, the

dilator pupillae and the Muller muscles are left without motor control and result in miosis (pupillary dilation) and ptosis (eyelid drooping) of the affected side (Ostergaard et al., 2005). Very rarely has amaurosis, or vision loss, been reported, and various mechanisms are postulated that involve anesthetic solution transported arterially into the central artery of the retina (Wilke, 2000) from mandibular block anesthesia, emboli, thrombus formation, vascular spasm, and chronic inflammation (Uckman, Cilasun, and Erkman, 2006).

Auditory complications

Although rare, total anesthesia of the branch of the trigeminal nerve, the auriculotemporal nerve can occur while performing the IANB or the Gow-Gates approach to anesthetizing the inferior alveolar nerve. The auriculotemporal nerve supplies somatosensory innervation to the auricle, external acoustic meatus, the outer side of the tympanic membrane, and the dermis of the temporal region. A rare report of broken needle during IANB by Ribeiro describes the migration of a needle fragment into the external auditory canal and subsequently piercing the tympanic membrane (Ribeiro et al., 2014).

Management of the aforementioned unintentional anesthesia

The sequelae of unintentional anesthesia generally persist for as long as the published duration of action for the injected local anesthetic. Facial nerve paralysis or even the more rare complication of ophthalmic involvement typically resolves after the local anesthetic has ceased its nerve blocking effects at the site of injection or regional block. For facial nerve paralysis, a relatively common injection complication, resolution occurs when the local anesthetic ceases its effects. Care must be taken to avoid injury to the ipsilateral eye in that lid closure is impeded with facial nerve anesthesia. Although the globe and cornea are at risk for injury due to the lack of protection from the eyelid, the corneal reflex remains. Consideration should be given to protecting the eye with artificial tears, lubricants, and possibly a shield taped over the lid and orbit. The clinician must communicate the effects of the complication to the patient to alleviate any undue worry. However, in the case of persistent and prolonged anesthesia of the facial nerve, or involvement of oculomotor, vision, or auditory innervation, immediate referral to an appropriate specialist is warranted for further evaluation (Glass and Tzafetta, 2014).

Hematoma

Hematomas, a bruise or discoloration resulting from blood entering an extravascular space, is a common complication following extra and intraoral local anesthesia administration. Certain injection techniques and locations have higher incidences of hematoma development than others. Predictably, areas that are more highly vascularized tend to result in hematomas than areas less vascularized. The PSA nerve block, anterior superior alveolar (ASA) nerve block, infraorbital (IO) nerve block, incisive (mental) nerve block, and IANB are common areas for hematoma development. Rarely will hematomas produce significant pain, swelling, or trismus, yet the extraoral development of a bruise and discoloration should be documented and explained to the patient that the condition is a fairly common complication of local anesthesia administration and is self-resolving in 7–14 days. Although most reports of this complication are benign, careful attention should be placed upon any intraoral swelling that could result in the loss of an airway to the patient (Cohen and Warman, 1989) (Figure 6.1).

Prevention

Any injection into a vascular area invariably carries risk of hematoma development, yet there are some practices that may reduce the incidence of this complication. When presented with alternative sites of injection, avoidance of multiple injections into a highly vascularized area as well as maintaining proper and consistent needle angulation throughout the advancement of the

needle may help prevent hematoma formation (Padhye *et al.*, 2011). The clinician should be aware of prior history of hematoma formation in a certain injection area and possibly consider an alternate, yet effective, injection technique. Also, certain medications and medical conditions, namely, antithrombotics (such as NSAIDs or other therapeutic anticoagulants) and the hemophilias or other disorders of coagulation, may increase the likelihood of hematoma sequelae (Piot *et al.*, 2002).

Management

For management of specific injection-related hematomas, see the following text. In general, direct and immediate pressure to the affected area will minimize the extent of swelling and discoloration due to the extravasation of blood into the soft tissue. Direct pressure may be extended if the patient is on antithrombotic or anticoagulant therapy. If possible, application of cold compresses after immediate recognition may help promote vasoconstriction and further growth of the hematoma, but intraoral application may prove difficult. Later management, generally accepted as after 6 h, includes frequent warm compresses to the affected area to promote vasodilation and increased perfusion to the discolored area to speed return to normal pigmentation. Pain and discomfort are generally addressed with over-the-counter analgesic formulations, and the clinician should consider alternatives to the anticoagulant effect of certain analgesics in the management of hematomas.

For the ASA or IO nerve block, direct application of pressure to the area below the inferior border of the orbit will help to prevent spread of a hematoma. Note that a true ASA nerve block technique requires direct digital pressure directly over the IO foramen that makes hematoma development unlikely. Cold compresses can be readily applied to the area to further promote vasoconstriction once the hematoma has been recognized. Later management can be left to patient directives of continuous applications of warm compresses to aid in dispersing areas of discoloration in a highly visible area.

For the PSA nerve block, where multiple vascular structures are involved in a region that can accommodate a large volume of extravascular blood, immediate swelling is often recognized followed by discoloration in a highly visible area of the face (Padhye *et al.*, 2011). When vessel integrity of the PSA artery and facial artery are compromised, the resulting extravasation of blood into the infratemporal fossa can be

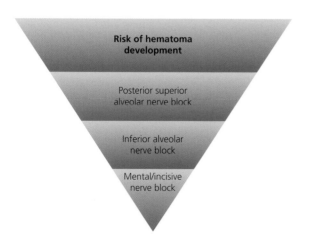

Figure 6.1 Anesthesia complications. Malamed (2013). Reproduced with permission from Elsevier.

significant and is a difficult area to apply direct pressure. It is often recommended to apply direct digital (finger) pressure intraorally in the mucobuccal fold region nearest to the maxillary tuberosity to control swelling. Intraoral and extraoral application of cold compresses, if possible, should be applied once a hematoma is recognized in this region.

For the IANB, direct pressure should be applied intraorally with direct digital pressure to the medial aspect of the ramus of the mandible of the affected side. In very small patients or those with limited airways, development of a significant hematoma may impinge upon maintaining an open airway (Hawthorne, Sim, and Acton, 2000) and should be managed with immediate intervention to reduce further swelling and possible securing of the airway (often involving emergent transport to a hospital facility) (Kitay, Ferraro, and Sonis, 1991).

Sublingual hematomas are generally reported to be sequelae from surgery or instrumentation involving the lingual aspect of the mandible and rarely involve only local anesthesia administration alone. However, because of the potential for life-threatening intraoral swelling and hematoma development, it is important for the clinician to be aware of the immediate concern of any rupture to the sublingual branch of the lingual artery and associated arterial branches to cause airway obstruction. Although pressure should be applied immediately, the measures for controlling significant hemorrhage of this area call for emergent transportation to a facility where surgical management and securing of the airway can be achieved as rapidly as possible (Tarakji and Nassani, 2012).

Toxicity and overdose

Local anesthetic toxicity and overdose is a serious and potentially life-threatening complication that can occur in the dental setting where local anesthetics are used in both topical and injected forms. Local anesthetics have maximum recommended dosages based on patient weight and the assumption that patients' dose/response curves fall within an average population. Various factors influence a patient's ability to redistribute, metabolize, and excrete various drugs, and very rarely is the rate of metabolism predictable in terms of dosing local anesthetics. Metabolites themselves may also be toxic. Nevertheless, the clinician's responsibility is to administer an appropriate amount of anesthesia to complete a procedure and to avoid administration of local anesthetics to the maximum recommended dose (MRD).

Understanding that local anesthetics are potent CNS depressants and are commonly used in medicine as antidysrhythmics to slow and correct myocardial electrical conduction, clinicians should consider the potency of these drugs in normal dental practice upon susceptible patients. Lidocaine, one of the most common dental local anesthetics used in North America, is an agent used in the American Heart Association's algorithm for Advanced Cardiac Life Support (ACLS) in the treatment of ventricular arrhythmias. Yet the metabolism and clearance of lidocaine from the body is heavily dependent upon hepatic function, and if liver function is compromised, the likelihood of toxicity increases (Ganzberg and Kramer, 2010).

Clinicians should be acutely aware of the amounts of local anesthetics delivered when using conventional dental cartridges. The standard convention of expressing concentration of local anesthesia contained within solution is by percentage. A 4% solution, for instance, contains 40 mg of local anesthesia per milliliter of solution. Likewise, a 3% solution contains 30 mg per milliliter, and a 2% solution contains 20 mg of drug in every milliliter of solution. Manufacturers accordingly publish maximum recommended dosages as milligrams per kilogram of body weight (Table 6.1).

Prevention

The single most important factor in preventing local anesthesia overdose and toxicity is slow injection technique (Malamed, 2013). Careful consideration of using local anesthetic agents with vasoconstrictors in patients

Table 6.1 Maximum recommended dosages.

Local anesthetic solution	Maximum recommended dose (mg/kg)
4% articaine with 1 : 100 000 epinephrine	7
2% lidocaine with 1 : 100 000 epinephrine	7
0.5% bupivacaine with 1 : 200 000 epinephrine	2
4% prilocaine plain	8
3% mepivacaine plain	6.6

able to tolerate the possible cardiac side effects of increased cardiac output—blood pressure and heart rate changes—can also prevent toxicity from limiting systemic uptake by vasoconstriction (Malamed, 2013). Inadvertent intravascular injection can lead to rapid serum levels of local anesthesia and resultant overdose and toxicity. Employing routine techniques of aspiration, or production of slight negative pressure in the dental local anesthesia cartridge by gentle thumb retraction of the plunger in an aspirating dental syringe, can effectively reduce the likelihood of high serum concentrations.

Choice of local anesthesia injection technique can also have profound effects upon systemic uptake and possibly systemic toxicity. Of the local anesthetic techniques commonly used in dentistry, intraosseous administration results in the most rapid uptake into systemic circulation (Wood *et al.*, 2005). Supraperiosteal infiltration followed by maxillary nerve blocks, while not at the degree of intraosseous administration, can also result in rapid systemic absorption because of the highly vascularized region and cancellous bone distinctly located in this region. Of the techniques used in dentistry, mandibular block local anesthesia administration, periodontal ligament injection, intrapulpal, and other intraoral nerve block techniques requiring minimal amounts of local anesthesia volume are at less risk to develop toxicity in the adult patient (Becker and Reed, 2012).

Clearly, the administered amount of local anesthetics needed for restorative or surgical procedures can have profound effects upon toxicity and systemic absorption. Simply put, the more local anesthesia administered to a patient, the greater the potential for toxicity. Clinicians should consider the length of treatment as well as the anesthetic coverage needed for a procedure and choose a local anesthetic agent accordingly. Reinjection with a short to moderate duration of action local anesthetic agent for a procedure that demands an extensive amount of time to complete puts patients at risk for development of toxicity. Alternatively, the choice of using a longer-acting, or long duration of action, local anesthetic agent for a procedure that may consume a shorter amount of time than expected decreases the likelihood of overdose and toxicity but may put the patient at risk for soft tissue injury as a result of prolonged anesthesia (see section "Soft Tissue Injury").

If the clinician chooses to use two or more local anesthetic agents during an appointment, modification to the calculation of MRD is required. The toxic effects of the drugs are presumed to be additive. Simply, if one half of the maximum dose of the first local anesthetic is given, then the clinician can administer up to one half of the maximum dose of the second local anesthetic, as calculated per kilogram of body weight (Weaver, 2007).

Management

Recognition of the signs and symptoms of overdose is of paramount concern in the emergent treatment of toxicity and overdose. Generally, local anesthesia overdose presents initially as excitation in the CNS followed by depression of the CNS. Patients may at first exhibit excitability, nervousness, and incoherence. Reports have also noted increased depth of respiration and even tremor and involuntary movement as various aspects of the CNS are inhibited. As the toxicity progresses, tinnitus (ringing of the ears), nausea, vomiting, and seizure activity may present. As the CNS becomes further depressed, respiratory function may diminish and eventually cease leading to cardiovascular collapse and/or hypoxic injury.

Management of local anesthesia toxicity requires immediate management in the form of basic life support. Because of the potential for respiratory depression, the clinician must prioritize supportive respiratory measures to ensure proper oxygenation and ventilation despite the onset of CNS depression. Transport to a hospital-based care facility should be considered immediately if the patient is suspected of having a local anesthetic overdose as progression of toxicity can occur rapidly. In-hospital management includes the aforementioned measures to maintain adequate oxygenation and a patent airway, seizure suppression, supportive measures to stabilize cardiovascular function, and consideration to provide lipid emulsion therapy (Intralipid™) to reverse neurological and cardiovascular effects (Cave and Harvey, 2009).

Methemoglobinemia

Hemoglobin, the molecule in human blood primarily responsible for oxygen delivery to tissues, generally exists in a ferrous form where all of the iron atoms have an atomic valence of +2. In acquired methemoglobinemia, any one of the iron atoms is oxidized to its ferric form where its atomic valence exists in a +3 state. Two of the most likely oxidizing agents used in dentistry are the topical anesthetic benzocaine and the injectable local anesthetic prilocaine. Both agents have been extensively studied for their potential in acquired methemoglobinemia whereby the hemoglobin (ferrous) molecule's oxygen-carrying capacity is markedly reduced in the methemoglobin (ferric) form. Although blood levels of methemoglobin exist normally in healthy individuals at a level approaching 2%, concentrations higher than 15% can produce frank cyanosis and symptoms of hypoxia that can include dizziness, headache, lethargy, loss of consciousness, and, in severe cases, death (Trapp and Will, 2010).

Prevention

Ample evidence exists that demonstrates benzocaine and prilocaine as the common anesthetic agents used in dentistry that produce methemoglobinemia (Taleb *et al.*, 2013). Because both formulations available to the dental clinicians are in relatively high concentrations (20% benzocaine topical and 4% prilocaine injectable), care must be taken to ensure excessive amounts of these agents are not delivered to patients. Moreover, if another anesthetic agent is available as an alternative, consideration should be given to using alternate agents in patients that are susceptible to methemoglobinemia or other oxygen-carrying compromise (sickle cell, anemia, kidney failure, chronic hypoxemia, etc.).

Management

Methemoglobinemia is difficult to diagnose in a typical dental setting but should be on the differential if the oxidizing substances of prilocaine or benzocaine are employed in patient care. Patients can display a range of symptoms that are consistent with hypoxemia: headache, fatigue, exercise intolerance, dizziness, syncope, confusion, seizures, etc. (Taleb *et al.*, 2013). Onset can be delayed and can occur hours after administration of local anesthesia. Access to pulse oximetry will often be misleading as significant methemoglobinemia will erroneously present with an oxygen saturation of 85% despite supplemental oxygen administration. Newer monitors are available that specifically target methemoglobin levels in the bloodstream, but they remain specialized monitoring devices outside the scope of many dental and ambulatory medical settings. Thus, in the absence of immediate co-oximetry blood sampling and

specific monitoring, the dental setting diagnosis of methemoglobinemia is reliant upon classical methods of observing the patient for cyanosis, shortness of breath, and the presence of "chocolate-brown" colored blood (Gutenberg, Chen, and Trapp, 2013). Methemoglobinemia can be life threatening, and as such, any cases of suspected methemoglobinemia should necessitate immediate transport to a care facility where the patient can be treated.

Acquired methemoglobinemia is treated with the administration of an intravenous (IV) infusion of methylene blue, 1–2 mg/kg of body weight, up to 50 mg. In the treatment of symptomatic methemoglobinemia, methylene blue is enzymatically reduced to leucomethylene blue and then reduces methemoglobin back into the oxygen-carrying hemoglobin—effectively reversing the effects of acquired methemoglobinemia (Lo, Darracq, and Clark, 2014). During the management of suspected acquired methemoglobinemia, the patient should be administered supplemental oxygen by means of a nonrebreather facemask to increase the amount of inspired fraction of oxygen to the remaining and functional hemoglobin. Other therapies such as hyperbaric oxygen, oral or parenteral ascorbic acid administration, and blood transfusion may also be considered (Gray and Hawkins, 2004).

Soft tissue injury

Masticatory or other soft tissue trauma as a result of residual local anesthesia is a common complication seen in dentistry. Oftentimes, inadvertent lip, cheek, or tongue biting occurs in the pediatric and patients with special-needs populations (Malamed, 2013). Injuries can range from minor and not requiring therapeutic intervention to severe and requiring extensive repair of lacerated soft tissue. Several etiologies have been explored for this relatively common and usually minor complication. Recent studies have reported obesity, IANB, and long-acting local anesthetic solutions as being the major contributors to soft tissue injury. In the pediatric and special-needs population, inadvertent lip biting results from curiosity of an unfamiliar sensation that elicits no pain. Nevertheless, the complications of inadvertent soft tissue injury resulting from local anesthesia administration can pose a risk to dental patients that require serious consideration in terms of prevention and management (Boynes, Riley, and Milbee, 2014).

Prevention

Awareness on the part of the clinician, patient, parent, or caregiver is of primary importance in relation to soft tissue injury. Effectively communicating risk and potential injury can decrease the incidence and unneeded intervention of an injury with varying presentation. Second, using local anesthetics with a shorter durations of action can potentially restore normal sensation to an area prone to mastication, yet even using a shorter-acting solution without a vasoconstrictor, such as the commonly available 3% mepivacaine plain solution, can yield postoperative soft tissue anesthesia that can last several hours in duration (Chi *et al.*, 2008). Lastly, the clinician should strongly consider mechanical measures to prevent accidental tissue trauma in postoperative planning that anticipates a high likelihood of injury. Large, rolled cotton gauze packs inserted halfway into the oral cavity that are large enough to make aspiration unlikely can prevent a patient from biting or trapping the cheek, lip, or tongue.

Management

The assessment and diagnosis of soft tissue injury related to dental local anesthesia administration can be elusive to caretaker or healthcare providers unaware of recent dental treatment—especially for patient populations that have difficulties in communication. Pointed and direct history taking should include not only recent dental and oral/maxillofacial treatment but also specific intraoral areas that were anesthetized. Once the assessment has been made that the presenting injury is indeed soft tissue trauma from mastication, further assessment should follow to expose any other areas of ipsilateral or contralateral involvement. Most often, ulceration will be present and should be evaluated for infection. Palliative treatment with over-the-counter preparations of nonsteroidal anti-inflammatory medications or acetaminophen will generally provide adequate analgesia for the duration of a minor injury. Some recommend the gentle debridement of the injured area with 0.12% chlorhexidine gluconate (Chi *et al.*, 2008). If severe infection, laceration, or loss of function is present, systemic antibiotics should be dispensed and referral to an appropriate specialist is indicated for possible surgical intervention and wound closure.

Resolution of soft tissue trauma generally occurs within days to weeks from the initial time of injury. However, final healing can be protracted if lip biting recurs in the same location as the initial injury, if the wound requires surgical intervention, or if the presence of infection is detected.

Complications of inhalation sedation

The use of nitrous oxide inhalation sedation has a revered history in the practice of dentistry. This colorless, sweet-smelling inhalational agent provides not only an anxiolytic effect, but it also provides a dose-related degree of analgesia reported by Jastak to be equivalent to 10–15 mg of the opioid morphine (Jastak and Donaldson, 1991). Its routine use in dentistry has proven to be a safe and effective modality to provide treatment with fast initial onset, ease of titratability, and rapid elimination from the body. Complications with nitrous oxide administration are fortunately rare. However, complications can arise in gas delivery, equipment, and psychogenic side effects, and previous studies have demonstrated nitrous oxide suitability across a wide range of patient types. More recent investigations have implicated nitrous oxide in increased complication risk for certain individuals with existing comorbidities and metabolic deficiencies.

Standard precautions in the administration of nitrous oxide–oxygen inhalation sedation include a thorough and regularly updated medical history, avoiding use in those with severe chronic obstructive pulmonary disease (COPD), severe emotional disturbances or drug-related dependencies, first trimester of pregnancy, treatment with bleomycin sulfate chemotherapy for neoplasms, recent retinal surgery with introduction of an intraocular gas bubble, methylenetetrahydrofolate reductase (MTHFR) deficiency, and cobalamin deficiency (AAPD, 2013).

Complications in equipment

Contemporary dental nitrous oxide–oxygen inhalational sedation units provide multiple safeguards from delivering potentially harmful hypoxic gas mixtures: Low oxygen flow alarms, oxygen fail-safes, and the inability to deliver nitrous oxide concentrations greater than 70%. Nevertheless, problems arise from misuse and lack of routine inspection and maintenance. In some cases with central supply lines, severe morbidity and death have been reported when nitrous oxide and oxygen supply lines were crossed (Herff *et al.*, 2007).

Prevention

Clearly, regular inspection and maintenance of flexible rubber apparatus on nitrous oxide–oxygen inhalation equipment will prevent breathing circuit leaks, issues with inadequate delivery, and possibly patient safety problems associated with equipment malfunction. In clinical practice areas unfamiliar to the operator, close inspection and verification (using oxygen analyzers on mobile anesthesia gas monitors or a rudimentary "smell" test) of nitrous oxide and oxygen supply lines can prevent delivery of potentially life-threatening hypoxic mixtures to patients (Malamed, 2010). It is important to note that oxygen fail-safe mechanisms, which prevent delivery of nitrous oxide gas when oxygen supply is depleted or falls below a minimum delivery pressure, will be *overridden* in the case of switched supply lines.

Regular inspection of nitrous oxide–oxygen inhalation sedation units should include the following:

1 Inspection of the pin index or diameter index safety system to ensure gas supplies cannot be or have not been interchanged.
2 Inspection of the tank or supply line high-pressure line to the tank yokes or manifold for leaks. A leak on either the oxygen or nitrous high-pressure supply side is generally an audible "hiss."
3 Inspection of the reservoir bag for tears and leaks to ensure a consistent gas mixture and avoid occupational exposure and environmental contamination. An intact gas reservoir bag, coupled with appropriate gas patient gas flow and a good mask seal, also becomes an additional monitoring device for patient ventilation (Malamed, 2010).
4 Inspection of flexible gas conduction tubing and breathing apparatus for leaks, cracks, or blockage (flattening or "kinking" of hoses) ensures adequate delivery of the nitrous oxide–oxygen gas supply without occlusion or interruption and may prevent occupational exposure and environmental contamination.
5 Inspection of scavenging system to include one-way exhalation valve on the nasal hood and scavenging tubing. Adequate scavenging of waste gas ensures a decreased occupational exposure to clinicians and assistants. Adjustments should be made to the vacuum supply to ensure reservoir bag and breathing circuit is not overscavenged to impair sedative gas mixture delivery (Malamed and Clark, 2003).

Management

Fortunately, modern nitrous oxide–oxygen inhalation sedation units will include safeguards to prevent hypoxic gas mixture delivery to the patient. However, in the case of suspected equipment malfunction, recognition remains the primary step in order to initiate intervention. Replacement of damaged or degraded equipment and a thorough check of proper function and delivery will rectify most equipment problems. Gas supply sources, whether via compressed gas tanks or gas manifold ("wall" or "pipeline") supply, must be checked periodically for evidence of leaks, valve malfunction, or even source switching. Ideally, supplies should be checked whenever the system is replenished (Herff *et al.*, 2007).

Inadequate sedation

Primarily, the root cause of inadequate sedation is inappropriate patient selection. Various factors such as patients of young age, the extremely fearful or apprehensive, those with special needs, or patients with a high tolerance to CNS depressants are poor candidates for nitrous oxide sedation. Additionally, some patients present with limitations, either permanent or temporary, to normal nasal breathing. This precludes usual and standard in-office dental nitrous oxide–oxygen sedation techniques using a nasal hood. Oftentimes in the young patient less than 5 years of age, nitrous oxide fails to provide adequate sedation and analgesia. Frequent crying, intolerance to the nitrous oxide delivery hood, and a patient breathing primarily through his or her mouth can lead to inadequate delivery of a concentrated dose of nitrous oxide. Nevertheless, despite careful patient selection and absence of predisposing factors, Malamed (2010) explains that nitrous oxide sedation "hyporesponders," or those that do not derive a therapeutic effect from average doses of an agent, represent about 15% of patients.

Prevention

Reliable predictors to foretell inadequate sedation are elusive. Reliable medical and social history taking, along with the clinician and patient's clear expectations of the therapeutic limitations of nitrous oxide–oxygen inhalation sedation, may provide for more favorable outcomes. The goal of nitrous oxide–oxygen inhalation sedation is to provide anxiolysis, a mild degree of analgesia, and possibly amnesia for a more comfortable and tolerable dental procedure. Unrealistic expectations of unconsciousness, complete amnesia, and profound analgesia simply cannot be provided by nitrous oxide–oxygen inhalation sedation exclusively.

Careful consideration should be given to offering the patient or their caretaker alternate forms of pain and anxiety control if the patient is unable to reasonably follow verbal requests or presents with a high level of fear and anxiety. Patients who have a low pain threshold and a high degree of apprehension also are not ideal candidates for inhalation sedation. Nitrous oxide–oxygen inhalation sedation may be inadequate for those patients with diagnosed or undiagnosed psychiatric or psychosocial disorders and may require more complex therapeutic treatment needs that may involve collaboration with other mental healthcare providers.

Treatment

Inadequate sedation can occur at any time to any patient undergoing dental procedures with nitrous oxide–oxygen sedation. Given the variables of dental treatment, patient temperament, psychological and social stressors, as well as variations in human behavior and perception (see prior definition of "pain"), even a patient who has completed a dental procedure previously without sedation can suffer from inadequate sedation in subsequent procedures. Clinicians who recognize that the patient is not experiencing the sedative effects of nitrous oxide after 5–15 min from the start of the administration (mild analgesia, peripheral vasodilation, mild euphoria, and/or decreased anxiety) should stop treatment, allow the patient to recover fully, and reappoint with an alternative strategy for anxiety and pain control.

Nausea and vomiting with nitrous oxide sedation

Although commonly attributed to only oversedation, the etiology of nitrous oxide sedation-related nausea and vomiting is multifactorial. Oversedation, a full or empty stomach, excessive patient movement, type of dental surgery, prolonged length of inhalation sedation, middle ear infection, inadequate sedation, local anesthesia administration, and a predisposition to emesis can all be contributory to this complication. Active vomiting by a patient during dental treatment can be a serious complication due to the presence of various

barrier and isolation techniques normally present during restorative dentistry, and the risks of pulmonary aspiration of vomitus and possibly even dental instruments can be life threatening. Because nitrous oxide–oxygen inhalation sedation depresses the CNS, protective laryngeal reflexes to prevent accidental aspiration of foreign objects and liquids into the tracheal may be impaired.

Prevention

Close attention paid in preparing the patient prior to nitrous oxide–oxygen inhalation sedation will prevent most instances of nausea and vomiting. Malamed (2010) recommends avoidance of large meals preceding nitrous oxide sedation and instead suggests a light, carbohydrate-rich meal 4–6 h before the appointment. Additionally, patient history may include a predisposition to nausea and vomiting that must be considered in length and type of appointment. Avoiding inhalation sedation administration to patients with upper respiratory tract infections (URI) can also decrease the incidence of both nausea and vomiting. Becker and Rosenberg (2008) suggest that middle ear infections, which are often associated with occluded Eustachian tubes, may present an area in which nitrous oxide fills the inner ear space due to nitrous oxide diffusing more readily into closed spaces than nitrogen. The resulting increase in pressure, and tension upon the tympanic membrane ("ear drum"), and then negative pressure has been implicated as a contributor to nausea and vomiting (Becker and Rosenberg, 2008). This low blood/gas partition coefficient can also lead to bowel distention and, consequently, potential gastrointestinal discomfort and nausea and vomiting (Ostergaard et al., 2005). It is important to note that increased duration of nitrous oxide inhalation sedation provides more time for closed spaces to fill with nitrous oxide gas. Some investigators also postulate that the metabolic disturbances of inhibited methionine synthetase, folate depletion, and resultant homocysteine increase contribute to nausea and vomiting (Peyton and Wu, 2014).

Local anesthesia, with its distinctive bitter taste, should be carefully administered during nitrous oxide inhalation sedation to patients that may be sensitive to its taste.

When the patient is seated in the dental chair, avoidance of excessive chair and patient movement can possibly prevent nausea and vomiting. The patient should be situated in a position that allows for unhindered dental treatment with nitrous oxide–oxygen inhalation sedation when equipment is placed on the patient, and the patient should also be comfortable in the chair prior to beginning inhalation sedation to minimize movement during the procedure.

Oversedation and associated nausea and vomiting are often preceded by report by the patient of "feeling sick." Oftentimes, vomiting is immediately preceded by sweating, salivation, agitation, and pallor change (Malamed, 2010). Careful and slow titration technique, with close communication with the patient in regard to therapeutic effects, can prevent the sudden onset of nausea and vomiting.

Pretreatment with oral and rectal antiemetics has been suggested as a preventative measure to avoid the complications of nausea and vomiting during nitrous oxide–oxygen inhalation sedation. Various preparations are available and some are available by prescription only (Malamed, 2010). Many antiemetic agents are also potent sedatives, so the clinician must consider levels of permitting in regard to oral and parenteral dosing of such drugs. Selective serotonin (5-HT$_3$) receptor agonists, such as oral dolasetron and ondansetron, do not have sedative effects (GlaxoSmithKline, 2014).

Management

Immediate management of the actively vomiting patient includes removal of the nasal hood and nitrous oxide delivery equipment, dental instruments, barrier and isolation devices, and loose restorative materials in the patient's mouth and oropharyngeal area. The clinician and assistant must provide active suction of the oropharynx and turn the patient onto the right side (right lateral decubitus position) or simply turn the patient's head to the side to prevent and minimize pulmonary aspiration. If possible, the dental chair should be placed in a Trendelenburg position to promote drainage out of the bronchi if pulmonary aspiration is suspected. After active vomiting has occurred, replacing the nitrous oxide hood to only administer 100% oxygen concentration for 3–5 min may minimize continued nausea and vomiting.

Metabolic disturbances

Recent studies have investigated nitrous oxide's effects upon metabolic processes. Specifically, the increased levels of serum homocysteine, the reduction of methionine synthetase, and folate deficiencies were extensively studied to determine cardiovascular risk to patients subject to nitrous oxide in noncardiac surgery. Certain patients with MTHFR deficiency, a genetic mutation that results in increased blood levels of homocysteine, have been postulated to have significant risk in developing venous and arterial thrombosis (Shay, Frumento, and Bastien, 2007). As of this writing, it remains unclear whether nitrous oxide conclusively poses an increased risk for experiencing an untoward cardiac event despite large-scale studies (Myles *et al.*, 2014).

The use of nitrous oxide–oxygen inhalation sedation is commonplace in pediatric dentistry (Udhya *et al.*, 2014). With the increasing rates of children diagnosed with autism spectrum disorder (ASD), several hypotheses explored exposure to nitrous oxide as an initiating event. However, any causal relationship has yet or will ever be established linking the methionine deactivating effect of nitrous oxide, prevalence of cobalamin deficiencies in children with autism, and genetic risk factors with nitrous oxide exposure (Rossignol, Genuis, and Frye, 2014).

Prevention

Patients diagnosed with hyperhomocysteinemia or mutations in the MTHFR gene should not receive nitrous oxide as part of their anesthetic regimen. Patients diagnosed with a cobalamin (vitamin B12) deficiency should also not receive nitrous oxide sedation since cobalamin is a cofactor in the conversion of homocysteine and methylenetetrahydrofolate to methionine and tetrahydrofolate (Baum, 2007). Patients who do not have the MTHFR deficiency can safely receive nitrous oxide as part of their anesthetic regimen without increased risk of untoward myocardial effects (Myles *et al.*, 2014).

Oversedation

Although unconsciousness is an extremely rare complication of nitrous oxide sedation, administration of nitrous oxide sedation past therapeutic levels is relatively common. When the patient no longer remains comfortable, cooperative, coherent, and cognizant to dental treatment, the clinician needs to recognize this as oversedation and rectify the situation before other complications arise. Ideal sedation, as Malamed (2010) describes, includes the symptoms of a wave of warmth over the patient's body, tingling of the extremities, numbness of the oral cavity and other parts of the body, and a general feeling of heaviness. Clinical signs of ideal nitrous oxide inhalation sedation include a slow and regular respiratory rate, decreased heart rate and blood pressure to resting levels, peripheral vasodilation, and decreased muscle tone. As oversedation develops, a patient may report sleepiness, agitation, inappropriate laughing and weeping, sweating, or even dreaming and hallucinations. Observable signs by the clinician when patient becomes oversedated include increases in heart rate and blood pressure, lacrimation, an increased rate of respiration, and increased patient movement. Obvious oversedation by nitrous oxide presents with nausea and vomiting, unresponsiveness, and possible loss of consciousness (Malamed, 2010).

Prevention
Careful and slow titration prevents oversedation. This entails continual verbal communication with a patient to assess levels of CNS depression and patient comfort. If the patient becomes incoherent because of repeated mouth closure, agitation, or any other signs or symptoms listed previously, efforts should be initiated to decrease levels of nitrous oxide until the patient displays signs and symptoms of ideal nitrous oxide inhalation sedation. Careful patient history documentation may also reveal the use of other anxiety-reducing medications that can contribute to unpredictable oversedation.

Management
Oversedation, when recognized early by the clinician, is completely avoidable in most patients. However, particular priority should always be placed upon the possibility of nausea and vomiting with oversedation. Access to high-volume suction and a saliva ejector should always be readily available during patient sedation to suction the oropharynx of vomitus and prevent possible pulmonary aspiration. Be advised that even the same patient may respond to differing levels of nitrous oxide concentrations at subsequent appointments and that titration of the sedation is always recommended.

Reports of inappropriate sensory experiences
Both Malamed (Malamed, 2010) and Kaufman (Kaufman, Galili, and Furer, (1990) report instances of heightened sensory stimulation and even accusations of sexual abuse during the administration of nitrous oxide–oxygen inhalation sedation. With the nitrous

apparatus in close contact with the patient's body and possibility of profound euphoria, accusations against the clinician or auxiliaries of impropriety can and do arise. Reports of sexual phenomena, dreaming, and imagery also are associated with IV administration of sedatives with nitrous oxide (Brandner et al., 1997).

Prevention
Malamed (2010) reports three common criteria that place clinicians at risk:
1 Treatment of a patient alone without another witness in the operatory or dental setting
2 Administration of a high concentration of nitrous oxide
3 Failure to titrate the patient to prevent sedation beyond the range of therapeutic effect

Therefore, it is recommended that clinicians render treatment with another auxiliary or practitioner in the operatory or setting, avoid administration of high concentrations of nitrous oxide to patients, and avoid patient oversedation. Careful adherence to ensuring the presence of a reliable and objective witness to any form of treatment is prudent practice. Additionally, concise documentation of each sedation performance can provide reliable defense against false accusation.

Management
Unfortunately, once an accusation has been filed, matters will most likely demand legal counsel for clinicians and staff involved in the instance. Prioritizing prevention should be the goal of management (Malamed, Serxner, and Wiedenfeld, 1988).

Common complications: moderate sedation and general anesthesia

Advanced forms of anxiety and pain control techniques in dentistry include enteral (oral) and parenteral moderate sedation. General anesthesia, or a drug-induced loss of consciousness during which patients are not arousable, even by painful stimulation (ADA, 2012), is a readily employed technique of anxiety and pain control that often finds utility in pediatric dentistry, hospital dentistry, office-based restorative and surgical procedures, and oral and maxillofacial surgery. Along with the complications listed previously for minimal and moderate sedation pertaining to nitrous oxide–oxygen inhalation techniques, a multitude of complications can arise that extend beyond the scope of this discussion. However, the most common and significant complications and management thereof will be outlined in the following.

Failure of moderate and deep sedation

Like the failure of inhalation sedation discussed previously, techniques that do not render patients unconscious carry a degree of unreliability and unpredictability in terms of providing adequate anxiety and pain control. Simply, not all procedures and surgical interventions are tolerated by all patients and a greater degree of anxiety and pain control may be required. Medicine acknowledges the unpredictability of the technique and even defines an insurance billing code—"Failed moderate sedation during procedure, initial encounter" that, as of this writing, has no counterpart in dentistry (ICD-10 T88.52XA). In most cases, however, the use of moderate and deep sedation coupled with local anesthesia administration for office-based dental procedures results in less morbidity and faster recoveries than general anesthesia. In some patients where general anesthesia techniques cannot be tolerated, a moderate or deep sedation technique is a viable anesthesia technique for performing dentistry and oral and maxillofacial surgery (Svrakic *et al.*, 2014).

Prevention

Again, careful patient selection and a thorough medical history are paramount in ensuring success with particular sedation techniques. In addition, most procedures in office-based dentistry rely on successful local anesthesia to augment pharmacologic depression of the CNS. Failure to achieve adequate local anesthesia in sedation techniques that do not produce significant amounts of analgesia will result in less than ideal patient comfort and acceptance. Some surgical procedures are simply too large in scope and exceed patient tolerance in terms of pain, discomfort, and duration.

The enteral route of administration of sedative medication can be unpredictable. Unlike the parenteral routes of administration where blood levels do not undergo hepatic first-pass metabolism, oral dosing of sedative medications are subject to varying rates of gastric emptying, variations in splanchnic circulation, biological variation in hepatic metabolism, and delayed onset of action. Attempts to "orally titrate" sedatives for patients undergoing dental procedures (incremental dosing) can result in over- or undersedation and therapeutic endpoints that are less than ideal. More importantly, the onset of multiple doses after an unpredictable period of time may result in an unintended loss of consciousness. In regard to patient safety and practitioners being able to "rescue" patients from unintended loss of consciousness, various authors have recommended additional training in various techniques of airway management and emergency response if multiple oral doses of sedative medications are planned (Dionne *et al.*, 2006). The American Dental Association (ADA), in its 2012 Guidelines for the Use of Sedation and General Anesthesia by Dentists, in reference to the unpredictable nature of incremental and supplemental dosing in enteral minimal and moderate sedation, advises practitioners to not exceed the MRD or 1.5 times the MRD for minimal to moderate sedation, respectively (ADA, 2012).

Management

When moderate to deep sedation fails, several options can be considered. If the clinician is permitted and trained to do so, converting the sedation technique to general anesthesia will provide a predictable level of anesthesia and analgesia. If general anesthesia is not a viable option, limiting procedure length and complexity should be considered. Additionally, alternate forms of anxiety and pain control must be considered with modifications to proposed treatment.

Unintended loss of consciousness

According to Weaver, the most common emergency in sedated patients is related to airway and respiratory problems (Weaver, 2010). When a moderately sedated patient, regardless of the route of drug administration, becomes unresponsive and enters a level of sedation that is unintended, it is imperative for the clinician to rescue and manage that patient from potential loss of airway reflexes and possible respiratory depression. The American Society of Anesthesiologists, in their Guidelines, recommends that moderate sedation practitioners have the capability to rescue patients who enter deep sedation, and those clinicians who administer deep sedation be able to rescue a patient entering general anesthesia (ASA, 2002).

Prevention

Clinicians utilizing enteral or parenteral moderate sedation for office-based dental procedures are advised to use sedative medications with a wide margin of safety or a wide therapeutic index that would make it unlikely to render a patient unconscious. These include medications such as oral benzodiazepines, parenteral benzodiazepines, and mild or moderately potent opioid analgesics. An added margin of safety is afforded by these two classes of drugs having reversal agents that act as antidotes to their actions. Drugs such as methohexital, ketamine, propofol, alfentanil, and remifentanil are not recommended for practitioners permitted to the level of providing moderate sedation because of their narrow therapeutic index and, with certain drugs, an inability for their CNS depressant effects to be reversed pharmacologically. Nevertheless, clinicians providing any level of sedation should be current in basic life support techniques that include the management of patients who are unconscious and not breathing (ADA, 2012). In operatory resuscitation equipment (bag-valve-mask resuscitators, supplemental oxygen, airway adjuncts, and automatic external defibrillator) should be immediately available, and clinicians and staff must be familiar with summoning emergency medical services.

Patient monitoring remains at the forefront of prevention of sedation disasters. With the advent of pulse oximetry in the mid-1980s, early recognition of hypoxia and decreases in oxygenation are rapidly determined. The regular use of exhaled carbon dioxide monitoring, capnography, is encouraged as an additional monitoring parameter to assess a patient's quality of respiration and to provide a quantitative value for exhaled gases. Pretracheal stethoscopes serve as immediate indicators of a patient's respiratory quality, and it can serve as a direct monitor of airway patency or obstruction through direct auscultation (Figures 6.2 and 6.3).

Management

Rescuing a patient from an unintended level of sedation requires rapid recognition and prior development of a treatment plan. Priority must be placed upon ensuring adequate ventilation and oxygenation in a patient that has diminished respiratory effort or an obstructed airway. The recommended AHA guidelines on performing rescue breathing—including positioning, head-tilt/chin-lift or jaw-thrust maneuvers, and attempts at positive pressure ventilation—should be accompanied by consideration of administering reversal medications such as naloxone for opioid-induced respiratory depression and flumazenil for benzodiazepines. Management is best handled with a team approach, and various members of that team should be designated for certain tasks such as summoning EMS, obtaining rescue equipment, and patient monitoring.

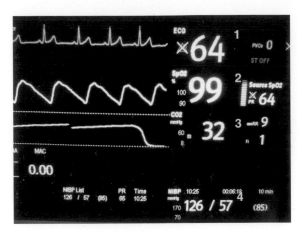

Figure 6.2 Pictured are (from top to bottom) (1) electrocardiogram (ECG) displaying normal sinus rhythm (NSR) and a cardiac rate of 69 beats per minute (bpm), (2) plethysmograph showing regular pulsatile waveform and oxyhemoglobin saturation at 99%, (3) capnograph displaying data from a sampling nasal cannula with a reading of 31 cm H_2O of exhaled carbon dioxide and a respiratory rate of 11 bpm, and (4) a noninvasive blood pressure (NIBP) reading of 126/57 and a mean arterial pressure of 85 mmHg. Photos (Capnography, Pulse Oximetry, Pre-tracheal stethoscope).

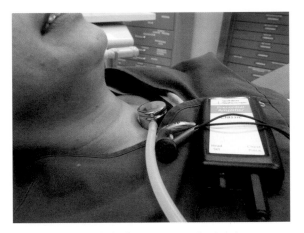

Figure 6.3 An amplified, electronic pretracheal stethoscope to monitor breath-to-breath respirations in a sedated patient. Photos (Capnography, Pulse Oximetry, Pre-tracheal stethoscope).

Intravenous access complications

The clinician utilizing the parenteral route of drug administration via peripheral IV access must be aware of the potential complications that can range from minor irritation to long-term injury and permanent damage.

Extravasation, infiltration, and phlebitis are common complications of IV access that can be managed effectively in an office-based setting. Unintended intra-arterial injection is a relatively rare complication that can lead to permanent tissue damage and possible loss of a peripheral limb or digit.

Extravasation and infiltration

Extravasation of a peripheral IV has been defined as the inadvertent administration of a vesicant medication or solution into the surrounding tissues. Infiltration is the leakage of a nonvesicant drug into the surrounding tissues (Dougherty, 2008). A vesicant drug, in these definitions, is a medication or solution that can cause blisters with subsequent tissue necrosis (Goolsby and Lombardo, 2006). During dental treatment under parenteral moderate sedation or deep sedation, it is not uncommon for a patient to move while an IV line is connected to a peripheral vein. This movement can contribute to loss of patency to an established peripheral IV access point. At best, this complication leads to minor irritation if managed accordingly, yet serious complications such as full-thickness skin loss and muscle and tendon necrosis have been reported (Dychter *et al.*, 2012).

Prevention

Preventing extravasation or infiltration first requires consideration of an IV access site. Avoiding areas that are joints or sites prone to patient movement will aid in preventing mechanical dislodgment of the cannula. Forearms or large straight veins on the dorsum of the hand are preferred over joints, such as the antecubital fossa, because of the potential for movement in this area. Rigid arm board fixation devices also aid in preventing unwanted patient movement. It is advisable to also choose an appropriate gauge of cannula to accommodate good fluid flow and rapid drug administration without compromising vessel integrity. Dougherty also recommends avoidance of using a steel-winged infusion device, also known as a "butterfly" needle (Dougherty, 2008). Generally, this implies using the smallest possible flexible indwelling cannula to accommodate the intended therapy and potential for emergency intervention. Second, choosing an access site not directly distal to a previous venipuncture site or a failed attempt site can prevent extravasation from previous or existing vessel wall injuries. Firmly securing and adequately dressing the IV cannula and attached fluid lines also

contribute to lowering the risks of infiltration and leakage at the site of access.

Recognition and management

Various signs and symptoms of extravasation and infiltration may present clinically. Initial recognition most often begins with a noticeable reduction in IV fluid flow despite an earlier well-flowing access site. If the patient is still able to perceive painful stimuli, reports of pain and discomfort may accompany the extravasation or infiltration site. The cannulation site may be swollen with blanched, taut skin due to the fluid invading the interstitial space. IV fluid and medications may also leak from the IV insertion site. If the patient is able to report symptoms, extravasation will be accompanied by symptomatic burning and stinging, followed by blistering, tissue necrosis, and ulceration (Dychter *et al.*, 2012).

The clinician should check for the presence of a tourniquet inadvertently left on the patient's limb as well as checking for clothing that can act as a tourniquet as this can impede fluid flow. Once this complication has been identified, fluid flow should be stopped and the IV tubing should be disconnected and the catheter left in place if the infusate is irritating to tissues. Aspiration of irritating drugs can be accomplished through the still-intact catheter if needed. Raising the affected limb and placing warm compresses can promote vasodilation and enhance dispersion of the extravasated drug. Conversely, application of cold to the affected area can help isolate a vesicant that may cause further tissue damage (Dychter *et al.*, 2012). Infiltration may be accompanied by bruising and additional bleeding into the extravascular space that can be controlled with direct pressure until bleeding stops. If significant tissue damage is anticipated or is encountered, immediate referral to an appropriate specialist is recommended. If the safety of the procedure is contingent upon vascular access, another IV access site should be considered and thorough documentation of the complication, intervention, and management entered into the patient record.

Intra-arterial injection

Iatrogenic intra-arterial injection of medications during sedation or general anesthesia can result in serious injury to the patient. Reports of gangrene, limb ischemia, skin necrosis, and amputations are direct consequences of drugs traveling distally from the site of cannulation (Sen, Chini, and Brown, 2005). The severe sequelae and drastic impairment often develop rapidly after the complication occurs, and intra-arterial injection can occur in any venue, including office-based dental settings, where IV access is commonplace.

Prevention

The accidental cannulation of peripheral arteries can be identified by observance of the following: presence of bright, red blood into the IV catheter, pulsatile movement of blood into the IV tubing, and backflow of blood into the IV tubing despite significant fluid column (IV fluid bag) height. Additionally, care must be taken to ensure arterial cannulation has not occurred in an anatomical area where arteries and veins are in close proximity to one another, such as in the antecubital fossa or the wrist (Ghouri, Mading, and Prabaker, 2002). Certain patient populations may carry a higher risk for accidental intra-arterial injection than others, and a higher degree of care must be exercised when obtaining IV access. These include patients who are morbidly obese, patients with dark skin pigmentation, patients with thoracic outlet syndrome (vanishing radial pulse with abduction/internal rotation of the arm), or patients with vascular abnormalities in the limbs. Additionally, patients who are unable to report symptoms of pain, such as those under deep sedation or general anesthesia, are at increased risk for intra-arterial injection (Sen, Chini, and Brown, 2005).

Recognition and management

If intra-arterial injection is identified prior to the administration of medications, the clinician must remove the catheter and apply direct pressure to the access site to minimize formation of a hematoma and prevent ecchymosis (bruising). If medications are infused, immediate reports of pain and severe discomfort distal to the site of injection are often expressed by patients. These symptoms may be followed by paresthesia and involuntary movement that may be accompanied by changes to the affected limb's skin. Finally, areas distal to the site of injection may be damaged by tissue necrosis and permanent alterations in motor control, sensory deficits, and the onset of chronic pain.

If intra-arterial injection is diagnosed in an office-based setting, the clinician must consider transporting the patient to an appropriate hospital-based setting for acute management and attempts to preserve the affected limb occur immediately. Management remains largely empirical and prospective studies regarding appropriate therapy are sparse. Sen, Chini, and Brown (2005) do, however, maintain a list of recommendations for managing this complication that include the following:

1 Maintain the intra-arterial catheter to provide access to therapeutic agents, allowing arterial sampling, and provide rapid access for angiography.
2 Identify the progress of the disease to provide a metric for further development of the injury.
3 Initiate anticoagulation to preserve circulation in the distal area.
4 Institute symptomatic relief and plan for rehabilitation.
5 Treat with antibiotics when indicated.
6 Perform specific interventions, such as local anesthesia intra-arterial injection with procaine or lidocaine to reperfuse the area, performance of sympatholysis (stellate ganglion or axillary plexus blocks) to decrease vasospasm, hyperbaric oxygen therapy, or initiate administration of arterial vasodilators and thrombolytics.

The authors have also reported comorbidities affecting the venous system after accidental intra-arterial injection. With the associated problems of vasospasm and immobility of the limb, deep vein thrombosis, compartment syndrome, and prolonged pain can warrant continued monitoring with ultrasound imaging (Hoehenstein *et al.*, 2014).

Phlebitis

Phlebitis is an inflammation of the wall of a vein. In the context of IV access in moderate sedation and general anesthesia, the usual etiology is from the IV access itself or the medications infused through the vein. Bacterial infection at the site of cannulation and entry of bacteria into the bloodstream via peripheral IV lines can also develop into phlebitis (Loftus *et al.*, 2012a). If the inflammation is caused by a blood clot, the condition is termed thrombophlebitis.

Prevention

According the US Centers for Disease Control, avoidance of a lower extremity IV site in adults will lower the risk of phlebitis (Grady *et al.*, 2011). Although rare in office-based and ambulatory surgical care settings, the CDC also recommends that the duration of catheterization should not exceed 72–96h to reduce the risk of developing phlebitis. Larger bore IV (16–20 gauge) cannulas inserted into a short, narrow lumen veins increase the risk of phlebitis as well as the choice of cannula material. Dychter *et al.* recommend catheters made of polyurethane (PEU) rather than those constructed from tetrafluoroethylene–hexafluoropropylene (Teflon™) to further reduce the risks of developing phlebitis (Dychter *et al.*, 2012). The common medications used as sedatives for dental treatment also contribute to the inflammation of peripheral veins. IV barbiturates, with their high pH, can irritate vessels. Diazepam, meperidine, beta-lactam antibiotics, barbiturates, etomidate, and propofol have also been implicated in the development of phlebitis due to various factors that include extremes in pH, osmolality, and size of particulate matter in solution (Dos Reis *et al.,* 2009). Proper and strict adherence to aseptic technique may also aid in preventing bacterial infection and entry of bacteria into the bloodstream due to catheter insertion and peripheral IV line establishment. Recent investigations into the use of stopcocks in IV lines point to an increased risk of bacterial reservoirs and infectious transmission to the patient (Loftus *et al.*, 2012b).

Recognition and management

Typically, a patient will develop redness, tenderness, erythema, and a palpable venous cord at the site of cannulation. The course of inflammation will travel along the trajectory of the affected vein and migrate proximal to the site of cannulation. When possible, the IV access site should be discontinued and no further medications infused through that vein. In some cases, cannulation and resultant tissue injury have resulted in chronic neuropathic pain (Gohil and Balasubramanian, 2012). Anti-inflammatory drugs, corticosteroids, and heparin have all been considered acceptable therapies, along with an application of heat to encourage vasodilation and increased perfusion to the site of inflammation (Dychter *et al.*, 2012). Topical nitroglycerin has also been suggested as a therapy to encourage increased perfusion to the site (Tjon and Ansani, 2000). If infection is suspected, aggressive and prompt administration of oral and parenteral antibiotics is warranted (Tagalakis *et al.*, 2002).

Negative pressure pulmonary edema

Negative pressure pulmonary edema (NPPE), a relatively rare complication of general anesthesia where inspiratory negative pressure generated during complete glottic closure produces significant pulmonary edema, can occur minutes to an hour after first presentation of laryngospasm. Intrathoracic negative pressures can reach up to −140 cm of H_2O and the resultant pulmonary edema is produced by multiple factors that include increased venous return, adrenergic and hypoxic pulmonary vasoconstriction, and increased interstitial pressure (Udeshi, Cantie, and Pierre, 2010). Clinical presentation includes frank hypoxia, tachypnea (rapid, shallow breathing), tachycardia (increased heart rate), rales (audible "crackles" upon inspiration), audible wheezing, and oftentimes the presence of pink, frothy secretions visible in the oropharynx.

Prevention, recognition, and management

Prevention of general anesthesia-related NPPE includes prompt treatment of laryngospasm or complete airway obstruction through several approaches. Paradoxical chest movement in response to airway obstruction, tracheal "tugging," frank hypoxia, absence of ventilatory patency, and absence of an end-tidal carbon dioxide waveform are all signs and symptoms of complete airway obstruction during sedation and general anesthesia (Louis and Fernandes, 2002). Early recognition is a key component in preventing NPPE, and efforts should be directed at ensuring adequate levels of anesthesia to prevent laryngospasm that may involve the use of depolarizing or nondepolarizing muscle relaxants, rapid increase in the depth of anesthesia for adequate mask ventilation, and, if employing an endotracheal or nasotracheal tube, a fully awake patient prior to extubation. Management includes positive pressure ventilation once the obstruction is removed or laryngospasm is managed. Careful consideration should be given to the use of diuretics to reduce pulmonary edema, although the use of diuretics can exacerbate hypovolemia and hypoperfusion. Steroids can also be considered to lessen the inflammation of damaged capillaries and alveoli (Udeshi, Cantie, and Pierre, 2010).

Malignant hyperthermia

Malignant hyperthermia is a heritable, hypermetabolic condition affecting the muscles. It is an autosomal dominant myopathy that produces sustained and prolonged muscle hypermetabolism and is characterized by increased body temperature, tachycardia, masseter muscle spasm, generalized muscle rigidity, hypercarbia, tachypnea, rapid increases in exhaled carbon dioxide, elevated creatine kinase, and respiratory and metabolic acidosis. The agents implicated in the triggering of malignant hyperthermia episodes in susceptible individuals are depolarizing muscle relaxants (succinylcholine) and volatile inhaled anesthetics used for general anesthesia (Larach *et al.*, 2010).

Recognition and management

Initial presentation after induction of general anesthesia and introduction of triggering agents can occur immediately to 90 min into the anesthetic. One of the first clinical signs of malignant hyperthermia is hypercarbia as evidenced by increases in end-tidal, or exhaled, carbon dioxide. The presentation pattern may also be followed or accompanied by masseter muscle spasm, generalized muscle rigidity, rhabdomyolysis, renal failure, hypotension, cardiac arrhythmias, and sinus tachycardia. New data has been presented that identifies temperature abnormalities can indeed be an early sign that typifies a malignant hyperthermia episode given that practitioners employ consistent and reliable temperature monitoring prior to and during general anesthesia (Larach *et al.*, 2014). Left untreated, the condition is often fatal and patient mortality usually results from lethal dysrhythmias and cardiac arrest.

Upon suspicion or recognition of a malignant hyperthermia episode, prompt treatment includes immediate discontinuation of triggering agents along with the administration of IV dantrolene at 2 mg/kg of patient weight and repeated every 5 min. Dantrolene, a hydantoin-derived skeletal muscle relaxant, is available as a powder that must be reconstituted with sterile water prior to IV administration. Normal saline or other diluents will not reconstitute this specific drug. If a closed anesthesia circuit was used to initiate general anesthesia, the breathing circuit and associated equipment should be switched out to circuits that contain no trace volatile anesthetics. Management of hypercarbia and acidosis will include increased mechanical ventilation rate and volume, initiating hyperventilation, and may also include consideration of the administration of IV sodium bicarbonate. Increased IV fluid loading, mannitol and furosemide diuresis, glucose and insulin administration, and adjunctive vasopressors and management of dysrhythmias have been shown to be effective in the treatment of malignant hyperthermia as well (Larach *et al.*, 2010). Active cooling with ice packs and gastric lavage is recommended, and immediate transport from an office-based or ambulatory care setting to a hospital is advised (Schneiderbanger *et al.*, 2014).

References

American Academy of Pediatric Dentistry (2013) *Guidelines of the Use of Nitrous Oxide for Pediatric Dental Patients*. Clinical Practice Guidelines. Reference Manual, Vol. 37, No. 6, 15/16, pp. 206–210, http://www.aapd.org/media/policies_guidelines/g_nitrous.pdf (accessed January 11, 2016).

Alhassani, A.A. and AlGhamdi, A.S.T. (2010) Inferior alveolar nerve injury in implant dentistry: diagnosis, causes, prevention, and management. *Journal of Implantology*, **XXXVI** (Five), 401–407.

Altay, M.A., Lyu, D.J.H., Collette, D., Baur, D.A., Quereshy, F.A., Teich, S.T. and Gonzalez, A.E. (2014) Transcervical migration of a broken dental needle: a case report and literature review. *Oral Surgery, Oral Medicine, Oral Pathology, Oral Radiology*, **118**, e161–e165.

American Dental Association (2012) *Guidelines for the Use of Sedation and General Anesthesia by Dentists*, American Dental Association, Chicago, IL.

American Society of Anesthesiologists (2002) Practice guidelines for sedation and analgesia by non-anesthesiologists. An updated report by the American Society of Anesthesiologists Task Force on sedation and analgesia by non-anesthesiologists. *Anesthesiology*, **96**, 1004–1017.

Baum, V.C. (2007) When nitrous oxide is no laughing matter: nitrous oxide and pediatric anesthesia. *Pediatric Anesthesia*, **17**, 824–830.

Becker, D.E. and Reed, K.L. (2012) Local anesthetics: review of pharmacological considerations. *Anesthesia Progress*, **59**, 90–102.

Becker, D.E. and Rosenberg, M. (2008) Nitrous oxide and the inhalation anesthetics. *Anesthesia Progress*, **55**, 124–131.

Beddis, H.P., Davies, S.J., Budenberg, A., Horner, K. and Pemberton, M.N. (2014) Temporomandibular disorders, trismus and malignancy: development of a checklist to improve patient safety. *British Dental Journal*, **217**, 351–355.

Belenguer-Guallar, I., Jimenez-Soriano, Y. and Claramunt-Lozano, A. (2014) Treatment of recurrent aphthous stomatitis. A literature review. *Journal of Clinical and Experimental Dentistry*, **6** (2), e168–e174.

Berkun, Y., Ben-Zvi, A., Levy, Y., Galili, D. and Shalit, M. (2003) Evaluation of adverse reactions to local anesthetics: experience with 236 patients. *Annals of Allergy, Asthma & Immunology*, **91**, 342–345.

Boynes, S., Riley, A. and Milbee, S. (2014) Evaluating complications during intraoral administration of local anesthetics in a rural, portable special needs dental clinic. *Special Care in Dentistry*, **34** (5), 241–245.

Brandner, B., Blagrove, M., McCallum, G. and Bromley, L.M. (1997) Dreams, images, and emotions associated with propofol anaesthesia. *Anaesthesia*, **52**, 750–755.

Brau, M.E., Branitzki, P., Olschewski, A., Vogel, W. and Hempelmann, G. (2000) Block of neuronal tetrodotoxin-resistant Na⁺ currents by stereoisomers of piperidine local anesthetics. *Anesthesia & Analgesia*, **91**, 1499–1505.

Cave, G. and Harvey, M. (2009) Intravenous lipid emulsion as antidote beyond local anesthetic toxicity: a systematic review. *Academic Emergency Medicine*, **16**, 815–824.

Chi, D., Kanellis, M., Himadi, E. and Asselin, M.E. (2008) Lip biting in a pediatric dental patient after dental local anesthesia: a case report. *Journal of Pediatric Nursing*, **23** (6 December), 490–493.

Chisci, G., Chisci, V. and Chisci, E. (2013) Ocular complications after posterior superior alveolar nerve block: a case of trochlear nerve palsy. *International Journal of Oral & Maxillofacial Surgery*, **42**, 1562–1565.

Ciancio, S.G., Hutcheson, M.C., Ayoub, F., Pantera, E.A., Pantera, C.T., Garlapo, D.A., Sobieraj, B.D. and Almubarak, S.A. (2013) Safety and efficacy of a novel nasal spray for maxillary dental anesthesia. *JDR Clinical Research Supplements*, **92** (7 Supplement), 43s–48s.

Clark, K., Reader, A., Beck, M. and Meyers, W.J. (2002) Anesthetic efficacy of an infiltration in mandibular anterior teeth following an inferior alveolar nerve block. *Anesthesia Progress*, **49**, 49–55.

Cohen, A.F. and Warman, S.P. (1989) Upper airway obstruction secondary to warfarin-induced sublingual hematoma. *Archives of Otolaryngology—Head and Neck Surgery*, **115** (June), 718–720.

Dionne, R.A., Yagiela, J.A., Cote, C.J., Donaldson, M., Edwards, M., Greenblatt, D.J., Haas, D., Malviya, S., Milgrom, P., Moore, P.A., Shampaine, G., Silverman, M., Williams, R.L. and Wilson, S. (2006) Balancing efficacy and safety in the use of oral sedation in dental outpatients. *The Journal of the American Dental Association*, **146**, 502–513.

Dos Reis, P.E., Silveira, R.C.V., Asques, C.I. and de Carvalho, E.C. (2009) Pharmacological interventions to treat phlebitis. *Journal of Infusion Nursing*, **32** (2), 74–79.

Dougherty, L. (2008) IV Therapy: recognizing the differences between infiltration and extravasation. *British Journal of Nursing*, **17** (14), 896–901.

Dychter, S.S., Gold, D.A., Carson, D. and Haller, M. (2012) Intravenous therapy: a review of complications and economic considerations of peripheral access. *Journal of Infusion Nursing*, **35** (2), 84–91.

Faix, D.J. (2001 September–October) Horner syndrome from the dentist's chair. *The Journal of the American Board of Family Practice*, **14** (5), 386–388.

Gambarini, G., Plotino, G., Grande, N.M., Testarelli, L., Prencipe, M., Messineo, D., Fratini, L. and D'Ambrosio, F. (2011) Differential diagnosis of endodontic-related inferior alveolar nerve paraesthesia with cone beam computed tomography: a case report. *International Endodontic Journal*, **44**, 176–181.

Ganzberg, S.I. and Kramer, K.J. (2010) The use of local anesthetic agents in medicine. *Dental Clinics of North America*, **54**, 601–610.

Garisto, G.A., Gaffen, A.S., Lawrence, H.P., Tenenbaum, H.C. and Haas, D.A. (2010) Occurrence of paresthesia after dental local anesthetic administration in the United States. *The Journal of the American Dental Association*, **141**, 836–844.

Gerbino, G., Zavattero, E., Berrone, M. and Berrone, S. (2013) Management of needle breakage using intraoperative navigation following inferior alveolar nerve block. *Journal of Oral and Maxillofacial Surgery*, **71**, 1819–1824.

Ghouri, A.F., Mading, W. and Prabaker, K. (2002) Accidental intraarterial drug injection via intravascular catheter placed on the dorsum of the hand. *Anesthesia & Analgesia*, **95**, 487–491.

Glass, G.E. and Tzfetta, K. (2014) Bell's palsy: a summary of current evidence and referral algorithm. *Family Practice*, **31** (6), 631–642.

GlaxoSmithKline (2014) *Prescribing Information: ZOFRAN (Ondansetron Hydrochloride)*, GlaxoSmithKline, Research Triangle Park, NC.

Gohil, S. and Balasubramanian, S. (2012) Case report and literature review of chronic neuropathic pain associated with peripheral venous cannulation. *Anaesthesia*, **67**, 1395–1397.

Goolsby, T.V. and Lombardo, F.A. (2006) Extravasation of chemotherapeutic agents: prevention and treatment. *Seminars in Oncology*, **33** (1), 139–143.

Grady, N.P., Alexander, M., Burns, L.A., Dellinger, P., Garland, J., Heard, S.O., Lipsett, P.A., Masur, H., Mermel, L.A., Pearson, M.L., Raad, I.I., Randolph, A., Rupp, M.E., Saint, S. and HICPAC (2011) *CDC Guidelines for the Prevention of Intravascular Catheter-Related Infections, 2011*, Centers for Disease Control, Atlanta, GA.

Gray, T.A. and Hawkins, S. (2004) A PACU crisis: a case study on the development and management of methemoglobinemia. *Journal of PeriAnesthesia Nursing*, **19** (4 August), 242–253.

Gutenberg, L.L., Chen, J.-W. and Trapp, L. (2013) Methemoglobin levels in generally anesthetized pediatric dental patients receiving prilocaine versus lidocaine. *Anesthesia Progress*, **60**, 99–108.

Hawthorne, M., Sim, R. and Acton, C.H.C. (2000) Quinine induced coagulopathy – a near fatal experience. *Australian Dental Journal*, **454**, 282–284.

Heller, A.A. and Shankland, W.E., II (2001) Alternative to the inferior alveolar nerve block anesthesia when placing mandibular dental implants posterior to the mental foramen. *Journal of Implantology*, **XXVII** (Three), 127–133.

Herff, H., Paal, P., von Goedecke, A., Lindner, K.H., Keller, C. and Wenzel, V. (2007) Fatal errors in nitrous oxide delivery. *Anaesthesia*, **62**, 1202–1206.

Hohenstein, C., Herdtle, S., Hoyme, M., Lauten, A. and Chaudhary, T. (2014) Rescue of the limb after accidental injection of diazepam into femoral artery. *American Journal of Emergency Medicine*, **32** (1149), e5–e6.

Huang, R.Y., Chen, Y.J., Fang, W.H., Mau, L.P. and Shieh, Y.S. (2013) Concomitant Horner and Harlequin syndromes after inferior alveolar nerve block anesthesia. *Journal of Endodontics*, **39** (12), 1654–1657.

International Association for the Study of Pain (IASP) (2015) *Taxonomy*, http://www.iasp-pain.org/Taxonomy#Pain (accessed December 29, 2015).

Jastak, J.T. and Donaldson, D. (1991) Nitrous oxide. *Anesthesia Progress*, **91**, 1401–1407.

Kanaa, M.D., Whitworth, J.M. and Meechan, J.G. (2012) A prospective randomized trial of different supplementary local anesthetic techniques after failure of inferior alveolar nerve block in patients with irreversible pulpitis in mandibular teeth. *Journal of Endodontics*, **38** (4 April), 421–425.

Kaufamn, E., Galili, D. and Furer, R. (1990) Sensory experience induced by nitrous oxide analgesia. *Anesthesia Progress*, **37**, 282–285.

Kim, J.W., Cha, I.H., Kim, S.J. and Kim, M.R. (2012) Which risk factors are associated with neurosensory deficits of inferior alveolar nerve after mandibular third molar extraction? *Journal of Oral and Maxillofacial Surgery*, **70**, 2508–2514.

Kitay, D., Ferraro, N. and Sonis, S.T. (1991) Lateral pharyngeal space abscess as a consequence of regional anesthesia. *The Journal of the American Dental Association*, **122** (6), 56–59.

Larach, M.G., Gronert, G.A., Allen, G.C., Brandom, B.W. and Lehman, E.B. (2010) Clinical presentation, treatment, and complications of malignant hyperthermia in North America from 1987 to 2006. *Anesthesia & Analgesia*, **110**, 498–507.

Larach, M.G., Brandom, B.W., Allen, G.C., Gronert, G.A. and Lehman, E.B. (2014) Malignant hyperthermia deaths related to inadequate temperature monitoring, 2007–2012: a report from the North American Malignant Hyperthermia Registry of the Malignant Hyperthermia Association of the United States. *Anesthesia & Analgesia*, **119**, 1359–1366.

Liberman, D.B. and Teach, S.J. (2008) Management of anaphylaxis in children. *Pediatric Emergency Care*, **24** (12), 861–869.

Lo, J.C.Y., Darracq, M.A. and Clark, R.F. (2014) A review of methylene blue treatment for cardiovascular collapse. *The Journal of Emergency Medicine*, **46** (5), 670–679.

Loftus, R.W., Patel, H.M., Huysman, B.C., Kispert, D.P., Koff, M.D., Gallagher, J.D., Jensen, J.T., Rowlands, J., Reddy, S., Dodds, T.M., Yeager, M.P., Ruoff, K.L., Surgenor, S.D. and Brown, J.R. (2012a) Prevention of intravenous bacterial injection from health care provider hands: the importance of catheter design and handling. *Anesthesia & Analgesia*, **115**, 1109–1119.

Loftus, R.W., Brown, J.R., Koff, M.D., Reddy, S., Heard, S.O., Patel, H.M., Fernandez, P.G., Beach, M.L., Corwin, H.L., Jensen, J.T., Kispert, D., Huysman, B., Dodds, T.M., Ruoff, K.L. and Yeager, M.P. (2012b) Multiple reservoirs contribute to intraoperative bacterial transmission. *Anesthesia & Analgesia*, **114** (6), 1236–1248.

Louis, P.J. and Fernandes, R. (2002) Negative pressure pulmonary edema. *Oral Surgery, Oral Medicine, Oral Pathology, Oral Radiology, and Endodontology*, **93**, 4–6.

Macy, E. (2003) Local anesthetic adverse reaction evaluations: the role of the allergist. *Annals of Allergy, Asthma & Immunology*, **91**, 319–320.

Malamed, S.F. (2004) Local complications, in *Handbook of Local Anesthesia*, 5th edn, Elsevier Mosby, St. Louis, MO, pp. 55–81.

Malamed, S.F. (2006) Nerve injury caused by mandibular block analgesia by Professors Hillerup and Jensen, Letter to the editor. *International Journal of Oral and Maxillofacial Surgery*, 2006, 876–877.

Malamed, S.F. (2010) *Sedation: A Guide to Patient Management*, 5th edn, Elsevier Mosby, St. Louis, MO.

Malamed, S.F. (2013) *Handbook of Local Anesthesia*, 6th edn, Elsevier Mosby, St. Louis, MO.

Malamed, S.F. and Clark, M.S. (2003) Nitrous oxide–oxygen: a new look at a very old technique. *Journal of the California Dental Association*, **31** (5), 397–403.

Malamed, S.F., Serxner, K. and Wiedenfeld, A.M. (1988) The incidence of sexual phenomena in females receiving nitrous oxide and oxygen inhalation sedation. *Journal of American Analgesic Society*, **22**, 9.

Malamed, S.F., Reed, K. and Poorsattar, S. (2010) Needle breakage: incidence and prevention. *Dental Clinics of North America*, **54**, 745–756.

Mason, R., Drum, M., Reader, A., Nusstein, J. and Beck, M. (2009) A prospective, randomized, double-blind comparison of 2% lidocaine with 1:100,000 and 1:50,000 epinephrine and 3% mepivacaine for maxillary infiltrations. *Journal of Endodontics*, **35** (9), 1173–1177.

Moore, P.A. and Haas, D.A. (2010) Paresthesias in dentistry. *Dental Clinics of North America*, **54**, 715–730.

Myles, P.S., Leslie, K., Chan, M.T.V., Forbes, A., Peyton, P.J., Paech, M.J., Beattie, W.S., Sessler, D.J., Devereaux, P.J., Silbert, B., Schricker, T., Wallace, S. and ANZCA Trials Group for the ENIGMA-II Investigators (2014) The safety of addition of nitrous oxide to general anesthesia in at-risk patients having major non-cardiac surgery (ENIGMA-II): a randomized, single-blind trial. *Lancet*, **384**, 1446–1454.

Nusstein, J.M., Reader, A. and Drum, M. (2010) Local anesthesia strategies for the patient with a "hot" tooth. *Dental Clinics of North America*, **54**, 237–247.

Ostergaard, C., Orhan-Sungur, M., Apfel, C. and Akça, Ö. (2005) Effects of nitrous oxide on intraoperative bowel distension. *Current Opinion in Anaesthesiology*, **18**, 620–624.

Padhye, M., Gupta, S., Chandiramani, G. and Bali, R. (2011) PSA block for maxillary molar's anesthesia – an obsolete technique? *Oral Surgery, Oral Medicine, Oral Pathology, Oral Radiology, and Endodontology*, **112**, e39–e43.

Park, Y.T., Kim, S.G. and Moon, S.Y. (2012) Indirect compressive injury to the inferior alveolar nerve caused by dental implant placement. *Journal of Oral and Maxillofacial Surgery*, **70**, e258–e259.

Peyton, P.J. and Wu, C.Y. (2014) Nitrous oxide-related post-operative nausea and vomiting depends on duration of exposure. *Anesthesiology*, **120** (5), 1137–1114.

Piot, B., Sigmund-Fiks, M., Huet, P., Fressinaud, E., Trossaert, M. and Mercier, J. (2002) Management of dental extractions in patients with bleeding disorders. *Oral Surgery, Oral Medicine, Oral Pathology, Oral Radiology, and Endodontology*, **93**, 247–250.

Preeti, L., Magesh, K.T., Rajkumar, K. and Karthik, R. (2011) Recurrent aphthous stomatitis. *Journal of Oral and Maxillofacial Pathology*, **15** (3), 252–256.

Ribeiro, L., Ramalho, S., Geros, S., Ferreira, E.C., Almeida, A.F. and Conde, A. (2014) Needle in the external auditory canal: an unusual complication of inferior alveolar nerve block. *Oral Surgery, Oral Medicine, Oral Pathology and Oral Radiology*, **117** (6), e436–e437.

Rossignol, D.A., Genuis, S.J. and Frye, R.E. (2014) Environmental toxicants and autism spectrum disorders: a systematic review. *Translational Psychiatry*, **4**, e360.

Schneiderbanger, D., Johannsen, S., Roewer, N. and Schuster, F. (2014) Management of malignant hyperthermia: diagnosis and treatment. *Therapeutics and Clinical Risk Management*, **10**, 355–362.

Sen, S., Chini, E.N. and Brown, M.J. (2005) Complications after unintentional intra-arterial injection of drugs: risks, outcomes, and management strategies. *Mayo Clinic Proceedings*, **80** (6), 783–795.

Shay, H., Frumento, R.J. and Bastien, A. (2007) General anesthesia and methylenetetrahydrofolate reductase deficiency. *The Journal of Anesthesia*, **21**, 493–496.

Shojaei, A.R. and Haas, D.A. (2002) Local anesthetic cartridges and latex allergy: a literature review. *Journal of the Canadian Dental Association*, **68** (10), 622–626.

Simon, R.A. (1996) Adverse reactions to food and drug additives. *Immunology and Asthma Clinics of North America*, **16** (1), 228.

Svrakic, M., Pollack, A., Huncke, T.K. and Roland, J.T., Jr (2014) Conscious sedation and local anesthesia for patients undergoing neurotologic and complex otologic procedures. *Otology & Neurology*, **35**, e277–e285.

Tagalakis, V., Kahn, S.R., Libman, M. and Blostein, M. (2002) The epidemiology of peripheral vein infusion thrombophlebitis: a critical review. *American Journal of Medicine*, **113**, 146–151.

Taleb, M., Ashraf, Z., Valavoor, S. and Tinkel, J. (2013) Evaluation and management of acquired methemoglobinemia associated with topical benzocaine use. *American Journal of Cardiovascular Drugs*, **13**, 325–330.

Tarakji, B. and Nassani, M.Z. (2012) Factors associated with hematoma of the floor of the mouth after placement of dental implants. *Saudi Dental Journal*, **24** (1), 11–15.

Tjon, J.A. and Ansani, N.T. (2000) Transdermal nitroglycerin for the prevention of intravenous infusion failure due to phlebitis and extravasation. *Annals of Pharmacotherapy*, **34** (10), 1189–1192.

Trapp, L. and Will, J. (2010) Acquired methemoglobinemia revisited. *Dental Clinics of North America*, **54**, 665–675.

Uckman, S., Cilasun, U. and Erkman, O. (2006) Rare ocular and cutaneous complication of inferior alveolar nerve block. *Journal of Oral and Maxillofacial Surgery*, **64**, 719–721.

Udeshi, A., Cantie, S.M. and Pierre, E. (2010) Postobstructive pulmonary edema. *Journal of Critical Care*, **25** (508), 508.e1–508.e5.

Udhya, J., Varadharaja, M.M., Pathiban, J. and Srinivasan, I. (2014) Autism disorder (AD): an updated review for paediatric dentists. *Journal of Clinical and Diagnostic Research*, **8** (2), 275–279.

Von Arx, T., Lozanoff, S. and Zinkernagel, M. (2014) Ophthalmologic complications after intraoral local anesthesia. An analysis of 65 published case reports. *Swiss Dental Journal*, **124**, 7–8.

Weaver, J.M. (2007) Calculating the maximum recommended dose of local anesthetic. *Journal of the California Dental Association*, **35** (1), 61–63.

Weaver, J.M. (2010) The ADA's new emergency airway course for sedationists. *Anesthesia Progress*, **57**, 137–138.

Wilke, G.J. (2000) Temporary uniocular blindness and ophthalmoplegia associated with a mandibular block injection: a case report. *Australian Dental Journal*, **45**, 131.

Wood, M., Reader, A., Nusstein, J.M., Beck, M., Padgett, D. and Weaver, J. (2005) Comparison of intraosseous and infiltration injection for venous lidocaine blood concentrations and heart rate changes after injection of 2% lidocaine with 1:100,000 epinephrine. *Journal of Endodontics*, **31**, 435–438.

CHAPTER 7

Implant complications

Deborah A. Termeie[1] and Daniel W. Nelson[2]

[1] Department of Periodontics, School of Dentistry, University of California, Los Angeles, CA, USA
[2] UCSF School of Dentistry, Division of Periodontology, San Francisco, CA, USA

Preoperative complications

Treatment planning complications
Compromised interdental space

It is important to take accurate measurements of the intertooth space to plan for the appropriate size implant. A minimum intertooth space of 7 mm is required to place a standard 3.75–4.1 mm diameter implant. There are times when the interdental space is too small to place an implant or too large for one implant but too small for two implants. Some studies (Tarnow *et al.*, 2003) have found that the distance between two implants should be at least 3 mm in order to preserve the interdental bone. It is also recommended that there be 1.5 mm between the implant and the tooth to maintain bone adjacent to the teeth and 1 mm between the implant and the tooth when using platform-switched implants (Vela *et al.*, 2012). Inability to perform good oral hygiene, compromised papilla on the adjacent tooth, persistent inflammation, bone loss, and pain may arise when the implants are placed in a compromised intertooth space (Figure 7.1).

It is also important to not only measure the distance between the roots but also at the crowns. The crowns may encroach into the edentulous space and make it difficult to maneuver instruments.

Prevention and management

Proper planning with diagnostic images (e.g., with a radiographic stent made from a diagnostic wax-up) and study casts can prevent placing an implant in an inadequate space. If there is insufficient space to place a standard-sized implant, other options should be considered such as:

1 Insert an implant with a narrower diameter.
2 Place a fixed partial denture instead of an implant.
3 Enlarge the space by orthodontically moving the adjacent teeth. If the distance between the crowns is minimal, reducing the proximal surfaces of the crowns can sometimes create enough space to allow placement of the implant (Greenstein and Cavallaro, 2010, p. 406). This reduction can also flatten the convexity of the proximal surfaces, broaden the contact with the implant-supported prosthesis, and minimize food impaction.

Malposition of the implant in the esthetic area

Malposition of an implant can lead to compromised esthetics. When teeth are lost in the esthetic zone, there are many factors that the clinician must evaluate (Belser, Bernard, and Buser, 2003):

- Mesiodistal dimension of the edentulous area:
  ○ It is more difficult to gain a papilla between two adjacent implants than a natural tooth and an implant. It is not recommended to place a central and lateral implant adjacent to one another.
- Three-dimensional radiographs of the site:
  ○ Cone-beam scans allow for three-dimensional radiographic examination of the implant site, which can reveal facial bone thickness, bone density, bone contours, presence of pathology on adjacent teeth, and proximity of adjacent anatomical structures such as nerves, vessels, bony undercuts, and the

---

Avoiding and Treating Dental Complications: Best Practices in Dentistry, First Edition. Edited by Deborah A. Termeie.
© 2016 John Wiley & Sons, Inc. Published 2016 by John Wiley & Sons, Inc.

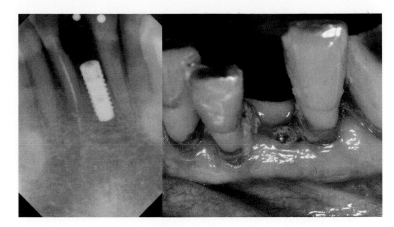

Figure 7.1 An implant placed less than 1.5 mm from the adjacent surface has lost bone on that surface. The patient's poor oral hygiene has also likely contributed to the bone loss.

proximity of the maxillary sinus and nasal floor. The aforementioned information can allow for more predictable treatment planning and presurgical preparation.

- Neighboring teeth (e.g., tooth dimensions, interproximal bone levels, restorative status, endodontic pathology, form, position, and orientation; periodontal/endodontic status; length of roots; bone level that will affect papilla fill; and crown-to-root ratio):
  ○ They help dictate where the implant will be placed.
  ○ Does site development need to be done before implant placement?
- Interarch relationships (e.g., vertical dimension of occlusion, interocclusal space, choosing between screw-retained or cement-retained implant crown, and necessity of odontoplasty of adjacent or opposing teeth).
- Esthetic parameters (e.g., height of upper smile line, lower lip line, occlusal plane orientation, dental and facial symmetry, and esthetics of contralateral tooth).
- Patient expectations:
  ○ Problems arise when the patient does not have ideal conditions for implant placement (e.g., bone quality) and still has high expectations (Klokkevold, 2006, p. 1182).
- Plaque control.
- Infection at or near the site where the implant will be placed.
- There is a greater chance of postoperative complications.
- Immunocompromised patient (i.e., any general health issue that lowers resistance to infection).

- Are the patient's anterior teeth triangular or highly scalloped with a thin biotype?
  ○ These cases are harder to manage because there is a greater risk of midfacial recession and loss of the interdental papilla.
  ○ Phonetic problems may result when the implant prosthesis is made with unusual palatal contours due to malpositioning of the implant (Klokkevold, 2006, p. 1189).

Prevention

A surgical stent and CT scans are essential in the prevention of implant malpositioning (Figure 7.2). A parallel pin can be placed in the osteotomy and an X-ray taken to ensure proper angulation of the implant after the pilot drill has been used. If a correction is needed, it can be done before further drilling is done.

Thin (≤1 mm) buccal walls are found in most extraction sites in the anterior maxilla (Huynh-Ba *et al.*, 2010). In most clinical situations, if less than 2 mm of facial bone thickness is predicted, augmentation procedures are necessary to attain sufficient bony contours around the implant (Chen and Buser, 2010, p. 142). Studies have also found that the insertion of a soft tissue graft at the time of immediate implant placement in the esthetic zone can be advantageous (Grunder, 2011).

Implant positioning

Apicocoronally the implant should be placed 1 mm apical to the cementoenamel junction of the adjacent tooth in patients who do not have gingival recession (Table 7.1) or 3 mm apical to the final buccal gingival margin of the

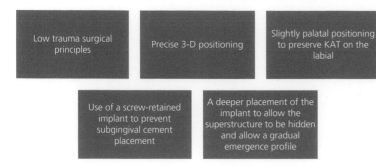

Figure 7.2 Principles for preventing malpositioning errors in the esthetic zone. (Termeie (2013). Reproduced with permission from Quintessence Publishing Group Inc., Chicago, IL).

Table 7.1 Consequences of deep and shallow implant placement.

Deep (more common)	Shallow
Bone loss and soft tissue recession because the load is supported by the weaker trabecular bone	Poor emergence profile
Increased crown height	Decreased crown height
Compromised papilla because the papilla is 100% present when the measurement from the interproximal point to the crest of bone is 5 mm or less. When the implant is placed subcrestal (>5 mm), the interproximal papilla may be absent (Tarnow *et al.*, 2003)	Cover screw, implant, or abutment exposure → esthetic issues
Cement removal may be difficult	
The bone above the implant may prevent complete seating of the prosthetic components	

Data from Al-Faraje (2011), p. 74.

implant restoration. If the implant is placed too deep, recession may occur and the gingival harmony may be disrupted. If the implant is too shallow, the metal margin may be visible. Deep implant placement may be caused by the surgeon wanting to ensure he achieves primary stability in immediate loading situations. Studies show that immediately loaded implants are placed 0.3 mm deeper than early loaded implants (Ganeles *et al.*, 2008).

The implant should not be placed too facially to prevent soft tissue recession. If the implant is placed too palatally, a ridge-lap crown would need to be fabricated, which may be difficult for the patient to clean (Chen and Buser, 2010, p. 138). When the occlusion allows, the surgeon should place the implant using the cingulum of the adjacent tooth as a guide, not the incisal edge. It may be prudent to avoid wide-diameter implants in the esthetic area to reduce the likelihood of recession and allow for a more esthetic emergence profile.

Treatment
Depending on the extent of malpositioning, the implant may need modification of the restoration design. If the implant is severely malpositioned, it is

favorable to remove the implant, start over, and inform the patient of the potential need for one or more regenerative procedures to prevent failure of the implant components.

A preparable ceramic abutment can be used in shallow placement situations. The ability to modify the crown-implant margin for subgingival placement can help when there is inadequate soft tissue thickness with a poor emergence profile (Al-Faraje, 2011, p. 74).

If recession has occurred, a connective tissue graft can be placed. However, once papillae have been lost, there are no predictable methods to regenerate them.

Limited jaw opening
The range of opening is 36 to 60 mm in women and 38 to 65 mm in men without regard to overlap and overbite (Misch, 2008, p. 250). Temporomandibular joint disorders can lead to limited jaw opening. The condyles are not able to move downward and forward the height of the articular eminence and therefore cause limited opening. Trismus causes limited jaw opening due to spasm of the muscles of mastication. Limited opening can complicate or prevent implant placement.

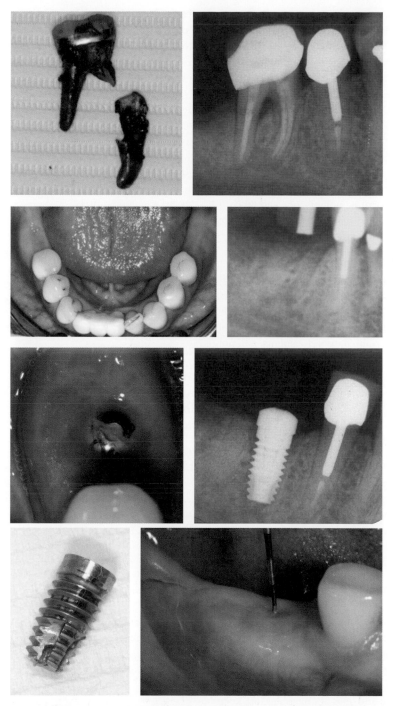

Figure 7.3 A root fragment resulting in implant failure. From left to right, in descending rows—Row 1: tooth #30 was extracted and was removed in multiple pieces. A ridge preservation bone graft was placed in the socket. Row 2: after 4 months of healing, the clinical and radiographic views. An implant was placed. Row 3: 4 months after implant placement, the implant was mobile and inflamed, with bone loss. Row 4, left: the implant was removed and the socket was debrided. Row 4, right: a fistula persisted after healing. A subsequent surgery revealed a thin root fragment on the buccal aspect of the mesial root socket. After removal of the fragment, an implant was later placed and was successful.

Management

In cases where there is limited jaw opening, tilting the implants mesially allows easier access for the dentist. The dentist may want to use the indirect coping technique that needs less vertical space (Greenberg and Prein, 2002). If access for screw placement is limited, a cement-retained implant prosthesis might be indicated (Rosen and Gornitsky, 2004).

Depending on the situation, control of symptoms of temporomandibular disorders with warm compresses, premedication with nonsteroidal anti-inflammatory drugs, and muscle relaxants may be considered. In the placement of multiple dental implants, one should consider starting with the most posterior implant so as the patient gets tired, the clinician is not "locked" out.

Retained root tips in the implant location

A retained root tip can lead to infection and peri-implantitis (Al-Faraje, 2011) or even implant failure (Figure 7.3). However, it is important to note that a study in baboons found that the unintentional placement of dental implants into retained root fragments did not cause any clinical problems or histological signs of inflammation (Gray and Vernino, 2004). A retained root tip or fragments may also result in poor bone healing, resulting in a fibrous-osseous defect. This will cause the dentist to abort the implant placement and have the implant placement procedures be delayed by 2–3 months.

Prevention

If a root tip is suspected at a dental implant site, a CT scan should be performed to help determine its location. In many cases an implant can be placed 2–4 months after the root tip has been removed. Sometimes it is possible to remove the tip and perform the osteotomy in the same procedure (Al-Faraje, 2011, p. 40).

Management/treatment

The implant site must be monitored for inflammation if the implant has been placed near a root tip.

Factors to consider are as follows:

1 If the root tip has had a previous endodontic procedure or shows sign of a periradicular lesion, it should be extracted, grafted, and replaced.
2 If the root tip is small and does not have a lesion, keep the osteotomy away from it. If the root tip is directly in the way of the osteotomy, remove the root tip and place the implant at the same time (if possible).
3 If the root is too close to the nerve and it can lead to more complications, keep the root tip as it is.

Periodontal considerations

Poor bone quality

Leckholm and Zarb (Brånemark, 1985; (Misch, 2008, p. 647)) classified the jaws according to bone quality and quantity (Table 7.2).

According to the Misch bone density scale, there are five types of bone (Figure 7.4):

Studies show that the greatest implant failure is in areas of the softest bone, especially in the maxilla (Misch, 2008, p. 645). Studies have found that the highest risk factor for implant failure is in type 4 bone found in the maxilla (Hutton *et al.*, 1995 and Goiato *et al.*, 2014). Another study found that of the 10% of the 1054 implants placed in type 4 bone, 35% failed (Jaffin and Berman, 1991). However, another study found no difference in survival rates in marginal bone level between implants positioned in the bone of various densities after 1 year (Bergkvist *et al.*, 2010).

Possible causes of poor quality of the bone are as follows:

1 Older patients with osteoporosis
2 Denture patients with maxillary resorption

Prevention

Avoid overheating the bone and allow the site to be irrigated. The use of internally irrigated drills can decrease heat.

Treatment

Use of surface-treated implants was found in a systematic review to have lower failure rates than machined surface implants (Goiato *et al.*, 2014). Additionally, there is the possibility of overengineering

Table 7.2 Classification of bone quantity and quality.

Bone quantity	Bone quality
A: The alveolar ridge is intact	1: Entire jaw is cortical bone
B: Moderate ridge resorption has occurred	2: Thick cortical bone surrounds a core of dense trabecular bone
C: Advanced residual ridge resorption has occurred	3: Thin layer of cortical bone surrounds a core of dense trabecular bone
D:Some resorption of the basal bone has occurred	4: Thin layer of cortical bone surrounds low-density trabecular bone
E: Extreme resorption of the basal bone has transpired	

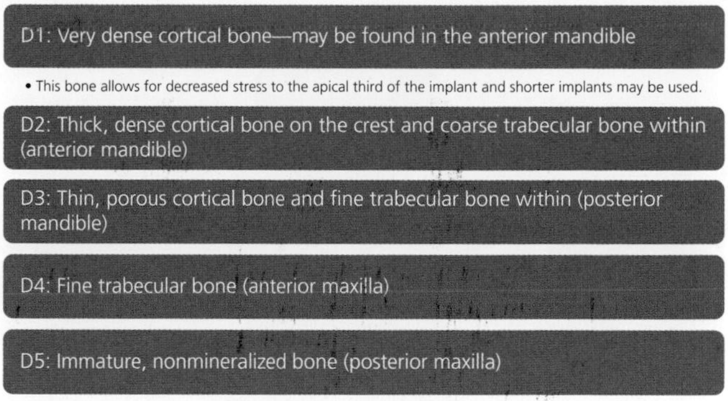

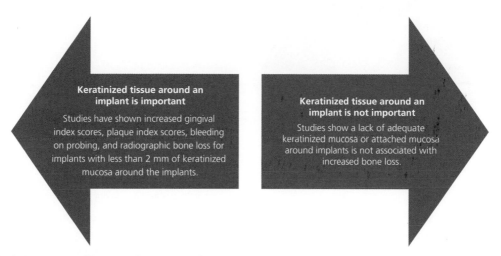

Figure 7.4 Five types of bone in the Misch bone density scale.

D1: Very dense cortical bone—may be found in the anterior mandible

• This bone allows for decreased stress to the apical third of the implant and shorter implants may be used.

D2: Thick, dense cortical bone on the crest and coarse trabecular bone within (anterior mandible)

D3: Thin, porous cortical bone and fine trabecular bone within (posterior mandible)

D4: Fine trabecular bone (anterior maxilla)

D5: Immature, nonmineralized bone (posterior maxilla)

Keratinized tissue around an implant is important

Studies have shown increased gingival index scores, plaque index scores, bleeding on probing, and radiographic bone loss for implants with less than 2 mm of keratinized mucosa around the implants.

Keratinized tissue around an implant is not important

Studies show a lack of adequate keratinized mucosa or attached mucosa around implants is not associated with increased bone loss.

Figure 7.5 The importance of keratinized tissue around implants. (Data from Bouri *et al.* (2008) and Chung *et al.* (2006)).

the case with more implants in type 4 bone. For example, if a case was planned to restore to the maxillary first molar, the clinician can consider placement of an additional implant in the second molar position.

Mucogingival defects around implants

Soft tissue grafting around implants is a controversial topic as depicted in Figure 7.5.

The etiology includes the following (Chu and Tarnow, 2013):

1 Poor implant spatial placement
2 Horizontal biologic width creation
3 Incorrect abutment contour
4 Excessive implant diameter
5 Thin biotype

Soft tissue defects are common in patients with a thin biotype. Figure 7.6 describes the characteristics of a thin biotype.

Prevention

Recognition that a patient has a thin biotype will help the clinician plan for a more gentle extraction that facilitates ridge preservation. Immediate implants are not recommended in these patients. Studies showed that sites with a thin gingival biotype had greater changes in facial gingival levels than sites with a thick gingival biotype (Kan *et al.*, 2011; Evans and Chen, 2008).

The implant should be placed with the buccal surface 1.5 mm from the dental arch curvature (Chen and Buser, 2010, p. 151). If the implant is placed too far facially, soft tissue grafting cannot remedy the recession.

Treatment

A connective tissue graft with a coronally advanced flap may be used to correct recession on the buccal mucosa. Studies have shown clinically significant improvement, but after 6 months the coverage shrank to a mean of

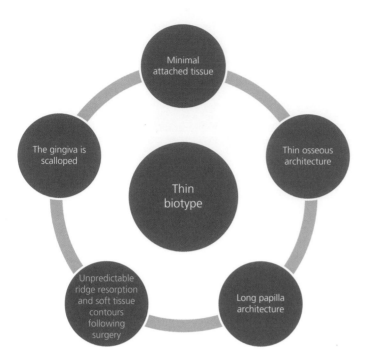

Figure 7.6 Characteristics of thin biotype. (Data from Al-Faraje, 2011, p. 72).

66% (Burkhardt, Joss, and Lang, 2008). Another option is to remove the suprastructures and bury the implant by advancing the flap. Once healing has occurred, a small opening can be made, and the excess soft tissue can be moved to the buccal when replacing the abutment and crown (Chen and Buser, 2010, p. 150). To maintain the tissues in a healthy and stable position over the long term, the abutment-crown contour should be flat or even undercontoured (Chu and Tarnow, 2013).

In cases where an immediate implant must be placed in thin biotype situations, a technique combining subepithelial connective tissue graft and immediate implant placement and provisionalization is recommended to gain a more predictable soft tissue contour (Kan, Rungcharassaeng, and Lozada, 2005).

Patients with periodontitis
The topic is controversial. Figure 7.7 describes the opposing viewpoints on this topic.

Management
In patients with aggressive periodontitis, dental implants should be considered in the overall treatment plan (Klokkevold and Nagy, 2006, p. 700). However, there is a possibility of progressive bone loss around implants in regenerated bone in patients treated for aggressive periodontitis (Mendel and Flores-de-Jacoby, 2005). Hopeless teeth can be used to develop the site for implant placement. With patients who lack papilla and bone, an orthodontist can use forced eruption to regenerate the bone with up to 70% efficacy and soft tissues with up to 60% efficacy (Amato *et al.*, 2012).

The surgeon must consider the following when assessing implant placement in patients with periodontal attachment loss (Rose and Minsk, 2004, p. 621):

1 Loss of attached gingiva
2 Deformities of the osseous structure
3 Poor contour of the soft and hard tissue
4 Change in embrasure space and papilla height

Poor patient compliance
Poor oral hygienc is a major risk factor for implant failure, and it should be addressed prior to dental implant treatment. The oral hygiene of the patient impacts the marginal bone stability around the implant (Quirynen and Teughels, 2003). One of the most important factors for long-term success is good oral hygiene and maintenance care. Plaque control by the patient with manual or powered toothbrushes as well as professional intervention (oral hygiene instruction and mechanical debridement) has been shown to be effective in reducing clinical signs of inflammation (Jepsen *et al.*, 2015).

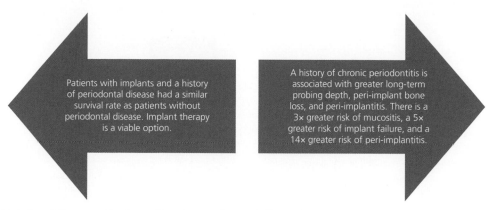

Figure 7.7 Periodontal disease and implants. (Data from Baelum and Ellegaard (2004), Karoussis, Kotsovilis, and Fourmousis (2007), and Swierkot *et al.* (2012)).

Management

Implants should not be an option for patients who appear uncooperative and are not compliant with oral hygiene instructions. If implants have already been placed and the patient is noncompliant, the risks and consequences must be explained to the patient and documented in the chart. Patients must understand and learn how to clean and care for their implants on a daily basis. It is the dentist's responsibility to teach patients effective plaque control skills. If the skills have been mastered by the patient, but are not routinely practiced, then it is a compliance problem. Periodic maintenance visits are essential to remove plaque subgingivally. Three-month cleaning recalls are recommended, especially for patients who have difficulties in performing the necessary plaque control skills (Armitage and Lundgren, 2008, p. 645).

Intraoperative complications

Damage to adjacent teeth

It is devastating when an implant hits an adjacent tooth. It not only compromises the tooth but also the implant. It may be caused by a lack of parallelism or incorrect positioning while inserting the implants (Lamas Pelayo *et al.*, 2008). The adjacent tooth may be devitalized, need endodontic treatment, or even removal (Greenstein and Cavallaro, 2010, p. 405).

Prevention

Meticulous treatment planning with a surgical guide and cone-beam CT images can help the clinician evaluate the space needed to place the implant. It is important to

identify if the roots of adjacent teeth angulate into the space of the planned implant. Furthermore, it is helpful to take periapical radiographs with a guide pin (5 mm depth) during implant placement to ensure that the angulation is correct (Greenstein and Cavallaro, 2010, p. 406).

Treatment

Depending on the amount of damage to the adjacent tooth, the adjacent tooth may have to be adjusted (smoothed, restored), endodontically treated, or removed. The implant will have to be removed and repositioned.

Complications related to flapless surgery

The indications for flapless surgery are the following:
1 Sufficient keratinized mucosa.
2 No bone graft is needed.
3 Good quality and quantity of bone (allow assessment of morphology).

The surgeon must understand the risks and benefits of flapless surgery, depicted in Figure 7.8 (Brodala, 2009).

The flapless technique is "often more demanding than the conventional surgical approach (Brodala, 2009). Therefore, the use of flapless implant placement as a 'routine' procedure in daily practice is not recommended." Another study found the flapless technique had more marginal bone resorption compared with the flap technique (Maló and Nobre, 2008).

Prevention

It is recommended that the surgeon use a surgical guide and three-dimensional radiographs to prevent unwanted clinical outcomes. The dentist should sound

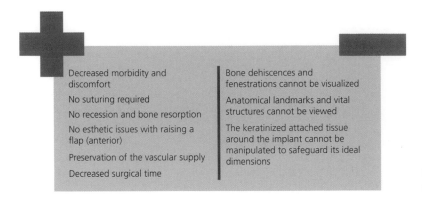

Figure 7.8 Risks and benefits of flapless surgery. (Data from Brodala (2009)).

Decreased morbidity and discomfort	Bone dehiscences and fenestrations cannot be visualized
No suturing required	Anatomical landmarks and vital structures cannot be viewed
No recession and bone resorption	The keratinized attached tissue around the implant cannot be manipulated to safeguard its ideal dimensions
No esthetic issues with raising a flap (anterior)	
Preservation of the vascular supply	
Decreased surgical time	

the bone to verify that the bone in the surgical area is consistently of good quality with no osseous or soft tissue defects. There should be plenty of bone in all three dimensions of the implant because it is easy to cause a dehiscence or fenestration. A good guideline before flapless implant surgery is to have 2 mm of bone around the implant.

Management

There is a possibility that a dehiscence or fenestration may result while drilling. A flap should be raised to cover the defect with guided bone regeneration. The implant may need to be removed or buried when there is an esthetic compromise or when removal of the implant is indicated (Wilson, 2010, p. 353).

Implant hits a vessel

Arteries in danger of being damaged during implant placement are as follows (Al-Faraje, 2011, p. 44):

1 Greater palatine
2 Nasopalatine/incisive
3 Lingual
4 Sublingual
5 Facial
6 Submental

Arterial damage at the floor of the mouth is usually a result of perforation of the lingual cortical plate.

Prevention

As previously mentioned, three-dimensional radiographs are essential in planning cases and preventing complications such as bleeding from a vessel following implant placement. The tip of periosteal elevators should always be placed on bone when reflecting flaps.

Management

Overall emergency management of bleeding from a damaged artery during surgery will depend on the skills and experience of the surgeon.

Bleeding from an artery can be managed in several ways (Al-Faraje, 2011, p. 43):

1 Compression of the vessel
2 Crushing of adjacent bone into the artery to reduce the size of the arterial lumen
3 Electrocautery
4 Hemostatic agents, such as bone wax

It is essential to stop the ongoing procedure, place gauze at the bleeding site, and reassure the patient. It is important to have a trained assistant that won't make comments to scare the patient. A local anesthetic (e.g., lidocaine) with epinephrine can be used temporarily to stop the bleeding.

Major bleeding from the floor of the mouth is a life-threatening situation with difficult access to the sublingual space (Al-Faraje, 2011, p. 47):

1 Call 911 at the first sign of swelling (possible respiratory compromise).
2 Apply pressure.
3 Explain the situation to the patient.
4 The vessel (if buried) should be ligated with the needle entering the tissue 6 mm away from the vessel on one side and exit 3 mm on the other side.
5 If the vessel can be isolated, close the lumen by placing a knot using sutures.

Implant hits a nerve

Nerve damage may arise intraoperatively (e.g., during osteotomy preparation or soft tissue manipulation) or postoperatively (e.g., from swelling of adjacent tissues, compression of the nerve). Postoperative nerve damage does not require immediate intervention (Pi-Anfruns, 2014). There are three types of nerve injuries (Greenstein and Cavallaro, 2010, p. 403):

- Neuropraxia:
  - The least serious. Sensation returns about 1 month after compression of the nerve. The axon is intact.
- Axonotmesis:
  - The nerve structure is not altered but there is ischemia, demyelination, and edema. Some sensation may return in 5–11 weeks with improvement within the next 10 months. Some axons may be damaged.
- Neurotmesis:
  - The nerve is altered (loss of continuity) and no signal can travel through the nerve. A surgery is needed to repair the nerve.

The following are symptoms of nerve injury (Al-Faraje, 2011, p. 25):

1 Paresthesia—atypical sensation
2 Hypoesthesia—reduced sensation
3 Hyperesthesia—increased sensation
4 Dysesthesia—painful (unpleasant) sensation
5 Anesthesia—absolute loss of sensation

The inferior alveolar nerve is the most commonly injured nerve (64.4%), followed by the lingual nerve (28.8%) for all types of oral and maxillofacial surgery (Tay and Zuniga, 2007).

More symptoms

1 Pain
2 Biting the cheek or tongue
3 Drooling

Prevention

Preventing nerve damage requires proper planning by the surgeon (i.e., cone-beam CT and knowledge of the anatomy at the implant site). A three-dimensional radiograph should be taken when important anatomical structures are in the area of the osteotomy. Drill guards can be used to prevent unwanted deep penetration in the osteotomy site (Greenstein and Cavallaro, 2010, p. 403).

Lingual nerve: The nerve can be as close as 5 mm apical to the distal lingual line angle of lower second and third molars. It is essential to place the elevator between the lingual plate and the flap. Any damage to the lingual nerve can cause a loss of sensation to the anterior two-thirds of the ipsilateral half of the tongue (Rateitschak and Wolf, 1995). Incisions should be in the retromolar pad area

(occlusal surface), and lingual vertical incisions should not be made distal to the first molar.

Inferior alveolar nerve: The implant should be placed 2 mm above the inferior alveolar canal. The following are some signs of inferior alveolar canal involvement when deciding to extract a tooth and place an implant (Farnad, 2014):

1 Darkening and notching of the root
2 Deflected roots at the region of the canal
3 Narrowing of the root
4 Interruption of the canal outline
5 Diversion of the canal from its normal course
6 Narrowing of the canal outline

Mental nerve: Clinicians should be mindful of the anterior loop of the mental nerve. It can be 3 mm anterior to the mental foramen (Al-Faraje, 2011, p. 27). The clinician should avoid incisions on the buccal aspect of the lower bicuspid area.

Anterior palatine/nasopalatine nerves: The chance for paresthesia is rare; however, the clinician should avoid incisions in the incisive papilla area and protect the flap with a periosteal elevator when doing surgery.

Management

The following tests need to be done by the dentist after a nerve injury has occurred:

1 Two-point discrimination.
2 Static light touch.
3 Brush stroke.
4 Vibrational test.
5 A map of the affected site must be drawn.

Patients should get a second opinion within the first 3 weeks of nerve injury. If a patient is numb for greater than 16 weeks, the nerve was likely disrupted and needs to be repaired (Greenstein and Cavallaro, 2010, p. 403)

Appropriate scans will be needed and the implant(s) will have to be removed. The patient needs to be carefully monitored following removal of the implants (Greenwood and Corbett, 2012). If the surgeon decides to let the implant remain without placing a crown, a traumatic neuroma may form, which can be painful (Greenstein and Cavallaro, 2010, p. 403).

Fractured jaw

The following are symptoms of mandibular fracture after implant placement (Al-Faraje, 2011, p. 81):

1 Fracture when there has not been trauma
2 Occlusal change

3 Swelling

4 Pain

Some studies found that mandibular fractures occurred 0.05% of the time in mandibles with a height of 10 mm or less, as measured at the mandibular symphysis. Other reasons fractures may occur 1 year or more after implant placement include peri-implantitis and trauma (Soehardi *et al.*, 2011).

Prevention

A cone-beam scan should be done on patients with atrophic mandibles to be able to determine the quality and quantity of bone at the site. After preparing the osteotomy, a few millimeters of cortical bone should remain on both the lingual and the labial sites (Chrcanovic and Custódio, 2009).

Bone grafting procedures (e.g., block graft or guided bone regeneration) may be done prior to the insertion of the implants to increase the bone strength and volume. Shorter abutments can minimize the stress on the implants, and the surgeon should refrain from excessive tightening of the implant (Al-Faraje, 2011, p. 81). Wide-diameter implants should be avoided in an alveolar ridge with significant horizontal resorption.

Treatment

There are a number of considerations that the surgeon must evaluate in deciding to whether remove or retain the implant (Al-Faraje, 2011, p. 81):

1 The stability of the implant

2 The importance of the implant to the overall treatment plan

3 Presence or absence of infection

4 Mobility of the fractured bone (Greenstein and Cavallaro, 2010, p. 412)

The following are treatment options for fractured mandibles (Soehardi *et al.*, 2011):

1 Closed reduction (immobilization)

2 Rigid fixation using osteosynthesis plates

3 Bone grafts with fixation

4 Occlusal restoration

Complications were found in 48% of the patients who had implant-associated fractures. These included non-union, osteomyelitis, screw loosening, plate fracture, and dehiscences with subsequent infections (Soehardi *et al.*, 2011). It is difficult to treat fractures because of the diminished blood supply to the site and the depressed vitality of the bone (Chrcanovic and Custódio, 2009).

These patients need to be placed on a soft diet and trained to limit jaw movements (Al-Faraje, 2011, p. 81).

Implant fracture

Implant fracture may occur during implant surgery or postoperatively. Studies have shown that the incidence of implant fractures in an implant-supported fixed partial denture after 5 years is 0.4% (Pjetursson *et al.*, 2004). The incidence of implant fracture in a combined tooth/implant-supported fixed partial denture is 0.9% after 5 years (Lang *et al.*, 2004a and 2004b).

Causes of implant fracture postoperatively include the following (Gealh *et al.*, 2011):

1 Bone loss around an implant can lead to fracture of the implant (below the abutment screw).

2 Design of the material: the crown's infrastructure made of nonprecious metal alloy.

3 Trauma (e.g., more with ceramic implants) (Spiekerman, 1995).

4 Nonpassive fit of the prosthetic structure—misfit or distortion.

5 Physiological or biomechanical overload (e.g., bruxism, clenching, or cantilevers).

6 Repeated gold screw or abutment loosening (Eckert and Salinas, 2010, p. 102).

Causes of implant fracture during surgery include the following:

1 Implant design: Small-diameter internal hex implants may not be able to withstand the torque applied when placed in dense bone (Al-Faraje, 2011, p. 83).

2 Dense bone was not tapped before placement of the implant.

Implant fracture is relatively uncommon. Studies have found 0.2% of 4045 implants had fractures in 5 years of service (Balshi, 1996). All patients with a fractured implant had parafunctional habits. The partially edentulous jaw encounters implant fractures more frequently than edentulous patients (Eckert and Salinas, 2010, p. 108).

Prevention

Patients with parafunctional habits should be given an occlusal guard to be worn at night. The surgeon may recommend a greater number and a wider diameter of implants to distribute the force to prevent implant fracture. It is also important for the surgeon to adjust lateral forces when screw loosening is encountered (Eckert and Salinas, 2010, p. 104).

Treatment

In most cases both fragments of a fractured implant will have to be removed with a trephine drill. However, if there is still adequate threads available, reversal tools can be used. If the implant is not to be replaced, the apical fragment may remain to prevent further bone loss (Spiekerman, 1995). The supraosseous portion may be ground down so it is flush with the osseous level. However, the fractured implant may become infected, and the patient must be monitored.

Surgical trauma

Overheating the bone can cause bone resorption and physiological damage to the bone.

Prevention

1 Studies have shown that the maximum drill speed of 2000 rpm with copious sterile saline irrigation should be used to prevent overheating. The threshold for bone damage is 47°C for 1 min (Eriksson and Albrektsson, 1984).
2 Sharp drills should always be utilized. In type 1 bone, the surgeon should use a drill 1–3 times, and about 10 times in type 2 bone. The surgeon can use the drill about 40 times in type 3 bone and 100 or more times with type 4 bone (Al-Faraje, 2011, p. 49).
3 The surgeon should use an in-and-out motion with the handpiece when preparing the osteotomy site to allow the irrigation to reach the bur's cutting edges.

Signs and symptoms (Piatelli *et al.*, 1998)

1 No regeneration of bone around the implant
2 Bone sequestra
3 Necrotic bone and bacteria around the implant
4 Inflammatory response in the area between the implant and the bone
5 No organization of the peri-implant bone clot
6 Presence of mature and compact bone around the implant

Treatment

The implant and necrotic bone needs to be removed. The patient may need antibiotics and pain medication if an infection is present. A new implant may be placed with a bone graft in 3–4 months (Al-Faraje, 2011, p. 50).

Compression necrosis

Compression necrosis is the overcompression of the adjacent bone during implant placement. An undersized osteotomy can cause compression necrosis. Areas of dense bone have a higher risk for this complication. Compression necrosis occurs within the first month, and the histology will show inflamed granulation tissue and nonviable bone sequestra with bacterial colonization (Bashutski, D'Silva, and Wang, 2009).

An initial torque of 20 N cm is ideal to achieve osseointegration. However, a higher torque of 30–45 N cm (bone necrosis may occur at higher torques in type 1 or 2 bone) is recommended for immediate loaded implants because of the stress they encounter from the provisional prosthesis (Al-Faraje, 2011, p. 85).

Prevention

1 Use drill in the correct order.
2 Use tapping drills in dense bone.
3 Before the implant is just short of its placement, a hand ratchet is recommended to have better control over the level of torque.

Broken instruments

Although it is rare for an instrument to break, it is possible and is a serious complication. Instruments are constantly sharpened and sterilized, and this can lead to fractures.

Treatment and management

If small fragments cannot be located, radiographs are necessary. There are special magnetic instruments that can attract the fragment and allow for retrieval. If there is a chance that the fragment has been aspirated, a chest radiograph is necessary. If the fragment was swallowed, periodic monitoring of feces is vital to make sure it passes through the digestive system.

Postoperative complications

Peri-implant mucositis

Peri-implant mucositis is the presence of inflammation in the soft tissue surrounding a dental implant without signs of any loss of supporting bone (Figure 7.9). This is a treatable and reversible plaque-induced inflammatory condition. A systematic review found that peri-implant mucositis arises in approximately 63.4% of the subjects and in 30.7% of the implants. Peri-implantitis was discovered in 18.8% of subjects and in 9.6% of implant sites. The incidence of peri-implant disease is higher in smokers (36.3%) compared to nonsmokers (Atieh *et al.*, 2013). Maintenance therapy reduces the rate of peri-implant

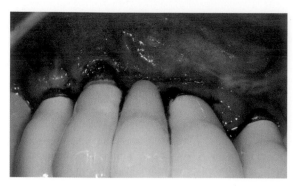

Figure 7.9 Peri-implant mucositis around implant restorations in the anterior maxilla. Note the lack of vestibular depth and keratinized attached gingiva, making oral hygiene difficult.

disease (Atieh *et al.*, 2013). In a 5-year systematic study, 6.3% of the implants had bone loss exceeding 2 mm over the 5-year observation period, and peri-implantitis and soft tissue complications occurred adjacent to 9.7% of the implant-supported single crowns (Jung *et al.*, 2008).

Clinical signs
1 Inflammation
2 Bleeding on probing (BOP)
3 Suppuration
4 Pockets that are greater than 4 mm

Possible etiology
1 Bacteria: The bacteria associated with gingivitis resemble the bacteria associated with mucositis (Lang, Wilson, and Corbet, 2000; Pontoriero *et al.*, 1994).
2 The sites that facilitate bacterial colonization and retention are the implant-abutment junction and the implant surfaces (Fletcher, 2014). Furthermore, switching abutments between companies result in greater risk for poor fit.
3 Excess or residual cement (Wilson, 2009).
4 Lack of keratinized gingiva (Block *et al.*, 1996).
   A consensus report (Lindhe and Meyle, 2008) found the following risk indicators:
1 Poor oral hygiene
2 A history of periodontitis
3 Diabetes
4 Smoking

Prevention
Oral hygiene by the professional and patient is required to minimize the bacterial load. The sooner peri-implant mucositis is diagnosed, the sooner treatment can be rendered. Peri-implant mucositis can be treated nonsurgically. Because of the problem of decontamination of the roughened, threaded surfaces of exposed implants, peri-implantitis is more difficult to treat (Khammissa *et al.*, 2012). Maintenance care should be conducted routinely based on the patient's susceptibility.

Management
Oral hygiene must be reviewed with the patient. Figure 7.10 describes the cumulative interceptive supportive therapy protocol for treating peri-implant mucositis and peri-implantitis.
   The main goals are as follows:
1 Disrupt the colonization of the plaque biofilm.
2 Dilute the bacterial load.
3 Detoxify the implant surface by mechanical and chemotherapeutic means (e.g., curettes, ultrasonics, abrasives, lasers, saline, citric acid, and chlorhexidine) (Fletcher, 2014).

Studies have found mechanical nonsurgical therapy and antimicrobial mouth rinses effective in the treatment of peri-implant mucositis lesions. However, in peri-implantitis lesions nonsurgical therapy was ineffective (Renvert, Roos-Jansåker, and Claffey, 2008).

Mechanical debridement (protocol A)
1 Curette: Must be soft because metal curettes can severely damage the implant surface. Carbon fiber curettes are sturdy enough to remove calculus yet they do not harm the implant surface (Eckert and Salinas, 2010, p. 104).
2 Ultrasonic scalers: Can cause a rough surface that attracts plaque (Rapley *et al.*, 1990); however, other studies found positive results for ultrasonic scalers with a nonmetal tip on polished and sand blasted, large grit, acid-etched surface (Louropoulou, Slot, and Van der Weijden, 2014).
3 Lasers: Some studies find them advantageous over conventional treatment and some studies do not (Kreisler *et al.*, 2003). A review article found no significant difference (in BOP, probing depth reduction of clinical attachment levels, or bone fill) between saline-soaked pellets at 12 and 24 months of follow-up and the use of the Er:YAG laser (Valderrama and Wilson, 2013).
4 Air abrasives: Studies have shown it to be a viable treatment option *in vitro* for implant surface cleaning in peri-implantitis treatment (Tastepe *et al.*, 2012).

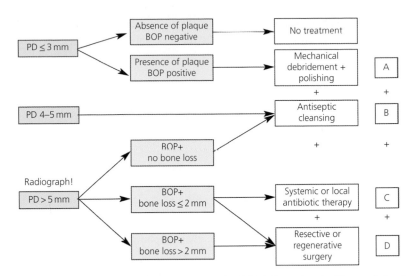

Figure 7.10 Management of mucositis and peri-implantitis. (Lang *et al.* (2004a). Reproduced with permission from Quintessence Publishing Group Inc., Chicago, IL). The protocol (cumulative interceptive supportive therapy) is additive, in that as pocketing and signs of inflammation progress, additional treatments are added.

5 Titanium brush: This brush is composed of a stainless steel shaft with titanium bristles that is inserted into an implant machine handpiece. It is recommended to protect the inner connection of the implant before debridement with a cover screw or healing abutment. It is for single patient use only. Studies have found it to be gentler to the implant surface and more effective in plaque removing capacity than steel curettes (John, Becker, and Schwarz, 2014). Randomized controlled studies are needed to further evaluate the efficacy of titanium brushes.

Chemotherapeutic (antiseptic protocol B) (Fletcher, 2014)

1 Chlorhexidine: It has high substantivity but it is not effective intracrevicularly. Studies have found no difference between patients receiving chlorhexidine irrigation and another group of patients receiving no treatment for 8 weeks (Lavigne *et al.*, 1994). Another study found the supplement of chlorhexidine (irrigation and gel) to mechanical debridement did not improve the effects as compared to mechanical debridement alone (Porras *et al.*, 2002).

2 0.25% sodium hypochlorite irrigation: Irrigation with 0.25% NaOCl results in an 80-fold decrease in bacterial endotoxin compared to water and reduces gingival inflammation and supragingival biofilm

accumulation (De Nardo *et al.*, 2012). This solution does not corrode titanium.

3 Citric acid: A review article found that citric acid is effective at decreasing the amount of lipopolysaccharide present on machined surface and hydroxyapatite-coated implants, but not on titanium plasma-sprayed implants (Valderrama and Wilson, 2013). Another study found citric acid conditioning of a peri-implantitis-affected surface improves nanohydroxyapatite-blended clot adhesion to the titanium implant surfaces (Gamal, Abdel-Ghaffar, and Iacono, 2013). More randomly controlled studies are needed to evaluate the clinical significance of citric acid.

Antibiotic protocol C

1 Minocycline microspheres are a bioabsorbable locally applied antibiotic. It has been found to improve bleeding scores and mean probing depth (from 5.0 to 4.1 mm) around peri-implant infections (Renvert *et al.*, 2004 and Salvi *et al.*, 2007).

2 Systemic antibiotics: Systemic administration of antibiotics has been shown to decrease the subgingival bacterial load and target the anaerobic segment in patients with peri-implantitis when used in conjunction with mechanical debridement (Mombelli and Lang, 1992; Renvert, Roos-Jansåker, and Claffey, 2008). However, systemic antibiotics do not remove biofilms, and it is unlikely that they are sufficient interventions for peri-implant disease.

If the patient has 4 mm pocket with BOP or 5 mm pockets with or without BOP, sodium hypochlorite irrigation in conjunction with debridement is recommended. If there is no resolution after 3 months, the treatment is repeated and minocycline microspheres are used and the restoration is removed and cleansed (remove plaque, detoxify the platform, and screw opening) (Lang *et al.*, 2004a, 2004b; Fletcher, 2014). The patient is encouraged to use antiseptic mouthwash and triclosan toothpaste at home. Studies have shown reductions in plaque index, gingival index, and bleeding index in the peri-implant gingival tissues (Ciancio *et al.*, 1995; Sreenivasan *et al.*, 2011), although long-term studies on the treatment of peri-implant disease are needed.

Regenerative or resective therapy (protocol D)

Once the infection has been controlled and treatment modalities A, B, and C have been tried, surgery can be considered. Regenerative therapy or resective therapy may be done based on the morphologic characteristics and size of the defect (Lang and Tonetti, 2010, p. 129).

Regenerative

1 Biologic mediators (e.g., enamel matrix derivative and platelet-derived growth factor): Their effects are debatable, but studies have shown that grown factors have positive effects on implant osseointegration (Qu *et al.*, 2011; Froum, Froum, and Rosen, 2012).
2 The defect configuration may have a big impact on the ability to regenerate the defect. Circumferential intrabony defects seem to be favorable in conjunction with a natural bone mineral and a collagen membrane. Defects with a buccal dehiscence (e.g., circumferential or semicircumferential) are not favorable (Schwartz *et al.*, 2010).

Resective therapy It is important to inform the patient that resective therapy, especially in the esthetic area, may lead to a poor esthetic outcome. It has been shown that the percentage of implants that turned out to be healthy subsequent to treatment (pocket reduction and bone recontouring) was higher for those with minimal initial bone loss (2–4 mm bone loss as evaluated during surgery) compared with the implants with a bone loss of ≥ 5 mm (74% vs. 40%) (Serino and Turri, 2011).

Combined resective and regenerative approach Implantoplasty, the removal of the suprabony implant threads affected by peri-implantitis, has been shown to be successful in combination with deproteinized bovine bone mineral and a collagen membrane. Regenerative and resective treatment of peri-implant defects produced positive outcomes in terms of radiographic defect bone fill and probing depth reduction after 12 months (Matarasso *et al.*, 2014).

Another study found that resective therapy with implantoplasty had a positive influence on the survival of oral implants involved with inflammatory processes (Romeo *et al.*, 2005).

Peri-implantitis

Peri-implantitis is a destructive inflammatory reaction affecting the soft and hard tissues, and it can result from peri-implant mucositis. Bleeding, suppuration, and loss of osseointegration of the coronal part of the implant, by increased probing depth, are some features of peri-implantitis. Treatment is not predictable for peri-implantitis (Khammissa *et al.*, 2012). The risk factors for periodontitis and peri-implantitis are similar. The progression from mucositis to peri-implantitis follows a very similar path of events as the progression of gingivitis to periodontitis. However, peri-implantitis has episodes of rapid progression and can be more pronounced than in cases of chronic periodontitis (Heitz-Mayfield and Lang, 2010). In most cases peri-implantitis-associated bone loss is characterized by a nonlinear progression, with the rate of loss increasing over time (Fransson *et al.*, 2010). Some of the differences between peri-implantitis and periodontitis are described in Table 7.3 (Figure 7.11).

Risk factors

1 Genetics:
   ○ Gene polymorphisms: It has been shown that there is a potential link between IL-1 genotype and peri-implantitis (Dereka *et al.*, 2012).
2 Poor oral hygiene:
   ○ Studies show that bacteria can be transmitted from the periodontal pocket to the peri-implant region (Sumida *et al.*, 2002). Periodontitis-enhancing factors such as poor oral hygiene and smoking also increase the risk for peri-implantitis (Quirynen, De Soete, and van Steenberghe, 2002).
3 History of periodontal disease:
   ○ Compared with periodontally healthy patients, subjects with a history of chronic periodontitis may

Table 7.3 Similarities and differences between periodontal disease and peri-implantitis.

	Periodontal disease	Peri-implantitis
Substructure	Enamel and dentin	Ceramic, acrylic, metal
Biofilm necessary	Yes	Yes
Microbiota	Gram-negative bacteria	Gram-negative bacteria and *Staphylococcus aureus* may be important bacteria in the initiation of peri-implantitis. A recent study (Aoki *et al.*, 2012) found colonization by bacteria at the implant sulcus was influenced by microorganisms in the gingival crevice of adjacent teeth as opposed to those on contralateral and occluding teeth
Host response	Inflammatory response	Persistent biofilm may cause a more pronounced inflammatory reaction; may involve the alveolar bone sooner (may be due to differences in vascularity and fibroblast-to-collagen ratios)
Therapy	Anti-infective	Anti-infective surgical access may be needed more frequently and sooner due to implant surface characteristics and microbial access limitations

Data from Heitz-Mayfield and Lang (2010).

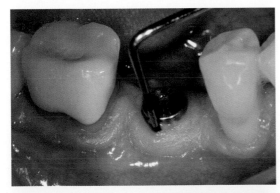

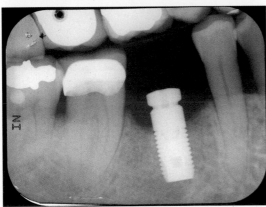

Figure 7.11 Peri-implantitis in a patient with partially treated periodontitis. The patient also had a history of implant loss in the #13 site.

exhibit significantly greater peri-implant marginal bone loss, long-term increases in probing depths, and incidence of peri-implantitis (Karoussis, Kotsovilis, and Fourmousis, 2007; Heitz-Mayfield and Lang, 2010). Peri-implantitis was a more frequent finding in patients with a history of periodontal disease and excess cement (Linkevicius *et al.*, 2012).

4 Smoking:
  o Smokers exhibit greater probing depth and pus around implants compared to nonsmokers (Fransson, Wennström, and Berglundh, 2008).

5 Diabetes:
  o There is evidence that diabetes is associated with peri-implantitis (Daubert *et al.*, 2015). Diabetes is considered a risk indicator for peri-implantitis (Lindhe and Meyle, 2008).

Etiology

1 Bacteria: Peri-implant mucositis can develop into peri-implantitis if it is not treated early. Bacteria can be a factor in the following situations:

  i) Contamination of the implant before placement (Al-Faraje, 2011, p. 108).

  ii) Preexisting bacteria at the time of surgery (e.g., bacteria from a previous infection) causing a retrograde infection (Quirynen *et al.*, 2005).

  iii) Fit of restoration: The gap should be minimal between the implant and the prosthesis.

2 Excess cement: Excess dental cement has been associated with signs of peri-implant disease. Studies have found that signs of inflammation were absent in 74% of implants after the removal of excess cement (Wilson, 2009).

3 Implant malpositioning: The deeper the position of the implant margin, the greater the amount of cement was found. Cement excess should not be evaluated using dental radiographs (i.e., it is not a reliable method) (Linkevicius *et al.*, 2013).

4 Local factors: Overcontouring the restoration can make plaque control difficult and lead to accumulation of plaque.

Figure 7.12 describes the advantages and disadvantages of cement-retained restorations.

Classification

Table 7.4 describes another classification system of peri-implantitis based on the severity of the disease. A combination of probing depth, extent of radiographic bone loss around the implant, and BOP and/or suppuration is used to classify the severity of peri-implantitis (Froum and Rosen, 2012).

Management

Figure 7.10 describes the protocol for management of peri-implantitis. Patients need to be instructed on proper oral hygiene techniques similar to methods used on natural dentition. It is imperative that the excess cement be removed and the implant surface detoxified. If regeneration is deemed necessary, it can be done with a soft tissue graft if there is a mucogingival defect. Some studies have found that in most cases, nonsurgical therapy achieved similar results to those of more complex therapies (Byrne, 2012) (Figure 7.13).

Postoperative bleeding

Please see postoperative bleeding in the periodontal chapter.

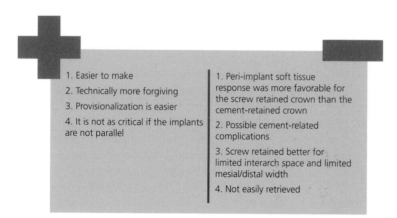

1. Easier to make
2. Technically more forgiving
3. Provisionalization is easier
4. It is not as critical if the implants are not parallel

1. Peri-implant soft tissue response was more favorable for the screw retained crown than the cement-retained crown
2. Possible cement-related complications
3. Screw retained better for limited interarch space and limited mesial/distal width
4. Not easily retrieved

Figure 7.12 The advantages and disadvantages of cement-retained crowns (Weber *et al.*, 2006).

Table 7.4 Classification of peri-implantitis.

	Early	Moderate	Advanced
Probing depth Bleeding and/or suppuration on probing noted on two or more aspects of the implant	Pocket depth is greater than 4 mm	Pocket depth is greater than 6 mm	Pocket depth is greater than 8 mm
Bone loss Measured on radiographs from the time of definitive prosthesis loading to current radiograph. If not available, the earliest available radiograph following loading should be used	Bone loss is less than 25% of the implant length	Bone loss is 25–50% of the implant length	Bone loss is greater than 25% of the implant length

Data from Froum and Rosen (2012).

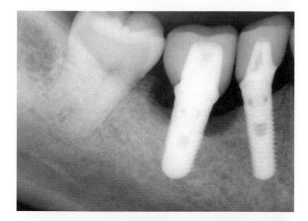

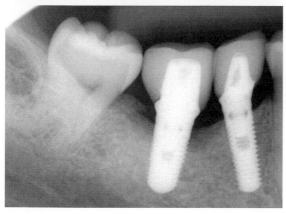

Figure 7.13 A case of peri-implantitis treated with mechanical debridement, 0.12% chlorhexidine, and oral hygiene instruction. The bottom radiograph shows increased radiopacity after only 5 weeks of treatment.

Bone growth over the cover screw at second-stage surgery

This complication may occur for several reasons (Al-Faraje, 2011, p. 106):

1 The implant is placed below the crestal bone.
2 Second-stage implant surgery is done after 8 months or longer.

It is imperative that the surgeon use extreme caution when removing bone to prevent damage to the platform of the implant.

Treatment/management

Always make sure the top of the implant is protected by placing the cover screw on top of the fixture. A bone mill or small chisels may be used to remove the

bony overgrowth (Al-Faraje, 2011, p. 106). A radiograph should be taken to make sure there is no space between the healing abutment and the fixture/platform.

Loss of a posterior implant in an all-on-four prosthesis

There are a number of risk factors that may cause a posterior implant to fail. According to Parel and Phillips (2011), these include the following:

1 Opposing natural dentition: Both existing opposing natural mandibular dentition (80%) and poor bone density (85%) presented the highest percentages of all failure scenarios.
2 Poor bone density (e.g., the posterior maxilla).
3 Male patient: Men are three times more likely to experience a primary implant failure.
4 Bruxism: About half of the failures in this study had a bruxing component. However, in none of these individuals was bruxing the only contributing factor.
5 Smoking: Patient compliance with smoking cessation can have a potentially significant role in the incidence of primary failures.
6 Bone volume: The evaluation of bone volume and bone density with a CAT scan was identified as important in planning maxillary implant therapy.
7 Cantilevers: Implants placed in the premolar–molar cantilever region are subjected to higher occlusal loads, even when the distal extension cantilever length was reduced in the provisional prosthesis.

Prevention

If the patient has one or more risk factors listed earlier, additional implants or delayed loading should be used. Because implants are more likely to fail in the maxillary arch, one or two additional implants can be placed. A pterygoid implant can also be placed to engage the pterygoid process without bone augmentation (Parel and Phillips, 2011). It is also important for the surgeon to limit the amount of cantilevers, stagger the implants (e.g., implants should not be placed in a straight line), use a wider diameter implant in molar sites, and see the patient more frequently for postoperative checks (Goodacre and Kattadiyil, 2010, p. 183). Patients who have a history of bruxism should use an occlusal guard.

Treatment/management

The failed implant should be removed and a replacement implant placed after adequate bony healing, approximately 6 months (Wang *et al.*, 2015). The replacement implant should not have any load placed on it until the surgeon deems that it is osseointegrated.

Implant mobility

Implant failure is defined as the state where the implant is no longer integrated after placement. Failure may occur early (i.e., before osseointegration and usually during the first year) or late (i.e., during and after the restorative treatment) (Rosenberg *et al.*, 2010, p. 111). Primary stability at the time of implant placement is necessary to ensure successful osseointegration. One meta-analysis found the failure rate at 7.7% over a 5-year period (bone graft excluded) (Esposito *et al.*, 1998). Another study (Berglundh, Persson, and Klinge, 2002) found implant failure of 2–3% when the implant was in function and a 2–3% failure rate of implants supporting fixed reconstructions. Patients with overdentures had a 5% failure rate during a 5-year period. No evident differences in implant survival were found between the different implant systems (Eckert *et al.*, 2005).

Possible causes of implant mobility

1 Infection
2 Host factors (smoking, autoimmune disorders)
3 Occlusion and loading
4 Poor bone quality
5 Poor prosthetic design (Rosenberg *et al.*, 2010, p. 111)
6 Inability of the surgeon to achieve primary stability
7 Trauma to the tissue (pressure necrosis and overheating of the bone) (Rosenberg *et al.*, 2010, p. 112)
8 Prior history of periodontitis
   Table 7.5 describes the characteristics associated with an infectious or traumatic cause of mobility.

Prevention

The cause of the failure must be diagnosed and addressed as soon as possible to make every effort to reverse the complication (Rosenberg *et al.*, 2010, p. 111). It is imperative that the surgeon plan the case thoroughly (e.g., cone-beam imaging, mounted study casts with diagnostic wax-ups, and review of systemic and local risk factors).

Table 7.5 Characteristics evaluated to determine the etiology of failure.

Condition	Infectious	Traumatic
Pain	Yes	Yes/no
Tissue inflammation	Yes	No
Broken implant parts/crown wear	No	Yes
Mobility	Yes	Yes
Bleeding on probing	Yes	No
Suppuration	Yes	No
Increased probing depth	Yes	No
Gingival index	High	Low
Plaque index	High	Low
Peri-implant radiolucency	Yes	Yes
Granulomatous tissue on removal	Yes	No

Rosenberg *et al.* (2010), p. 113. Reproduced with permission from Wiley.

Treatment

When the implant is found to be mobile, it needs to be removed. If there is adequate bone and minimal infection, an immediate implant may be an option (after thorough degranulation). A wider diameter implant with possible bone grafting may be necessary and antibiotics prescribed (Rosenberg *et al.*, 2010, p. 116). Studies have (Machtei *et al.*, 2008) found a survival rate of 83.5% for implants placed in previously failed sites. This is a much lower survival rate compared to implants placed in pristine sites.

Dental changes of adjacent natural teeth relative to the implant crown

When teeth and implants coexist and subtle adult craniofacial growth occurs, complications may occur. Throughout adulthood there is tooth drifting and change in arch length. The continuous eruption of the adjacent anterior teeth can cause great risk of a less favorable esthetic and/or functional implant outcome. The placement of an implant in patients with a normal facial profile should be postponed until growth has concluded. For patients with a long or short face type, further growth, particularly the continuous eruption of adjacent teeth, creates a crucial risk even after the age of 20 years (Heij *et al.*, 2006). When changes in tooth position relative to implant restorations secondary to long-term adult growth happens, they can cause complications that are difficult to treat (Daftary *et al.*, 2013).

Immediate implant placement

Implants placed in fresh extraction sockets, referred to as immediate implants, are a unique clinical challenge with a higher complexity and therefore a higher potential for complications. The most common complications associated with immediate implants are discussed in this section, with guidelines on prevention and management. The concepts and guidelines of prevention and management of implant complications still apply; only the complications unique to immediate implants will be discussed in this section.

Immediate implant failure

While immediate implants have a high survival rate, several studies show higher failure rates compared to more delayed implant placement protocols. A meta-analysis of seven randomized controlled trials comparing immediate implants with immediate-delayed implants and delayed implants did not show statistically significant differences of implant survival between the groups, but several preliminary conclusions were made that were not statistically significant, including a possibly higher implant failure rate in the immediate group (Esposito *et al.*, 2010). Individual randomized controlled trials either show no difference in implant survival (Siegenthaler *et al.*, 2007) or a higher failure rate with immediate implants (Schropp *et al.*, 2005; Lindeboom, Tjiook, and Kroon, 2006), with implant survival rates of as little as 91% in these studies. A cross-sectional analysis also identified immediate implant placement as a risk factor for implant failure (Daubert *et al.*, 2015).

Prevention

Although survival of the immediate implant is high, several studies show higher failure rates of immediate implants. Therefore, prevention of this complication encourages the use of a nonimmediate implant placement protocol.

The following list of requirements for success has been published for the prevention of complications with immediately placed implants (Wagenberg and Froum, 2010): (i) removal of all infectious material from the socket, (ii) adequate available bone and soft tissue, (iii) initial implant stability, (iv) patient cooperation with postsurgical maintenance, (v) apical or lateral stabilization, (vi) residual infection removed, (vii) careful determination of patient expectations, and (viii) consideration of final outcome after healing.

Midfacial gingival recession in the anterior maxilla

A systematic review by Chen and Buser (2014) showed that esthetic outcomes are achievable with immediate implants in the anterior maxilla, but the esthetic results are more variable, and there is a higher frequency of midfacial recession than implants placed in a delayed fashion. A literature review showed 0.5–0.9 mm of midfacial gingival recession with immediate implant placement (Chen and Buser, 2009).

Risk factors

The two major risk factors identified in midfacial recession are buccal implant positioning and thin periodontal biotype (Chen *et al.*, 2009). Buccal malposition of the immediate implant is a possibility because the extraction socket, which is more buccal than the ideal placement of the implant, tends to push the osteotomy and the implant into the empty socket.

Proper diagnosis and treatment planning can prevent poor esthetic outcome. The following factors are important to consider: medical status, smoking habit, patient's esthetic expectations, lip line, tissue biotype, shape of tooth crowns, infection at implant site, bone level of adjacent teeth, restorative status of neighboring teeth, width of edentulous span, soft tissue anatomy, and bone anatomy of alveolar crest.

Prevention

Ideal implant position in the anterior maxilla is palatal to the incisal edge, which will result in thicker hard and soft tissue buccal to the implant (Figure 7.14) and a slight buccal cantilever to the restoration.

Prevention first involves presurgical treatment planning with a three-dimensional imaging that shows the volume and position of the bone. The clinician must decide before extraction whether an immediate implant can be stabilized in an ideal position. Ideally, an

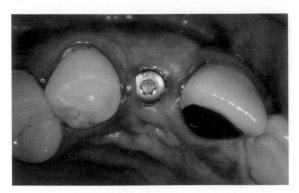

Figure 7.14 Anterior implants need to be placed palatal to the incisal edge in order to avoid gingival recession.

immediate implant in the anterior maxilla will have 5 mm of bone apical to the extraction socket to stabilize the implant.

If an implant can safely be placed into an extraction socket, the use of a tapered implant can allow for easier angulation of the implant for proper palatal emergence of the head of the implant. The narrower apex of the tapered implant reduces the incidence and severity of fenestration of the bony concavity of the anterior maxilla during the osteotomy, and it increases the primary stability of the implant.

To prevent buccal malposition, the surgeon usually must initiate the osteotomy in the palatal bone of the extraction socket in the anterior maxilla. This is facilitated by using a sharp implant drill to create a purchase point for ideal positioning of the initial twist drill. A Lindemann side-cutting drill can also be used (Al-Faraje, 2011, p. 13).

If the patient has thin bone or thin soft tissue, a bone and/or connective tissue graft can be placed at the implant surgery appointment to thicken the tissue. The crescent-shaped soft tissue graft has been described for flapless cases (Han and Jeong, 2009). It must be reemphasized that bone and/or soft tissue grafting cannot make up for buccal malpositioning of the implant.

Treatment

If an implant cannot be stabilized in an ideal position, the implant should not be placed, and the extraction socket and osteotomy should be filled with a ridge preservation bone graft to minimize alveolar resorption while the extraction socket heals, a process that takes 3–6 months. Alternatively, a delayed approach has been shown to be predictable and successful (Buser *et al.*, 2013).

If the implant is restored and midfacial recession has occurred, the clinician must evaluate the etiology of the recession and determine if reshaping of the restorative abutment or crown can reverse the recession. If an implant is poorly positioned, it must be removed.

Generally speaking, treatment of mucogingival defects around implants by soft tissue grafting is not predictable (Levine, Huynh-Ba, and Cochran, 2014), and it cannot overcome poor implant positioning.

Sinus floor bone graft complications

The edentulous posterior maxilla often has limited vertical bone height for dental implant placement. Sinus floor bone grafts, commonly referred to as sinus lifts, are predictable methods of increasing the vertical bone height for implant placement by raising the floor of the maxillary sinus and filling the space with a bone graft.

The maxillary sinus is a pyramid-shaped air space in the maxilla, above the roots of the maxillary posterior teeth, approximately 10–15 ml in volume. It is lined by the Schneiderian membrane, a pseudostratified ciliated columnar epithelium overlying a thin layer of connective tissue, between 0.45 and 1.40 mm thick (Katsuyama and Jensen, 2011, p. 14). The ostium drains the maxillary sinus high on the medial wall.

There are two approaches to accessing the sinus floor for bone grafting: through the lateral wall of the maxillary sinus and crestally through an implant osteotomy.

These procedures are advanced surgical procedures and should only be attempted by experienced surgeons with proper training. The reader is guided through the presentation, prevention, and management of the most common sinus floor bone graft complications. The surgeon can use this chapter as a guide to manage sinus lift complications that arise in the office.

Lateral approach for sinus floor bone graft

The lateral approach involves preparing an opening in the lateral bony wall of the maxillary sinus to allow access to elevate the Schneiderian membrane off of the bony floor. A bone graft is placed between the membrane and the bone, a membrane is placed over the window, and the site is closed. If sufficient height of native bone is available to stabilize an implant, an implant may be placed simultaneously. The lateral approach is appropriate for large bone grafts, for

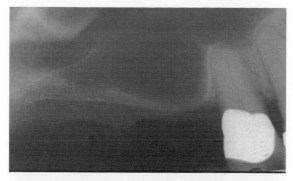

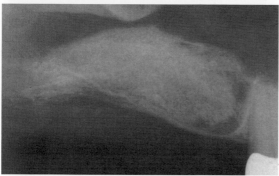

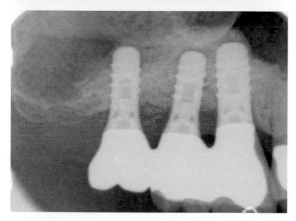

Figure 7.15 A case of the lateral approach sinus floor bone grafting (middle radiograph), with a 10-year follow-up after implant placement (bottom radiograph). (S. Nelson, San Mateo, CA. Reproduced with permission from S. Nelson).

significant increase in vertical height, and for visual access of the sinus (Figure 7.15).

The lateral approach sinus lift is a predictable way to increase the vertical bone height for implant placement in the posterior maxilla. Implants placed into bone-grafted sinuses have high predictability and well-documented long-term survival rates of greater than 95%

(Del Fabbro, Wallace, and Testori, 2013; Wallace and Froum, 2003; Aghaloo and Moy, 2007). The following are among the more common complications of the lateral approach to sinus floor bone grafting.

Membrane perforation

The most common intraoperative complication of the lateral approach is perforation of the Schneiderian membrane, with an incidence of approximately 10% (range 4.8–56%) (Chiapasco, Casentini, and Zaniboni, 2009). Wallace (2010) estimated that experienced surgeons have about 25% perforation rate with rotary instrumentation. If unrepaired, perforation can lead to loss of graft material, graft infection, reduced bone formation, and decrease in implant survival (Proussaefs *et al.*, 2004).

Perforation of the sinus membrane can occur during preparation of the lateral window, during elevation of the membrane with hand instruments, during placement and condensation of graft material, or even on flap elevation with thin or absent bone (Wallace, 2010). Thin Schneiderian membranes are more prone to perforation, and complex sinus anatomy, such as bony septa, are associated with membrane perforation (Wallace, 2010, pp. 286–287).

Prevention

Proper presurgical evaluation of the bony sinus anatomy through three-dimensional radiography, such as cone-beam scans, can assist the surgeon in planning the surgery (Figure 7.16). Preparation of the lateral window using a piezosurgery device that cuts bone but not soft tissue has been shown to reduce the perforation rate to as low as 7% (Wallace *et al.*, 2007). If rotary instrumentation is to be used, a diamond bur would be preferable to a carbide bur (Wallace, 2010). Preparation of a large enough window to allow access to the sinus and around septa can prevent perforations (Wallace, 2010, p. 287). Wallace (2010) recommends a window that is 3 mm above the floor of the sinus, 3 mm distal to the anterior border of the sinus, and 15 mm in height. When elevating the membrane, it is important that the elevating instruments stay in contact with the bone. Piezosurgery devices can remove septa without tearing the thin overlying membrane.

Management

Small perforations can be repaired with a collagen membrane. If a perforation is small enough, it can close spontaneously. If the perforation occurs before full

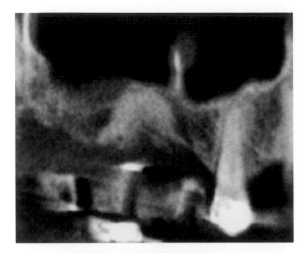

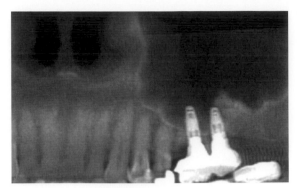

Figure 7.17 Cone-beam scan of implant placed in sites #14 and #15 three years ago by an inexperienced surgeon. The implant has perforated the floor of the maxillary sinus, and bone graft particles have migrated posterior to the distal implant.

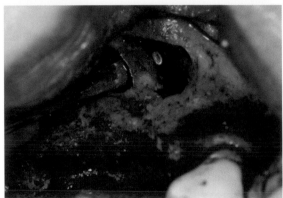

Figure 7.16 Radiographic and clinical views of a prominent septum in the right maxillary sinus.

elevation of the membrane, the elevation should be carefully completed without expansion of the perforation. Larger perforation repairs can be attempted using resorbable sutures, although this is difficult. Membrane stabilization and graft containment are required for repairs. Techniques have been reported for managing large perforations (Testori *et al.*, 2008). If containment and stability of the graft cannot be achieved, the procedure should be aborted, and the patient allowed to heal for 2–4 months before a subsequent attempt. This is an uncommon complication, occurring less than 1% of the time (Chiapasco, Casentini, and Zaniboni, 2009).

Intraoperative bleeding

The blood supply to the lateral maxillary sinus is provided by intraosseous and extraosseous branches of the maxillary artery, specifically the posterior superior alveolar artery, the greater palatine artery, and the infraorbital artery (Solar *et al.*, 1999). Preparation of the lateral window results in bleeding from the lateral wall of the sinus. This bleeding is usually minor and of relatively short duration but at times can be profuse and difficult to control (Wallace, 2010, p. 284).

Prevention

Preoperative medical history evaluation should be done to determine if the patient is on anticoagulants or has a clotting disorder. Cone-beam scans can identify intraosseous vessels in the lateral wall, allowing for presurgical planning of window placement and surgical technique (Figure 7.17). Elian *et al.* (2005) showed that 53% of sinuses have a radiographically visible intraosseous vessel by CT scan, and that 20% of these cases have the vessel in a position where it is likely to be cut or damaged by preparation of the lateral wall. Piezosurgery can reduce the incidence and severity of intraoperative bleeding by reducing soft tissue damage. With this knowledge, the surgeon can preoperatively plan window placement and surgical technique to reduce the likelihood of blood vessel damage.

Management

Bleeding during lateral window preparation and membrane elevation is flowy in nature and usually manageable (Wallace, 2010, p. 243). Use of a piezosurgery device will provide lavage with sterile saline, allowing better visualization. If bleeding is more severe, other measures may be needed, such as direct pressure on the bleeding site, use of local vasoconstrictors, bone wax, or crushing of bone surrounding an intraosseous vessel (Wallace, 2010).

Postoperative infection

Infection following lateral window sinus lifts has been reported to occur between 2 and 5.6% of cases (Testori *et al.*, 2012). Most infections occur in the early postoperative period, but some infections can show up after several months.

Prevention

Testori *et al.* (2012) recommended preoperative antibiotics of amoxicillin 875 mg and clavulanic acid 125 mg twice per day, beginning 24 h before surgery and three times per day for 7 days postoperatively. Patients with a penicillin allergy are recommended to take clarithromycin 250 mg twice per day and metronidazole 250 mg thrice per day, beginning 24 h before surgery and extending 7 days after surgery.

Infections can be reduced with aseptic surgical technique.

Evaluation and treatment for preoperative sinusitis, especially microbial in origin, can help prevent infections, especially if a perforation occurs.

Management

If a postoperative infection develops, it must be treated quickly with antibiotics. If unsuccessful, consider referral to an otolaryngologist and/or surgical debridement of the infected tissues.

Postoperative sinusitis

Postoperative sinusitis has been reported following lateral window sinus lifts, with reports of mild discomfort, stuffiness, and difficulty breathing through the nose (Wallace, 2010, p. 305). The average incidence of postoperative sinusitis has been reported to be 2.5%, with different studies reporting a range of 0–27% (Chiapasco, Casentini, and Zaniboni, 2009). Postoperative sinusitis is correlated with presurgical chronic sinusitis, membrane hypertrophy, and postextraction timing of the surgical procedure (Timmenga *et al.*, 1997). More moderate to severe sinusitis following sinus lifts is most likely from blockage of the ostium, preventing proper drainage of the sinus (Wallace, 2010, p. 305). Sinusitis can be of inflammatory or infectious in nature and be caused by postoperative edema, bleeding from a sinus perforation, and exfoliation of graft particles into the sinus. Figure 7.18 shows a case of sinusitis caused by implants sticking through the Schneiderian membrane.

Prevention

Because many incidents of postoperative sinusitis are correlated with presurgical sinusitis, proper medical evaluation and assessment of the health of the sinus are important. If the patient has any sinus pathology, or if radiographs or three-dimensional imaging show sinus pathology, it is prudent to refer for evaluation and treatment by an otolaryngologist. Antibiotics and/or anti-inflammatory medication may be needed.

Proper surgical management is necessary to prevent postoperative sinusitis. If a perforation occurs, the repair must be stable and contain the graft.

Treatment

Decongestants and saline rinses can be performed to manage mild postoperative sinusitis. If the etiology is microbial, antibiotics may be needed. More severe cases of sinusitis should be referred to an otolaryngologist.

Osteotome/crestal approach sinus lift complications

The crestal approach, first described by Tatum (1986) and later modified by Summers (1994), involves preparation of the implant osteotomy to within 1 mm of the sinus floor, then elevating the bone and soft tissue by fracturing the floor of the maxillary sinus and elevating the Schneiderian membrane. An implant is placed simultaneously. Later techniques included addition of bone graft into the osteotomy and using the graft to elevate the membrane with osteotomes (Figure 7.19). More recent variations employ different methods of reaching the sinus floor and lifting the Schneiderian membrane.

The crestal approach is less invasive than the lateral approach, but it does not allow for visualization of the membrane and can achieve only limited increases in bone height. Fugazzotto (2005) reports that the maximum amount of predictable bone height with a crestal approach sinus lift is $2x-2$ mm, where x is the preoperative bone height. Several authors suggest a minimum of 5 mm bone height to be able to stabilize an implant placed simultaneously (Rosen, 2010; Summers, 1994).

The primary disadvantage of this technique is that it is not possible to visualize perforation of the Schneiderian membrane.

It has been recommended that the crestal approach sinus lift only be attempted by surgeons properly

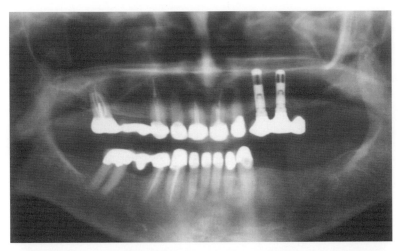

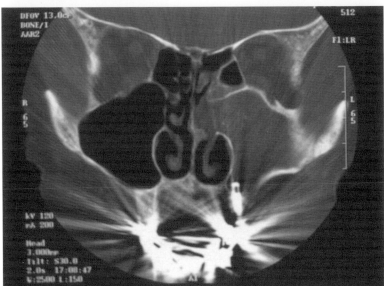

Figure 7.18 Severe maxillary sinusitis caused by implants placed into the sinus in an 83-year-old woman. The implants were placed 12 years prior to the radiographs. The patient's entire left maxillary sinus was occluded.

trained in performing a lateral window sinus lift (Katsuyama and Jensen, 2011, p. 6).

Perforation

Perforation of the Schneiderian membrane is the most common intraoperative complication of the crestal approach sinus lift (Fugazzotto, Melnick, and Al-Sabbagh, 2015). A systematic review by Tan *et al.* (2008) showed a range of perforation of 0–21.4%, with a mean of 3.8%. Perforation can be caused by overzealous elevation of the membrane, extending the

osteotomes beyond the sinus floor, or the presence of sinus anatomy such as septa.

Prevention

Prevention of perforation includes proper case selection with a minimum of 5 mm of crestal bone height, a flat sinus floor, following the 2x–2 rule (Fugazzotto, 2005) to prevent overstretching of the sinus membrane, cone-beam scans to evaluate bony anatomy of the sinus, radiographic verification of the osteotome 1 mm below the sinus floor, and gentle surgical technique and tapping.

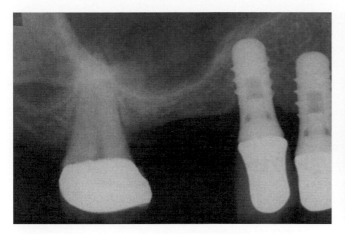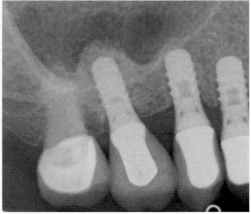

Figure 7.19 Radiographs showing a 12-year postoperative result of a crestal approach sinus lift. (S. Nelson, San Mateo, CA. Reproduced with permission from S. Nelson).

Management

After preparation of the osteotomy and sinus floor elevation, a Valsalva maneuver can be performed. If air passes from the maxillary sinus through the osteotomy, a perforation is present and must be managed with either repair using tissue fibrin glue (Pjetursson *et al.*, 2004), repair from opening a lateral window, or by allowing the site to heal for 4–6 months, and then attempting the procedure again.

Inadequate primary stability

With limited bone height and porous type 4 bone in the posterior maxilla, there is potential for compromised primary stability of implants. Implants with less primary stability are more likely to be lost (Rosen, 2010).

Prevention

Proper case selection, with adequate buccopalatal bone width and at least 5 mm of native vertical bone height, is necessary for implant stability. The use of a tapered implant or tulip-shaped implant can improve primary stability of the implant. If the bone is porous, the osteotomy can be undersized to improve primary stability. Finally, a provisional restoration must not have any contact with the implant during the healing period.

Poor patient experience and vertigo

The most well-documented technique for crestal approach sinus lifts involves tapping for the elevation of the sinus floor, and this is perceived by patients as a

negative experience (Diserens *et al.*, 2006). This malleting technique has also been associated with benign paroxysmal positional vertigo (BPPV), with symptoms of dizziness, imbalance, lightheadedness, and nausea. BPPV is not progressive and symptoms subside or disappear within 6 months (Rosen, 2010, p. 316).

Prevention

Prevention of the poor patient experience includes patient education (Rosen, 2010, p. 319), conscious sedation (Fugazzotto, Melnick, and Al-Sabbagh, 2015), and surgical planning to minimize tapping, including drilling to within 1 mm of the sinus floor, and preparation of the osteotomy with drills rather than osteotomes. Fugazzotto, Melnick, and Al-Sabbagh (2015) also recommend a gentle, intermittent malleting technique. Recent techniques and products can reduce or eliminate the need to fracture the sinus floor, with either special drills or piezosurgery devices that do not cut soft tissue.

Management

Management of BPPV should include referral to an otolaryngologist for evaluation. Management by the otolaryngologist may include an Epley maneuver.

Infection

Infection following a crestal approach sinus lift is uncommon but has been reported to occur between 0 and 2.5% of cases, with a mean of 0.8% (Tan *et al.*, 2008). The most likely cause of infection is either poor oral hygiene, contamination of the implant or graft during insertion, or infection from a perforated Schneiderian membrane, especially one with untreated sinusitis (Rosen, 2010, p. 311). Prevention includes resolution of preexisting sinus disease, aseptic surgical technique, and preoperative and postoperative antibiotics as described by Testori *et al.* (2012). Management of a postoperative infection includes systemic antibiotics.

Acknowledgments

The authors wish to thank Dr. Richard Kao, Dr. Paul Fugazzotto, Dr. Gary Armitage, Dr. Mark Ryder, and Mrs. Melanie Nelson for reviewing this chapter.

References

Aghaloo, T.L. and Moy, P.K. (2007) Which hard tissue augmentation techniques are the most successful in furnishing bony support for implant placement? *Int J Oral Maxillofac Implants*, **22** (suppl), 49–70.

Al-Faraje, L. (2011) *Surgical Complications in Oral Implantology*, Quintessence, Chicago, IL.

Amato, F., Mirabella, A.D., Macca, U. and Tarnow, D.P. (2012) Implant site development by orthodontic forced extraction: a preliminary study. *Int J Oral Maxillofac Implants*, **27**, 411–420.

Aoki, M., Takanashi, K., Matsukubo, T., Yajima, Y., Okuda, K., Sato, T. and Ishihara, K. (2012) Transmission of periodontopathic bacteria from natural teeth to implants. *Clin Implant Dent Relat Res*, **14**, 406–411.

Armitage, G.C. and Lundgren, T. (2008) Risk assessment of the implant patient, in *Clinical Periodontology and Implant Dentistry*, 5th edn (eds J. Lindhe, N.P. Lang and T. Karring), Blackwell Munksgaard, Oxford, pp. 634–651.

Atieh, M.A., Alsabeeha, N.H., Faggion, C.M., Jr and Duncan, W.J. (2013) The frequency of peri-implant diseases: a systematic review and meta-analysis. *J Periodontol*, **84**, 1586–1598.

Baelum, V. and Ellegaard, B. (2004) Implant survival in periodontally compromised patients. *J Periodontol*, **75**, 1404–1412.

Balshi, T.J. (1996) An analysis and management of fractured implants: a clinical report. *Int J Oral Maxillofac Implants*, **11**, 660–666.

Bashutski, J.D., D'Silva, N.J. and Wang, H.L. (2009) Implant compression necrosis: current understanding and case report. *J Periodontol*, **80**, 700–704.

Belser, U.C., Bernard, J.-P. and Buser, D. (2003) Implants in the esthetic zone, in *Clinical Periodontology and Implant Dentistry*,
5th edn (eds J. Lindhe, N.P. Lang and T. Karring), Blackwell Munksgaard, Oxford, pp. 1146–1174.

Bergkvist, G., Koh, K.J., Sahlholm, S., Klintström, E. and Lindh, C. (2010) Bone density at implant sites and its relationship to assessment of bone quality and treatment outcome. *Int J Oral Maxillofac Implants*, **25**, 321–328.

Berglundh, T., Persson, L. and Klinge, B. (2002) A systematic review of the incidence of biological and technical complications in implant dentistry reported in prospective longitudinal studies of at least 5 years. *J Clin Periodontol*, **29**, 197–212.

Block, M.S., Gardiner, D., Kent, J.N., Misiek, D.J., Finger, I.M. and Guerra, L. (1996) Hydroxyapatite-coated cylindrical implants in the posterior mandible: 10-year observations. *Int J Oral Maxillofac Implants*, **11**, 626–633.

Bouri, A., jr, Bissada, N., Al-Zahrani, M.S., Faddoul, F. and Nouneh, I. (2008) Width of keratinized gingiva and the health status of the supporting tissues around dental implants. *Int J Oral Maxillofac Implants*, **23**, 323–326.

Brånemark, P.I. (1985) An introduction to osseointegration, in *Tissue-integrated Prostheses: Osseointegration in Clinical Dentistry* (eds P.-I. Brånemark and T. Albrektsson), Quintessence, Chicago, IL, pp. 11–53.

Brodala, N. (2009) Flapless surgery and its effect on dental implant outcomes. *Int J Oral Maxillofac Implants*, **24**, 118–125.

Burkhardt, R., Joss, A. and Lang, N.P. (2008) Soft tissue dehiscence coverage around endosseous implants: a prospective cohort study. *Clin Oral Implants Res*, **19**, 451–457.

Buser, D., Chappuis, V., Bornstein, M.M., Wittneben, J.G., Frei, M. and Belser, U.C. (2013) Long-term stability of contour augmentation with early implant placement following single tooth extraction in the esthetic zone: a prospective, cross-sectional study in 41 patients with a 5- to 9-year follow-up. *J Periodontol*, **84** (11), 1517–1527.

Byrne, G. (2012) Effectiveness of different treatment regimens for peri-implantitis. *J Am Dent Assoc*, **143**, 391–392.

Chen, S. and Buser, D. (2009) in *ITI Treatment Guide, Vol. 3: Implant Placement in Post-Extraction Sites: Treatment Options* (eds D. Buser, D. Wismeijer and U. Belser), Quintessence, Chicago, IL.

Chen, S.T. and Buser, D. (2010) Esthetic complications due to implant malpositions: etiology, prevention, and treatment, in *Dental Implant Complications: Etiology, Prevention and Treatment* (ed S.J. Froum), Wiley-Blackwell, Hoboken, NJ, pp. 134–155.

Chen, S.T. and Buser, D. (2014) Esthetic outcomes following immediate and early implant placement in the anterior maxilla: a systematic review. *Int J Oral Maxillofac Implants*, **29** (suppl), 186–215.

Chen, S.T., Darby, I.B., Reynolds, E.C. and Clement, J.G. (2009) Immediate implant placement postextraction without flap elevation. *J Periodontol*, **80** (1), 163–172.

Chiapasco, M., Casentini, P. and Zaniboni, M. (2009) Bone augmentation procedures in implant dentistry. *Int J Oral Maxillofac Implants*, **24** (suppl), 237–259.

Chrcanovic, B.R. and Custódio, A.L. (2009) Mandibular fractures associated with endosteal implants. *Oral Maxillofac Surg*, **13**, 231–238.

Chu, S.J. and Tarnow, D.P. (2013) Managing esthetic challenges with anterior implants. Part 1: Midfacial recession defects from etiology to resolution. *Compend Contin Educ Dent*, **34**, 26–31.

Chung, D.M., Oh, T.J., Shotwell, J.L., Misch, C.E. and Wang, H.L. (2006) Significance of keratinized mucosa in maintenance of dental implants with different surfaces. *J Periodontol*, **77**, 1410–1420.

Ciancio, S.G., Lauciello, F., Shibly, O., Vitello, M. and Mather, M. (1995) The effect of an antiseptic mouthrinse on implant maintenance: plaque and peri-implant gingival tissues. *J Periodontol*, **66**, 962–965.

Daftary, F., Mahallati, R., Bahat, O. and Sullivan, R.M. (2013) Lifelong craniofacial growth and the implications for osseo-integrated implants. *Int J Oral Maxillofac Implants*, **28**, 163–169.

Daubert, D.M., Weinstein, B.F., Bordin, S., Leroux, B.G. and Flemming, T.F. (2015) Prevalence and predictive factors for peri-implant disease and implant failure: a cross-sectional analysis. *J Periodontol*, **86** (3), 337–347.

De Nardo, R., Chiappe, V., Gómez, M., Romanelli, H. and Slots, J. (2012) Effects of 0.05% sodium hypochlorite oral rinse on supragingival biofilm and gingival inflammation. *Int Dent J*, **62**, 208–212.

Del Fabbro, M., Wallace, S.S. and Testori, T. (2013) Long-term implant survival in the grafted maxillary sinus: a systematic review. *Int J Periodontics Restorative Dent*, **33** (6), 773–783.

Dereka, X., Mardas, N., Chin, S., Petrie, A. and Donos, N. (2012) A systematic review on the association between genetic predisposition and dental implant biological complications. *Clin Oral Implants Res*, **23**, 775–788.

Diserens, V., Mericske, E., Schäppi, P. and Mericske-Stern, R. (2006) Transcrestal sinus floor elevation: report of a case series. *Int J Periodontics Restorative Dent*, **26** (2), 151–159.

Eckert, S.E. and Salinas, T.J. (2010) Implant fractures: etiology, prevention, and treatment, in *Dental Implant Complications: Etiology, Prevention, and Treatment*, Wiley-Blackwell, Chichester.

Eckert, S.E., Choi, Y.G., Sánchez, A.R. and Koka, S. (2005) Comparison of dental implant systems: quality of clinical evidence and prediction of 5-year survival. *Int J Oral Maxillofac Implants*, **20**, 406–415.

Elian, N., Wallace, S., Cho, S.C., Jalbout, Z.N. and Froum, S. (2005) Distribution of the maxillary artery as it relates to sinus floor augmentation. *Int J Oral Maxillofac Implants*, **20** (5), 784–787.

Eriksson, R.A. and Albrektsson, T. (1984) The effect of heat on bone regeneration: an experimental study in the rabbit using the bone growth chamber. *J Oral Maxillofac Surg*, **42**, 705–711.

Esposito, M., Hirsch, J.M., Lekholm, U. and Thomsen, P. (1998) Biological factors contributing to failures of osseointegrated oral implants. (I). Success criteria and epidemiology. *Eur J Oral Sci*, **106**, 527–551.

Esposito, M., Grusovin, M.G., Polyzos, I.P., Felice, P. and Worthington, H.V. (2010) Interventions for replacing missing teeth: dental implants in fresh extraction sockets (immediate, immediate-delayed and delayed implants). *Cochrane Database Syst Rev*, **8** (9), CD005968.

Evans, C.D. and Chen, S.T. (2008) Esthetic outcomes of immediate implant placements. *Clin Oral Implants Res*, **19**, 73–80.

Farnad, F. (2014) *Oral Surgery Complications*. Lecture in Alpha Omega Conference, March 2014, Los Angeles, CA, USA.

Fletcher, P. (2014) *Diagnosis, Prevention and Treatment of Peri-Implant Disease*. Lecture in Peri-implantitis, February 26, 2014, Los Angeles, CA, USA.

Fransson, C., Wennström, J. and Berglundh, T. (2008) Clinical characteristics at implants with a history of progressive bone loss. *Clin Oral Implants Res*, **19**, 142–147.

Fransson, C., Tomasi, C., Pikner, S.S., Gröndahl, K., Wennström, J.L., Leyland, A.H. and Berglundh, T. (2010) Severity and pattern of peri-implantitis-associated bone loss. *J Clin Periodontol*, **37**, 442–448.

Froum, S.J. and Rosen, P.S. (2012) A proposed classification for peri-implantitis. *Int J Periodontics Restorative Dent*, **32**, 533–540.

Froum, S.J., Froum, S.H. and Rosen, P.S. (2012) Successful management of peri-implantitis with a regenerative approach: a consecutive series of 51 treated implants with 3- to 7.5-year follow-up. *Int J Periodontics Restorative Dent*, **32**, 11–20.

Fugazzotto, P.A. (2005) Treatment options following single-rooted tooth removal: a literature review and proposed hierarchy of treatment selection. *J Periodontol*, **76** (5), 821–831.

Fugazzotto, P., Melnick, P.R. and Al-Sabbagh, M. (2015) Complications when augmenting the posterior maxilla. *Dent Clin North Am*, **59** (1), 97–130.

Gamal, A.Y., Abdel-Ghaffar, K.A. and Iacono, V.J. (2013) A novel approach for enhanced nanoparticle-sized bone substitute adhesion to chemically treated peri-implantitis-affected implant surfaces: an in vitro proof-of-principle study. *J Periodontol*, **84**, 239–247.

Ganeles, J., Zöllner, A., Jackowski, J., ten Bruggenkate, C., Beagle, J. and Guerra, F. (2008) Immediate and early loading of Straumann implants with a chemically modified surface (SLActive) in the posterior mandible and maxilla: 1-year results from a prospective multicenter study. *Clin Oral Implants Res*, **19**, 1119–1128.

Gealh, W.C., Mazzo, V., Barbi, F. and Camarini, E.T. (2011) Osseointegrated implant fracture: causes and treatment. *J Oral Implantol*, **37**, 499–503.

Goiato, M.C., dos Santos, D.M., Santiago, J.F., Jr, Moreno, A. and Pellizzer, E.P. (2014) Longevity of dental implants in type IV bone: a systematic review. *Int J Oral Maxillofac Surg*, **43** (9), 1108–1116.

Goodacre, C.J. and Kattadiyil, M.T. (2010) Prosthetic-related dental implant complications: etiology, prevention, and treatment, in *Dental Implant Complications: Etiology, Prevention and Treatment* (ed S.J. Froum), Wiley, Oxford, pp. 172–196.

Gray, J.L. and Vernino, A.R. (2004) The interface between retained roots and dental implants: a histologic study in baboons. *J Periodontol*, **75**, 1102–1106.

Greenberg, A.M. and Prein, J. (2002) *Craniomaxillofacial Reconstructive and Corrective Bone Surgery: Principles of Internal Fixation Using the AO/ASIE Technique*, Springer-Verlag, New York.

Greenstein, G. and Cavallaro, J.S. (2010) A potpourri of surgical complications associated with dental implant placement: 35 case reports – common problems, avoidance, and management, in *Dental Implant Complications: Etiology, Prevention and Treatment* (ed S.J. Froum), Wiley-Blackwell, Hoboken, NJ, pp. 388–414.

Greenwood, M. and Corbett, I. (2012) *Dental Emergencies*, Wiley-Blackwell, Oxford.

Grunder, U. (2011) Crestal ridge width changes when placing implants at the time of tooth extraction with and without soft tissue augmentation after a healing period of 6 months: report of 24 consecutive cases. *Int J Periodontics Restorative Dent*, **31**, 9–17.

Han, T. and Jeong, C.W. (2009) Bone and crescent shaped free gingival grafting for anterior immediate implant placement: technique and case report. *The Journal of Implant & Advanced Clinical Dentistry*, (July/August), 23–32.

Heij, D.G., Opdebeeck, H., van Steenberghe, D., Kokich, V.G., Belser, U. and Quirynen, M. (2006) Facial development, continuous tooth eruption, and mesial drift as compromising factors for implant placement. *Int J Oral Maxillofac Implants*, **21**, 867–878.

Heitz-Mayfield, L.J. and Lang, N.P. (2010) Comparative biology of chronic and aggressive periodontitis vs. peri-implantitis. *Periodontology*, **53**, 167–181.

Hutton, J.E., Heath, M.R., Chai, J.Y., Harnett, J., Jemt, T., Johns, R.B., McKenna, S., McNamara, D.C., van Steenberghe, D., Taylor, R. *et al.* (1995) Factors related to success and failure rates at 3-year follow-up in a multicenter study of overdentures supported by Brånemark implants. *Int J Oral Maxillofac Implants*, **10**, 33–42.

Huynh-Ba, G., Pjetursson, B.E., Sanz, M., Cecchinato, D., Ferrus, J., Lindhe, J. and Lang, N.P. (2010) Analysis of the socket bone wall dimensions in the upper maxilla in relation to immediate implant placement. *Clin Oral Implants Res*, **21**, 37–42.

Jaffin, R.A. and Berman, C.L. (1991) The excessive loss of Branemark fixtures in type IV bone: a 5-year analysis. *J Periodontol*, **62**, 2–4.

Jepsen, S., Berglundh, T., Genco, R., Aass, A.M., Demirel, K., Derks, J., Figuero, E., Giovannoli, J.L., Goldstein, M.,

Lambert, F., Ortiz-Vigon, A., Polyzois, I., Salvi, G.E., Schwarz, F., Serino, G., Tomasi, C. and Zitzmann, N.U. (2015) Primary prevention of peri-implantitis: managing peri-implant mucositis. *J Clin Periodontol*, **42** (Suppl 16), S152–S157.

John, G., Becker, J. and Schwarz, F. (2014) Rotating titanium brush for plaque removal from rough titanium surfaces: an in vitro study. *Clin Oral Implants Res*, **25** (7), 838–842.

Jung, R.E., Pjetursson, B.E., Glauser, R., Zembic, A., Zwahlen, M. and Lang, N.P. (2008) A systematic review of the 5-year survival and complication rates of implant-supported single crowns. *Clin Oral Implants Res*, **19**, 119–130.

Kan, J.Y., Rungcharassaeng, K. and Lozada, J.L. (2005) Bilaminar subepithelial connective tissue grafts for immediate implant placement and provisionalization in the esthetic zone. *J Calif Dent Assoc*, **33**, 865–871.

Kan, J.Y., Rungcharassaeng, K., Lozada, J.L. and Zimmerman, G. (2011) Facial gingival tissue stability following immediate placement and provisionalization of maxillary anterior single implants: a 2- to 8-year follow-up. *Int J Oral Maxillofac Implants*, **26**, 179–187.

Karoussis, I.K., Kotsovilis, S. and Fourmousis, I. (2007) A comprehensive and critical review of dental implant prognosis in periodontally compromised partially edentulous patients. *Clin Oral Implants Res*, **18**, 669–679.

Katsuyama, H. and Jensen, S.S. (2011) in *ITI Treatment Guide, Vol. 5: Sinus Floor Elevation Procedures* (eds S. Chen, D. Buser and D. Wismeijer), Quintessence, Chicago, IL.

Khammissa, R.A., Feller, L., Meyerov, R. and Lemmer, J. (2012) Peri-implant mucositis and peri-implantitis: clinical and histopathological characteristics and treatment. *S Afr Dent J*, **67** (122), 124–126.

Klokkevold, P.R. (2006) Implant-related complications and failures, in *Carranza's Clinical Periodontology*, 10th edn, Elsevier, St. Louis, MO.

Klokkevold, P.R. and Nagy, R.J. (2006) Treatment of aggressive and atypical forms of periodontitis, in *Carranza's Clinical Periodontology*, 10th edn (eds N. Takei and K. Carranza), Elsevier, St. Louis, MO, p. 700.

Kreisler, M., Kohnen, W., Marinello, C., Schoof, J., Langnau, E., Jansen, B. and d'Hoedt, B. (2003) Antimicrobial efficacy of semiconductor laser irradiation on implant surfaces. *Int J Oral Maxillofac Implants*, **18**, 706–711.

Lamas Pelayo, J., Peñarrocha Diago, M., Martí Bowen, E. and Peñarrocha, D.M. (2008) Intraoperative complications during oral implantology. *Med Oral Patol Oral Cir Bucal*, **13**, E239–E243.

Lang, N.P. and Tonetti, M.S. (2010) Peri-implantitis: etiology, pathogenesis, prevention, and therapy, in *Dental Implant Complications: Etiology, Prevention and Treatment* (ed S.J. Froum), Wiley-Blackwell, Hoboken, NJ, pp. 119–133.

Lang, N.P., Wilson, T.G. and Corbet, E.F. (2000) Biological complications with dental implants: their prevention, diagnosis and treatment. *Clin Oral Implants Res*, **11** (Suppl 1), 146–155.

Lang, N.P., Pjetursson, B.E., Tan, K., Brägger, U., Egger, M. and Zwahlen, M. (2004a) A systematic review of the survival and complication rates of fixed partial dentures (FPDs) after an observation period of at least 5 years. II. Combined tooth-implant-supported FPDs. *Clin Oral Implants Res*, **15**, 643–653.

Lang, N.P., Berglundh, T., Heitz-Mayfield, L.J., Pjetursson, B.E., Salvi, G.E. and Sanz, M. (2004b) Consensus statements and recommended clinical procedures regarding implant survival and complications. *Int J Oral Maxillofac Implants*, **19**, 150–154.

Lavigne, S.E., Krust-Bray, K.S., Williams, K.B., Killoy, W.J. and Theisen, F. (1994) Effects of subgingival irrigation with chlorhexidine on the periodontal status of patients with HA-coated integral dental implants. *Int J Oral Maxillofac Implants*, **9**, 156–162.

Levine, R.A., Huynh-Ba, G. and Cochran, D.L. (2014) Soft tissue augmentation procedures for mucogingival defects in esthetic sites. *Int J Oral Maxillofac Implants*, **29** (suppl), 155–185.

Lindeboom, J.A., Tjiook, Y. and Kroon, F.H. (2006) Immediate placement of implants in periapical infected sites: a prospective randomized study in 50 patients. *Oral Surg Oral Med Oral Pathol Oral Radiol Endod*, **101** (6), 705–710.

Lindhe, J. and Meyle, J. (2008) Group D of European Workshop on Periodontology. Peri-implant diseases: consensus report of the Sixth European Workshop on Periodontology. *J Clin Periodontol*, **35**, 282–285.

Linkevicius, T., Puisys, A., Vindasiute, E., Linkeviciene, L. and Apse, P. (2012) Does residual cement around implant-supported restorations cause peri-implant disease? A retrospective case analysis. *Clin Oral Implants Res*, **24**, 1179–1184.

Linkevicius, T., Vindasiute, E., Puisys, A., Linkeviciene, L., Maslova, N. and Puriene, A. (2013) The influence of the cementation margin position on the amount of undetected cement. A prospective clinical study. *Clin Oral Implants Res*, **24**, 71–76.

Louropoulou, A., Slot, D.E. and Van der Weijden, F. (2014) The effects of mechanical instruments on contaminated titanium dental implant surfaces: a systematic review. *Clin Oral Implants Res*, **25**, 1149–1160.

Machtei, E.E., Mahler, D., Oettinger-Barak, O., Zuabi, O. and Horwitz, J. (2008) Dental implants placed in previously failed sites: survival rate and factors affecting the outcome. *Clin Oral Implants Res*, **19**, 259–264.

Maló, P. and Nobre, M.D. (2008) Flap vs. flapless surgical techniques at immediate implant function in predominantly soft bone for rehabilitation of partial edentulism: a prospective cohort study with follow-up of 1 year. *Eur J Oral Implantol*, **1**, 293–304.

Matarasso, S., Iorio Siciliano, V., Aglietta, M., Andreuccetti, G. and Salvi, G.E. (2014) Clinical and radiographic outcomes of a combined resective and regenerative approach in the treatment of peri-implantitis: a prospective case series. *Clin Oral Implants Res*, **25**, 761–767.

Mengel, R. and Flores-de-Jacoby, L. (2005) Implants in regenerated bone in patients treated for generalized aggressive periodontitis: a prospective longitudinal study. *Int J Periodontics Restorative Dent*, **25**, 331–341.

Misch, C.E. (2008) *Contemporary Implant Dentistry*, 3rd edn, Mosby Elsevier, St. Louis, MO.

Mombelli, A. and Lang, N.P. (1992) Antimicrobial treatment of peri-implant infections. *Clin Oral Implants Res*, **3**, 162–168.

Parel, S.M. and Phillips, W.R. (2011) A risk assessment treatment planning protocol for the four implant immediately loaded maxilla: preliminary findings. *J Prosthet Dent*, **106**, 359–366.

Pi-Anfruns, J. (2014) Complications in implant dentistry. *Alpha Omegan*, **107**, 8–12.

Piattelli, A., Piattelli, M., Mangano, C. and Scarano, A. (1998) A histologic evaluation of eight cases of failed dental implants: is bone overheating the most probable cause? *Biomaterials*, **19**, 683–690.

Pjetursson, B.E., Tan, K., Lang, N.P., Brägger, U., Egger, M. and Zwahlen, M. (2004) A systematic review of the survival and complication rates of fixed partial dentures (FPDs) after an observation period of at least 5 years. *Clin Oral Implants Res*, **15**, 625–642.

Pontoriero, R., Tonelli, M.P., Carnevale, G., Mombelli, A., Nyman, S.R. and Lang, N.P. (1994) Experimentally induced peri-implant mucositis. A clinical study in humans. *Clin Oral Implants Res*, **5**, 254–259.

Porras, R., Anderson, G.B., Caffesse, R., Narendran, S. and Trejo, P.M. (2002) Clinical response to 2 different therapeutic regimens to treat peri-implant mucositis. *J Periodontol*, **73**, 1118–1125.

Proussaefs, P., Lozada, J., Kim, J. and Rohrer, M.D. (2004) Repair of the perforated sinus membrane with a resorbable collagen membrane: a human study. *Int J Oral Maxillofac Implants*, **19** (3), 413–420.

Qu, Z., Andrukhov, O., Laky, M., Ulm, C., Matejka, M., Dard, M. and Rausch-Fan, X. (2011) Effect of enamel matrix derivative on proliferation and differentiation of osteoblast cells grown on the titanium implant surface. *Oral Surg Oral Med Oral Pathol Oral Radiol Endod*, **111**, 517–522.

Quirynen, M. and Teughels, W. (2003) Microbiologically compromised patients and impact on oral implants. *Periodontology*, **33**, 119–128.

Quirynen, M., De Soete, M. and van Steenberghe, D. (2002) Infectious risks for oral implants: a review of the literature. *Clin Oral Implants Res*, **13**, 1–19.

Quirynen, M., Vogels, R., Alsaadi, G., Naert, I., Jacobs, R. and van Steenberghe, D. (2005) Predisposing conditions for retrograde peri-implantitis, and treatment suggestions. *Clin Oral Implants Res*, **16**, 599–608.

Rapley, J.W., Swan, R.H., Hallmon, W.W. and Mills, M.P. (1990) The surface characteristics produced by various oral hygiene instruments and materials on titanium implant abutments. *Int J Oral Maxillofac Implants*, **5**, 47–52.

Rateitschak, K.H. and Wolf, H.F. (1995) *Color Atlas of Dental Medicine*, Thieme, Stuttgart.

Renvert, S., Lessem, J., Lindahl, C. and Svensson, M. (2004) Treatment of incipient peri-implant infections using topical minocycline microspheres versus topical chlorhexidine gel as an adjunct to mechanical debridement. *J Int Acad Periodontol*, **6**, 154–159.

Renvert, S., Roos-Jansåker, A.M. and Claffey, N. (2008) Non-surgical treatment of peri-implant mucositis and peri-implantitis: a literature review. *J Clin Periodontol*, **35**, 305–315.

Romeo, E., Ghisolfi, M., Murgolo, N., Chiapasco, M., Lops, D. and Vogel, G. (2005) Therapy of peri-implantitis with resective surgery. A 3-year clinical trial on rough screw-shaped oral implants. Part I: Clinical outcome. *Clin Oral Implants Res*, **16**, 9–18.

Rose, L.F. and Minsk, L. (2004) Dental implants in the periodontally compromised dentition, in *Periodontics Medicine, Surgery, and Implants* (eds L.F. Rose and B.L. Mealey), Elsevier, St. Louis, MO.

Rosen, P.S. (2010) Complications with the bone-added osteotome sinus floor elevation: etiology, prevention, and treatment, in *Dental Implant Complications: Etiology, Prevention and Treatment* (ed S.J. Froum), Wiley-Blackwell, Hoboken, NJ, pp. 310–324.

Rosen, H. and Gornitsky, M. (2004) Cementable implant-supported prosthesis, serial extraction, and serial implant installation: case report. *Implant Dent*, **13**, 322–327.

Rosenberg, E.S., Evian, C.I., Stern, J.K. and Waasdorp, J. (2010) Implant failure: prevalence, risk factors, management, and prevention, in *Dental Implant Complications: Etiology, Prevention and Treatment* (ed S.J. Froum), Wiley, Oxford, pp. 110–118.

Salvi, G.E., Persson, G.R., Heitz-Mayfield, L.J., Frei, M. and Lang, N.P. (2007) Adjunctive local antibiotic therapy in the treatment of peri-implantitis II: clinical and radiographic outcomes. *Clin Oral Implants Res*, **18**, 281–285.

Schropp, L., Kostopoulos, L., Wenzel, A. and Isidor, F. (2005) Clinical and radiographic performance of delayed-immediate single-tooth implant placement associated with peri-implant bone defects. A 2-year prospective, controlled, randomized follow-up report. *J Clin Periodontol*, **32**, 480–487.

Schwarz, F., Sahm, N., Schwarz, K. and Becker, J. (2010) Impact of defect configuration on the clinical outcome following surgical regenerative therapy of peri-implantitis. *J Clin Periodontol*, **37**, 449–455.

Serino, G. and Turri, A. (2011) Outcome of surgical treatment of peri-implantitis: results from a 2-year prospective clinical study in humans. *Clin Oral Implants Res*, **22**, 1214–1220.

Siegenthaler, D.W., Jung, R.E., Holderegger, C., Roos, M. and Hämmerle, C.H. (2007) Replacement of teeth exhibiting periapical pathology by immediate implants: a prospective, controlled clinical trial. *Clin Oral Implants Res*, **18** (6), 727–737.

Soehardi, A., Meijer, G.J., Manders, R. and Stoelnga, P.J. (2011) An inventory of mandibular fractures associated with implants in atrophic edentulous mandibles: a survey of Dutch oral and maxillofacial surgeons. *Int J Oral Maxillofac Implants*, **26**, 1087–1093.

Solar, P., Geyerhofer, U., Traxler, H., Windisch, A., Ulm, C. and Watzek, G. (1999) Blood supply to the maxillary sinus relevant to sinus floor elevation procedures. *Clin Oral Implants Res*, **10** (1), 34–44.

Spiekerman, H. (1995) *Implantology*, Thieme, Stuttgart.

Sreenivasan, P.K., Vered, Y., Zini, A., Mann, J., Kolog, H., Steinberg, D., Zambon, J.J., Haraszthy, V.I., da Silva, M.P. and De Vizio, W. (2011) A 6-month study of the effects of 0.3% triclosan/copolymer dentifrice on dental implants. *J Clin Periodontol*, **38**, 33–42.

Sumida, S., Ishihara, K., Kishi, M. and Okuda, K. (2002) Transmission of periodontal disease-associated bacteria from teeth to osseointegrated implant regions. *Int J Oral Maxillofac Implants*, **17**, 696–702.

Summers, R.B. (1994) A new concept in maxillary implant surgery: the osteotome technique. *Compendium*, **15** (2), 152–158.

Swierkot, K., Lottholz, P., Flores-de-Jacoby, L. and Mengel, R. (2012) Mucositis, peri-implantitis, implant success, and survival of implants in patients with treated generalized aggressive periodontitis: 3- to 16-year results of prospective long-term cohort study. *J Periodontol*, **83**, 1213–1225.

Tan, W.C., Lang, N.P., Zwahlen, M. and Pjetursson, B.E. (2008) A systematic review of the success of sinus floor elevation and survival of implants inserted in combination with sinus floor elevation. Part II: Transalveolar technique. *J Clin Periodontol*, **35** (suppl), 241–254.

Tarnow, D., Elian, N., Fletcher, P., Froum, S., Magner, A., Cho, S.C., Salama, M., Salama, H. and Garber, D.A. (2003) Vertical distance from the crest of bone to the height of the interproximal papilla between adjacent implants. *J Periodontol*, **74**, 1785–1788.

Tastepe, C.S., van Waas, R., Liu, Y. and Wismeijer, D. (2012) Air powder abrasive treatment as an implant surface cleaning method: a literature review. *Int J Oral Maxillofac Implants*, **27**, 1461–1473.

Tatum, H. (1986) Maxillary and sinus implant reconstructions. *Dent Clin North Am*, **30**, 207–229.

Tay, A.B. and Zuniga, J.R. (2007) Clinical characteristics of trigeminal nerve injury referrals to a university centre. *Int J Oral Maxillofac Surg*, **36**, 922–927.

Termeie, D. (2013) *Periodontal Review*, Quintessence, Chicago, IL, p. 180.

Testori, T., Wallace, S.S., Del Fabbro, M., Taschieri, S., Trisi, P., Capelli, M. and Weinstein, R.L. (2008) Repair of large sinus membrane perforations using stabilized collagen barrier membranes: surgical techniques with histologic and radiographic evidence of success. *Int J Periodontics Restorative Dent*, **28** (1), 9–17.

Testori, T., Drago, L., Wallace, S.S., Capelli, M., Galli, F., Zuffetti, F., Parenti, A., Deflorian, M., Fumagalli, L., Weinstein, R.L., Maiorana, C., Di Stefano, D., Valentini, P., Giannì, A.B., Chiapasco, M., Vinci, R., Pignataro, L., Mantovani, M., Torretta, S., Pipolo, C., Felisati, G., Padoan, G., Castelnuovo, P., Mattina, R. and Del Fabbro, M. (2012) Prevention and treatment of postoperative infections after sinus elevation surgery: clinical consensus and recommendations. *Int J Dent*, **2012**, 1–5.

Timmenga, N.M., Raghoebar, G.M., Boering, G. and van Weissenbruch, R. (1997) Maxillary sinus function after sinus lifts for the insertion of dental implants. *J Oral Maxillofac Surg*, **55** (9), 936–939.

Valderrama, P. and Wilson, T.G., Jr (2013) Detoxification of implant surfaces affected by peri-implant disease: an overview of surgical methods. *Int J Dent*, **2013**, 740680.

Vela, X., Méndez, V., Rodríguez, X., Segalá, M. and Tarnow, D.P. (2012) Crestal bone changes on platform-switched implants and adjacent teeth when the tooth-implant distance is less than 1.5 mm. *Int J Periodontics Restorative Dent*, **32**, 149–155.

Wagenberg, B.D. and Froum, S.J. (2010) Implant complications related to immediate implant placement into extraction sites, in *Dental Implant Complications: Etiology, Prevention and Treatment* (ed S.J. Froum), Wiley-Blackwell, Hoboken, NJ, pp. 325–340.

Wallace, S.S. (2010) Complications in lateral window sinus elevation surgery, in *Dental Implant Complications: Etiology, Prevention and Treatment* (ed S.J. Froum), Wiley-Blackwell, Hoboken, NJ, pp. 284–309.

Wallace, S.S. and Froum, S.J. (2003) Effect of maxillary sinus augmentation on the survival of endosseous dental implants: a systematic review. *Ann Periodontol*, **8** (1), 328–343.

Wallace, S.S., Mazor, Z., Froum, S.J., Cho, S.C. and Tarnow, D.P. (2007) Schneiderian membrane perforation rate during sinus elevation using piezosurgery: clinical results of 100 consecutive cases. *Int J Periodontics Restorative Dent*, **27** (5), 413–419.

Wang, F., Zhang, Z., Monje, A., Huang, W., Wu, Y. and Wang, G. (2015) Intermediate long-term clinical performance of dental implants placed in sites with a previous early implant failure: a retrospective analysis. *Clin Oral Implants Res*, **26** (12), 1443–1449.

Weber, H.P., Kim, D.M., Ng, M.W., Hwang, J.W. and Fiorellini, J.P. (2006) Peri-implant soft-tissue health surrounding cement- and screw-retained implant restorations: a multi-center, 3-year prospective study. *Clin Oral Implants Res*, **17**, 375–359.

Wilson, T.G., Jr (2009) The positive relationship between excess cement and peri-implant disease: a prospective clinical endoscopic study. *J Periodontol*, **80**, 1388–1392.

Wilson, T.G. (2010) Complications associated with flapless surgery, in *Dental Implant Complications: Etiology, Prevention and Treatment* (ed S.J. Froum), Wiley-Blackwell, Hoboken, NJ, pp. 341–354.

CHAPTER 8

Pediatric dentistry complications and challenges

Rebecca L. Slayton and Elizabeth A. Palmer

Department of Pediatric Dentistry, University of Washington School of Dentistry, Seattle, WA, USA

Common complications associated with the treatment of dental caries

Posttreatment complications
Self-inflicted lip, tongue, or cheek trauma

The administration of local anesthesia to children, particularly those who are young or have special health-care needs, is associated with an increased risk of self-inflicted trauma to the lip, tongue, or cheek. One study (College *et al.*, 2000) found that 13% of children who receive an inferior alveolar nerve block in conjunction with their dental treatment experience postoperative tissue trauma. Children may bite themselves for a number of reasons. They cannot feel the pain associated with the action. Some children may be curious about the foreign feeling associated with local anesthesia. Other children may unintentionally bite themselves while eating or sleeping when the soft tissues are still anesthetized (Figure 8.1).

Prevention

Caregivers responsible for posttreatment supervision should be given clear instructions about how to observe their child and watch for any behavior that might suggest biting or sucking on the lip or cheek. Caregivers should also be given realistic time estimates as to how long the child will have soft tissue anesthesia after the dental appointment. A description of what this type of trauma looks like may also be helpful so that the parent is not overly alarmed if the trauma does occur. For an inferior alveolar nerve block, the use of 3% mepivacaine or 4% prilocaine without a vasoconstrictor does not significantly reduce the duration of soft tissue anesthesia produced in comparison with 2% lidocaine with 1:100 000 epinephrine. Therefore, 3% mepivacaine and 4% prilocaine are generally not recommended as alternatives to decrease the risk of self-inflicted soft tissue trauma (Hersh *et al.*, 1995). The use of bilateral inferior alveolar mandibular nerve blocks does not increase the risk of self-inflicted soft tissue trauma when compared to a unilateral mandibular block (College *et al.*, 2000). The authors hypothesize that children may be more likely to traumatize their soft tissue when only one side is anesthetized because it feels "different" to them, whereas with bilateral anesthesia, both sides feel the same. The incidence of soft tissue trauma was actually found to be higher in pediatric patients under the age of 4 years who received a unilateral mandibular block compared to bilateral mandibular blocks. Mandibular local infiltration instead of mandibular nerve blocks has not been found to be effective in decreasing the duration of soft tissue anesthesia; however, its use may decrease the amount of tissues anesthetized. As a caution, mandibular infiltration is not as effective in achieving profound anesthesia when compared to a mandibular nerve block for some procedures (Oulis, Vadiakas, and Vasilopoulou, 1996). Upon completion of the dental treatment, a cotton roll placed between the teeth on the anesthetized side may provide both a reminder and a barrier to the patient to avoid self-injury (Figure 8.2).

Avoiding and Treating Dental Complications: Best Practices in Dentistry, First Edition. Edited by Deborah A. Termeie.
© 2016 John Wiley & Sons, Inc. Published 2016 by John Wiley & Sons, Inc.

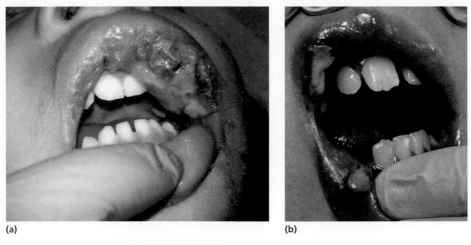

(a)   (b)

Figure 8.1 (a and b) Self-inflicted lip trauma after receiving dental treatment with local anesthesia.

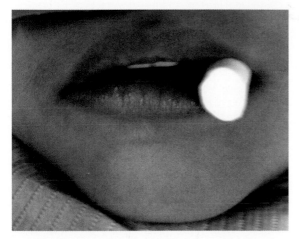

Figure 8.2 Placement of a cotton roll between teeth adjacent to an anesthetized area of the mouth.

Treatment

Most lesions resulting from self-induced soft tissue trauma are self-limiting and heal without complications, although bleeding and infection are possible. The child can be given over-the-counter analgesics as needed for pain. It is important that the injured area is kept clean to allow for optimal healing. Alcohol-free chlorhexidine gluconate (0.12%) may be prescribed with the following instructions: 1–2 times daily, apply a small amount to the affected area with cotton applicator. No antibiotics are recommended unless there are signs of soft tissue infection. The healing process may take several weeks (Chi *et al.*, 2008).

Nickel allergy

Dental alloys containing nickel are commonly found in restorative and orthodontic materials used in the dental treatment of children. However, nickel is a known allergen. One study (Kerusuo *et al.*, 1996) of Finnish adolescents observed that a nickel allergy identified with patch testing was present in 30% of girls and 3% of boys. This discrepancy between the sexes was found to be due to their different prevalence of pierced ears. Overall, 31% of adolescents had pierced ears compared to 2% with no piercing of ears. If an individual is already sensitized to nickel, small amounts of nickel being released from a dental material could elicit a Type IV hypersensitivity reaction that may present clinically as gingival overgrowth, angular cheilitis, and labial desquamation in the oral cavity (Setcos *et al.*, 2006).

Prevention

When planning to use either nickel-containing restorative materials or orthodontic appliances, it is important to review the patient's allergies. If the patient has a known nickel allergy, one must select alternative nickel-free materials (Pazzini *et al.*, 2011).

Treatment

Treatment of a suspected or known nickel allergy requires removal of the allergenic material and its replacement with a nickel-free alternative. Resolution of symptoms may occur over a short or delayed time period.

Premature loss of a primary tooth

A primary tooth may be prematurely lost due to several reasons, for example, caries, trauma, or ectopic eruption. A newly created space in the dental arch may result in the mesial migration or tipping of adjacent molars, distalization of anterior teeth, and/or the altered eruption path of permanent teeth. Thus, premature primary tooth loss may result in several possible orthodontic challenges including crowding, ectopic eruption, dental impaction, crossbite formation, and dental midline discrepancies (Laing *et al.*, 2009).

Prevention

Preventing caries and restoring carious tooth surfaces to proper contours are important to reduce the risk of space loss. When premature loss of a primary tooth is unavoidable, a dental space maintainer may be indicated. Referral to a pediatric dentist is recommended if the general dentist is not comfortable with fitting bands and fabricating space maintainers.

Management

According to the American Academy of Pediatric Dentistry (AAPD, 2014b), the following combinations of factors must be considered in determining the appropriateness and timing of treatment:

1 Specific tooth lost
2 Time elapsed since tooth loss
3 Preexisting occlusion
4 Favorable space analysis
5 Presence and root development of permanent successor
6 Amount of alveolar bone covering permanent successor
7 Patient's health status
8 Patient's cooperative ability
9 Active oral habits
10 Oral hygiene

Patients who are at a greater risk for infection, such as those who are immunocompromised, or are at risk for subacute infective endocarditis are not recommended to receive space maintainer therapy. Patients who are to receive space maintainer therapy must be established dental patients who would return for evaluations at regular intervals. In addition, they should be able to cooperate for the steps needed to fabricate, deliver, adjust, and remove the appliance. Because space maintainer appliances can trap food and debris, good oral hygiene is also important.

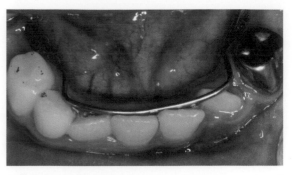

Figure 8.3 Lower lingual holding arch blocking the eruption of lateral incisor.

When a space maintainer is considered for a pediatric patient, an appropriate case selection is imperative as there are multiple potential adverse effects of space maintainer therapy including the following (Brothwell, 1997):

1 Dislodged, broken, and lost appliances
2 Plaque accumulation
3 Caries
4 Damage or interference with successor eruption (Figure 8.3)
5 Undesirable tooth movement
6 Inhibition of alveolar growth
7 Soft tissue impingement
8 Pain

If the patient's general health, oral hygiene, and ability to cooperate support the use of space maintainer therapy, the patient's dental development, occlusion, and the specific tooth lost are the next set of considerations. For example, a prematurely lost anterior tooth most often does not require space maintenance treatment. Space maintainer therapy for a prematurely missing primary molar should be considered in most cases, except when a primary first molar is prematurely lost after the first permanent molars have erupted in class I occlusion. Additionally, space maintenance is not indicated when the permanent successor is near eruption as long as there is an adequate spacing for the tooth to erupt. Lastly, space maintainer therapy will be most effective when the appliance is delivered at the time of the removal of the primary tooth or soon after as the majority of the tooth movement of the adjacent teeth occurs soon after the tooth is lost.

Thus, the dental provider must make decisions regarding the recommendation for space maintainer therapy on an individual need basis weighing the possible orthodontic challenges that may result without a space maintainer versus the patient's risk for adverse outcomes (Figure 8.4).

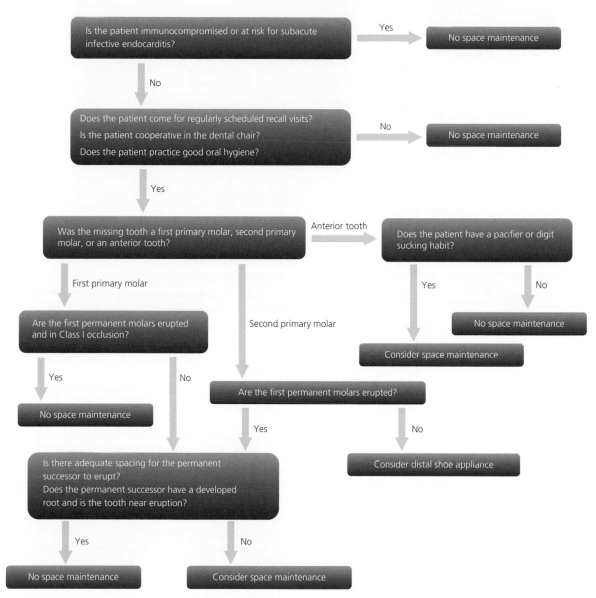

Figure 8.4 Decision tree for the consideration of a space maintainer.

Common complications associated with behavior guidance

Frequently, children and individuals with special health-care needs are unable to cooperate for dental care in the traditional setting. Pediatric dentistry training includes techniques, both nonpharmacologic and pharmacologic, to manage or guide the behavior of the patient so that treatment can be provided in a safe and effective manner. General dentists and other specialists may choose to refer patients to a pediatric dentist or use the techniques described in the succeeding text to manage behavior in the clinic or hospital setting.

Referral to a specialist

If the referring dentist does not feel confident that they can provide the standard of care in a safe manner, it is appropriate to refer a patient to a specialist such as a pediatric dentist. The referral should include the child's relevant demographic information, medical history, and the purpose of the referral. If any radiographs are available, they should be sent with the referral to avoid having to reexpose the patient. If the patient is being referred for a specific procedure with the expectation that the referring dentist will provide ongoing care for the patient, this should be made clear on the referral form. Most specialists have a referral form available on their website that can be filled out online and emailed or faxed to their office.

Complications associated with nitrous oxide

For children and adolescents who are anxious about dental treatment, nitrous oxide analgesia can be a very effective tool to relieve anxiety and facilitate care (AAPD, 2014a). There are a few known contraindications to the use of nitrous oxide, including vitamin B_{12} (cobalamin) deficiency, 5,10-methylenetetrahydrofolate reductase (MTHFR) deficiency, chronic obstructive pulmonary disease, and first trimester of pregnancy (Selzer et al, 2003; Sanders, Weimann, and Maze, 2008; AAPD, 2014a). High levels of nitrous oxide may cause nausea or vomiting, and inhalation of 100% nitrous oxide has been known to result in death from asphyxiation (Winek, Wahba, and Rozin, 1995). Although nitrous oxide has been used for decades in both medicine and dentistry, there have been questions about its safety recently, particularly in relation to the developing and the aging brain (Baum 2007; Sanders, Weimann, and Maze, 2008). Studies in immature and adult rats have shown that nitrous oxide has neurotoxic effects in the brain (Baum, 2007). The human brain matures at a slower rate than rodents' and current evidence does not support a similar action in humans. It is an area of continued research.

Prevention

Avoid using nitrous oxide when it is contraindicated. As patients might not be aware of vitamin B_{12} or MTHFR deficiency, reviewing family history is important. Vegetarians and vegans have a greater likelihood of having vitamin B_{12} deficiency. Asking questions about diet may reveal a possible deficiency in vitamin B_{12}. Nitrous oxide delivery systems (Pawlak, Lester, and Babatunde, 2014) should be tested and calibrated at the time of installation and on an annual basis to ensure that the gauge readings accurately reflect the quantity of nitrous

oxide and oxygen being delivered to the patient and to confirm that the scavenging system is functioning effectively. In a fail-safe delivery system, the delivery of nitrous oxide is always in combination with oxygen. The system should never be able to deliver less than 30% oxygen. Safe levels of nitrous oxide for children range from 20 to 50%. A well-fitted nasal hood will minimize the loss of nitrous oxide into the surrounding atmosphere and decrease its exposure to the chairside provider and assistant. Some state boards recommend the use of a pulse oximeter to monitor oxygen saturation during the use of nitrous oxide. Some states also require specific permits in order to administer nitrous oxide. Training on the proper use and monitoring of nitrous oxide is strongly encouraged.

Treatment

Nitrous oxide is titrated in specific volumes with oxygen to achieve the desired level of analgesia. At the end of treatment, it is important to have the child breathe 100% oxygen for 5 min to clear any residual nitrous oxide from their lungs. Other indications requiring suspension of nitrous oxide and delivery of 100% oxygen include any signs of respiratory distress, excitation, nausea, or vomiting.

Sedation complications

Sedation is defined by either the route or the level of sedation achieved. Recently, most professional organizations and state dental boards define the levels of sedation (minimal, moderate, and deep) regardless of the route used to deliver the drugs. Sedating patients of any age requires advanced education and training to be knowledgeable about appropriate drug doses and appropriate monitoring of vital signs and to be prepared to manage complications. In healthy children, most sedation-related complications are due to a compromised airway. Patient selection and compliance with guidelines from the AAPD (2014b) and the American Academy of Pediatrics are essential to minimize risk and maximize success. In young children, effective sedation may lead the dentist to attempt to provide more dental treatment than appropriate, resulting in either an overdose of local anesthetic or ineffective pain management. Local anesthetic dose should be based on the weight of the child and should not exceed 4.4 mg/kg for 2% lidocaine with 1:100000 epinephrine. Oral sedative medications are also weight based and once administered should not be redosed. Emergency drugs and reversal agents should be present in the clinic and kept current.

Complications may arise from the overdose of sedative medications, overdose of local anesthetic agent, aspiration of foreign objects related to the patient having diminished protective reflexes, airway obstruction due to poor head positioning, and unknown drug allergy. Any dental provider who sedates patients must have advanced education and training to be able to manage and rescue patients from these potential complications.

General anesthesia

For very young children, children, and young adults with severe anxiety or with special health-care needs, it is frequently necessary to provide treatment under general anesthesia in either a hospital or outpatient surgical center. Only providers with training in anesthesiology and appropriate licensure in the state that they are practicing in should administer general anesthesia. In most cases, all necessary dental treatment can be completed in one session because local anesthetic is not generally used and therefore is not a limitation. Guidelines from the AAPD recommend limiting treatment under general anesthesia in an office-based setting to children over 24 months of age and American Society of Anesthesiology (ASA) classification I or II (AAPD, 2014b, 2014c). However, the ultimate decision about which patients are safe and appropriate to be treated in an office-based setting under general anesthesia relies on the clinical judgment and evaluation of the anesthesia provider.

Protective stabilization or medical immobilization

This method of behavior guidance may involve the use of a "papoose board" or immobilization wrap (passive restraint) or the involvement of one or more individuals holding the patient's hands or head (active restraint). The purpose of this type of behavior guidance is to secure the patient for a short period of time to accomplish specific, often urgent treatment in a patient who is unable or unwilling to cooperate (AAPD, 2014d). Most commonly, this is used for a very young child with a traumatic injury or infection or for a patient with developmental disabilities who needs an oral assessment and urgent treatment. In some cases, protective stabilization is also used while a patient is sedated. The goal is to minimize harm to the patient and the health-care providers and facilitate evaluation or treatment in a safe way. Informed consent from the child's parent/guardian for the use of a stabilization wrap is essential.

Informed consent

Informed consent may be written or verbal. For legal reasons, it is best to have consent documents in writing (AAPD, 2014e). The purpose of informed consent is to provide the patient or parent/guardian (for underage patients) with information regarding the diagnosis and recommended treatment options so that they can make an informed decision about care. An informed consent document should also include the potential benefits and risks of all treatment alternatives including a risk of no treatment. For families whose first language is not English, an interpreter must be present to explain the consent document in the patient's and parent's primary language.

Common complications associated with developmental anomalies

By definition, developmental anomalies cannot be prevented. They are anomalies of tooth or jaw development that are influenced by genetics or by an interaction between genes and environment. Timely and appropriate treatment can minimize future complications.

Supernumerary teeth

Complications related to supernumerary teeth include interference with the eruption of permanent teeth, ectopic eruption, or crowding (Cameron and Widmer, 2003) (Figure 8.5a and b). Multiple supernumerary teeth are associated with syndromes such as cleidocranial dysplasia or Gardner syndrome (Slayton, 2013) (Figure 8.6).

Treatment

Supernumerary teeth are usually detected radiographically (Figure 8.5a). In some situations, the extra tooth erupts within the normal arch form or slightly out of the arch on the palate or lingual/buccal gingiva (Figure 8.5b). The timing of surgical excision of supernumerary teeth depends on their location, their stage of development, and the development of adjacent teeth. It is important to minimize damage to the developing permanent teeth. To help plan the surgical approach, multiple periapical

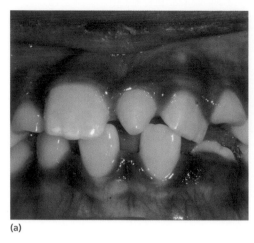
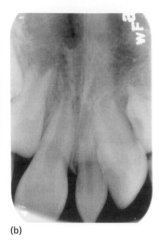

(a)   **(b)**

Figure 8.5 (a and b) Erupted mesiodens clinical and radiographic images.

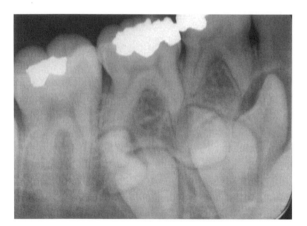

Figure 8.6 Multiple supernumerary teeth.

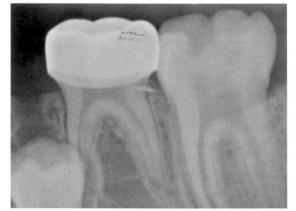

Figure 8.7 Hypodontia of premolars.

radiographs taken at different angles (same-lingual, opposite-buccal (SLOB) rule) or cone beam computed tomography should be used to locate the extra tooth or teeth in three dimensions.

Hypodontia

Developmentally missing teeth is a fairly common finding in children. Hypodontia is the term used to describe the absence of one or more teeth. The incidence of hypodontia in the primary dentition is less than 1%, while in the permanent dentition, it ranges from 1.5 to 10% (excluding third molars) (Slayton, Brickhouse, and Adair, 2011). The most frequently missing teeth are the third molars, followed by mandibular second premolars (Figure 8.7), maxillary lateral incisors, and then

maxillary second premolars. Hypodontia can occur as an isolated finding or associated with syndromes such as ectodermal dysplasia (Figure 8.8), orofaciodigital syndrome, or Williams syndrome, among others. There are over 150 different types of ectodermal dysplasia with every known inheritance pattern. Complications of one or more missing permanent teeth include esthetic concerns, excess spacing, and alveolar bone loss.

Treatment

The age of the patient, number and location of the missing teeth, and presence of other systemic findings are important considerations in terms of the treatment of hypodontia. When premolars are missing, every attempt should be made to maintain the primary molars until the

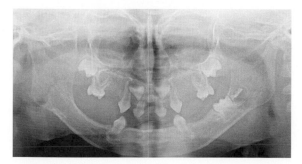

Figure 8.8 Multiple missing teeth in ectodermal dysplasia.

patient is old enough to consider placement of implants. Since ankylosis occurs more frequently in primary molars with no successors, it is important to monitor these teeth on a regular basis. Replacement of developmentally missing teeth may include removable partial dentures in the growing patient, orthodontic movement of teeth into the place of the missing teeth (e.g., canine replacement for lateral incisors), fixed bridges, or implants once the child has finished growing. When multiple teeth are missing, as in patients with ectodermal dysplasia, removable dentures can be made as soon as the child is able to tolerate impressions. For young children, in whom the primary objective is to improve esthetics, maxillary dentures are easier to tolerate than mandibular dentures. Because the mandibular alveolar ridge is often very underdeveloped in children with ectodermal dysplasia, fabrication of a functional mandibular denture is challenging. Once children with ectodermal dysplasia have finished growing, implants or implant-retained dentures are indicated, often following bone grafts to enhance the alveolar ridge. Referral to a prosthodontist is recommended. Resources for families and providers are available from the National Foundation for Ectodermal Dysplasias (www.nfed.org).

Dens invaginatus

This anomaly is described as an invagination of the inner enamel epithelium and can result in a carious communication between the occlusal environment and the pulp (Cameron and Widmer, 2003; Slayton, Brickhouse, and Adair, 2011). It is most commonly found in permanent maxillary lateral incisors but may also occur in permanent canines and premolars (Figure 8.9). This altered anatomy puts the tooth at risk for irreversible pulpitis and necrosis due to the communication between oral bacteria and pulp tissue.

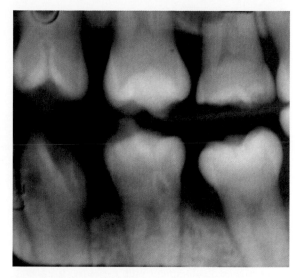

Figure 8.9 Radiograph of dens invaginatus in canine and premolar (taurodontism also present).

Treatment

This anomaly is generally detected radiographically during routine examinations. If detected prior to the development of irreversible pulpitis or pulp necrosis, a sealant is recommended to eliminate communication between the pulp and the oral microbial environment. If the tooth first presents with signs of irreversible pulpitis or necrosis, it is necessary to perform root canal therapy for a closed apex tooth or pulp regeneration therapy for an open apex tooth (Cohenca, Paranjpe, and Berg, 2013). Regenerative endodontics is a relatively new procedure intended to promote the continued development of immature roots and surrounding tissues by restoring health to the pulp tissue. This procedure is indicated for a tooth with pulp necrosis and an immature apex. It is an alternative to apexification or extraction. The regenerative procedure involves disinfection of the canal followed by induction of bleeding within the canal. Stem cells located in the apical papilla of immature teeth are stimulated by this process and aid in root development (Cohenca, Paranjpe, and Berg, 2013; Hargreaves, Diogenes, and Teixeira, 2013). More information about the procedure and access to the database of cases treated using this procedure is available on the website of the American Association of Endodontists (http://www.aae.org/regeneration/).

Dens evaginatus

There have been a variety of names used to describe this anomaly including enamel tubercle, odontome, occlusal enamel pearl, and evaginatus odontoma (Levitan and Himel, 2006). The preferred terminology recommended by Oehlers, Lee, and Lee in 1967 is dens evaginatus (DE) (Oehlers, Lee, and Lee, 1967). This developmental anomaly is caused by an evagination of the enamel epithelium and often results in the pulp chamber extending into an extra cusp (Cameron and Widmer, 2003; Slayton, Brickhouse, and Adair, 2011). The most commonly affected teeth are the mandibular premolars (Figure 8.10). The reported frequency varies from 0.5 to 4% and is more common in females and in persons of Asian descent (Cameron and Widmer, 2003; Levitan and Himel, 2006). The cusp is more susceptible to wear or fracture and subsequent pulp exposure, irreversible pulpitis, or necrosis.

Treatment

Treatment recommendations vary depending on the status of the tooth at the time of examination. Levitan and Himel (2006) describe six "types" of DE with specific recommendations for each type. The description of each type includes the pulpal status (normal, inflamed, or necrotic) and the development of the root apex (mature or immature). For teeth with normal pulpal status, the application of resin composite around and over the tubercle combined with occlusal adjustment of the opposing tooth is recommended. When the tooth is

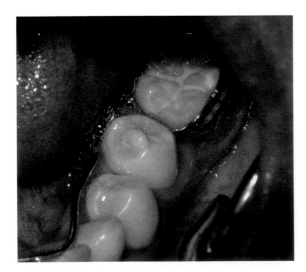

Figure 8.10 Clinical image of dens evaginatus in a premolar.

inflamed or necrotic with a mature apex, pulpotomy or root canal therapy is indicated. Often, this anomaly is not detected until after the tooth has become necrotic. When this happens in a tooth with an immature root apex, treatment options to consider are apexification, pulp regeneration, and extraction. Apexification is a procedure that involves debridement of the necrotic pulp tissue followed by placement of calcium hydroxide. The patient should be seen for evaluation and replacement of the calcium hydroxide every 3 months until root formation is complete. This may take an average of 8 months or more and will require close monitoring clinically and radiographically (Rafter, 2005). Once a calcific barrier has formed, traditional root canal treatment can be initiated. Pulpal regeneration is described in section "Dens invaginatus" and in Chapter 3 (Endodontic complications). Sequential reduction of the enamel portion of the extra cusp has been recommended in the past to decrease the risk of fracture and pulp exposure by stimulating reparative dentin (Levitan and Himel, 2006). There is limited evidence to support this approach, and the risk for causing a microscopic pulp exposure is significant.

Enamel hypoplasia

This term describes a defect in the quantity of enamel but is sometimes also used to describe defects in an enamel quality. There are many acquired, systemic causes of this anomaly including prenatal nutrition, prenatal or perinatal infections (rubella embryopathy, syphilis, cytomegalovirus), premature birth (Mast *et al.*, 2013; Nelson *et al.*, 2013), or dental trauma, among others. There are also genetic causes and associations with specific genetic syndromes such as Down syndrome, tuberous sclerosis, epidermolysis bullosa, and cleidocranial dysplasia (Wright, Carrion, and Morris, 2015).

Treatment

Teeth with enamel hypoplasia are at an increased risk for caries, have increased sensitivity to stimulation, and, in the anterior region, present an esthetic challenge (Figure 8.11). Depending on the extent of the defect and the quality of the enamel, restorative treatment is indicated to reduce the risk for caries and to decrease sensitivity and improve anterior esthetics. When there is a lack of enamel, but the quality is acceptable, sealants or composite restorations should be attempted. If the defect is extensive and the enamel appears chalky, full coverage is indicated (Figure 8.12). For young permanent molars,

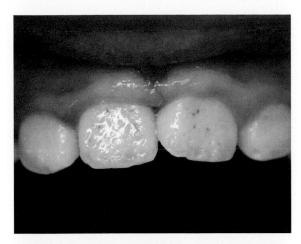

Figure 8.11 Incisor enamel hypoplasia.

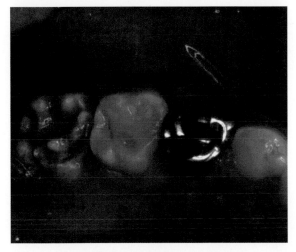

Figure 8.12 Molar enamel hypoplasia.

well-fitted stainless steel crowns are recommended using minimal reduction of tooth structure (Croll, 2000). When enamel hypoplasia is diagnosed when tooth eruption is incomplete, temporary glass ionomer restorations are indicated until the tooth has fully erupted. For older adolescents or young adults, permanent crowns are recommended. Frequently, adequate anesthesia may be difficult to achieve in molars with enamel hypoplasia that have been given local anesthesia. Sedation or general anesthesia may be needed to accomplish treatment.

Ankyloglossia

Also known as "tongue tie," this anomaly is relatively common in newborn babies and children. Ankyloglossia arises when the lingual frenum is shorter than normal, resulting in restriction of the movement of the tip of the tongue. In babies, it may interfere with the ability to latch on to the mother's nipple for an effective breastfeeding (Cameron and Widmer, 2003; Kupietsky and Botzer, 2005). In childhood, severe ankyloglossia may impede speech articulation (Webb, Hao, and Hong, 2013) and can limit the ability to clear food debris from the buccal vestibule and around the teeth (Figure 8.13a and b).

Treatment

For infants demonstrating difficulty with breastfeeding, the recommended treatment is a lingual frenotomy (Power and Murphy, 2015). This is a fairly simple procedure due to the very thin, relatively avascular nature of the lingual frenum in the first few months of age. The procedure involves retraction of the tongue

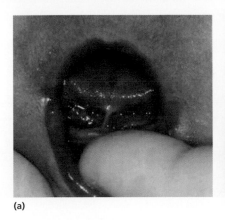

(a)

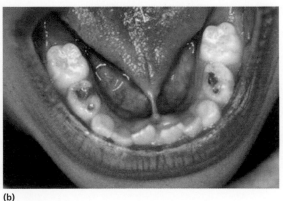

(b)

Figure 8.13 (a and b) Ankyloglossia in an infant and a young child.

with sterile gauze and then careful cutting of the frenum with sterile surgical scissors. Topical anesthetic may be used but is not required because the procedure is associated with little discomfort and must be balanced with the risk of benzocaine exposure in the infant (Ovental *et al.*, 2014).

Osteogenesis imperfecta

Osteogenesis imperfecta (OI) is a heterogeneous disorder with an autosomal dominant inheritance pattern, resulting in brittle bones. There are seven well-characterized types of OI, and overall, the prevalence is 1 in 15 000–20 000 births (Patel *et al.*, 2015). Most cases are due to a mutation in the COL1A1/COL1A2 genes, resulting in defects in the quality or quantity of Type I collagen (Willing *et al.*, 1996). In some cases, OI is associated with dentinogenesis imperfecta (DI), a defect in dentin development (discussed later). OI has variable expressivity including lethality in the perinatal period, extreme bone fragility, or a mild presentation with minimal fracture risk.

Treatment

Routine preventive dental care is recommended for patients with OI to minimize the risk for caries and the need for restorative treatment. Patients with mild (Type I) OI can be treated in the traditional dental setting. Patients with severe forms (Type III or Type IV) of OI are frequently nonambulatory and should either be examined in their wheel chair or carefully transferred to the dental chair by a family member who is familiar with the child's ability to tolerate this type of transfer. When children with OI also have DI, there is an increased risk for caries and dental abscess. The prevalence of OI with DI is not well documented, but a recent cross-sectional, multicenter study found that DI occurs in all types of OI and is most common in Type III OI (Patel *et al.*, 2015). In this case, it is recommended that the treatment be performed in the hospital under general anesthesia by a pediatric dentist or oral and maxillofacial surgeon who is familiar with this condition. The risk for fracture of the jaw during an extraction or fracture of other bones during an intubation or positioning on the treatment table is high (Slayton, 2013). Frequently, patients with OI are treated with intravenous bisphosphonates to increase bone density and decrease the risk of long bone fractures. There is some evidence to demonstrate the effectiveness of this therapy on bone mineral density (Kusumi *et al.*, 2015). To date, there is no evidence that treatment with bisphosphonates in children with OI puts them at an increased risk for osteonecrosis of the jaw (Maines *et al.*, 2012).

Dentinogenesis imperfecta

Developmental anomalies of tooth formation are uncommon but not rare. DI is caused by a genetic defect of dentin development and is inherited in an autosomal dominant manner. The most common documented genetic mutation is in dentin sialophosphoprotein (DSPP) (Li *et al.*, 2012). Frequently, multiple family members from multiple generations report having this disorder. In some cases, it is associated with OI. The presentation of this disorder varies considerably from one individual to the next. In some, the teeth are of a normal size and shape but have a bluish or grayish opalescent appearance. In others, the enamel appears to be missing, leaving a yellowish, brown dome of dentin (Figure 8.14a and b). The extreme wear leads to the loss of vertical dimension, tooth sensitivity, and an increased risk for an abscess.

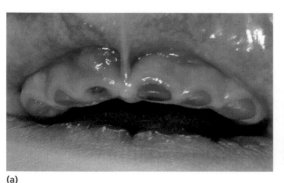

(a)

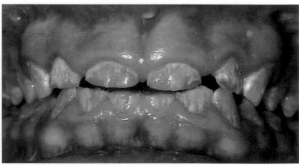

(b)

Figure 8.14 (a and b) Clinical images of dentinogenesis imperfecta in primary and permanent teeth.

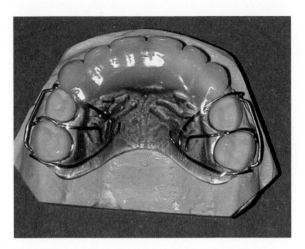

Figure 8.15 Partial overdenture to provide esthetics for young girl with dentinogenesis imperfecta.

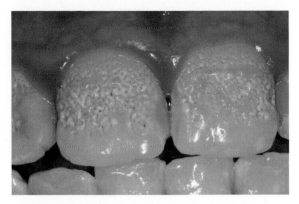

Figure 8.16 Amelogenesis imperfecta with incisor pitting.

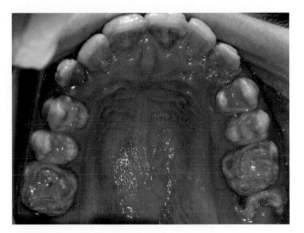

Figure 8.17 Amelogenesis imperfecta with significant loss of enamel and brown discoloration.

Treatment

Teeth affected by DI generally require full-coverage restorations both in the primary and permanent dentitions. In the primary dentition, posterior stainless steel crowns are recommended as soon as there are signs of occlusal wear. This often must be done under general anesthesia because of the extent of treatment needs and the young age of the child when this is indicated (2–3 years of age). If enough tooth structure is present in the anterior sextants, esthetic crowns are indicated. For children, these options include stainless steel crowns with esthetic resin facings or prefabricated zirconia crowns. When the primary anterior teeth show excessive wear, it may be impossible to restore them. Options for providing temporary esthetic solutions include a removable partial overdenture (Figure 8.15) or extraction and fabrication of a fixed pedo partial. Permanent incisors may be treated with composite veneers until the child is old enough for full-coverage porcelain crowns.

Amelogenesis imperfecta

Amelogenesis imperfecta (AI) is a genetic anomaly of tooth development. There are three primary types and 14 subtypes of this disorder (Slayton, 2013). To date, 10 genes have been identified that are responsible for this condition, and the inheritance patterns include autosomal dominant, autosomal recessive, and x-linked recessive (Wright, Carrion, and Morris, 2015). The phenotypes vary considerably but generally result in defects in the quality or quantity of enamel. Teeth appear

yellowish or brownish in color and may be pitted or chalky in texture (Figures 8.16 and 8.17). Frequently teeth with AI are very sensitive, making it difficult for children to eat or to maintain good oral hygiene without experiencing discomfort. Although these patients often present with caries, it should be recognized that the underlying condition has contributed to their increased susceptibility to plaque retention and subsequent caries lesions.

Treatment

Treatment options vary based on the type of amelogenesis and the symptoms the child is experiencing. Esthetics is a concern for all types of AI and usually requires full-coverage crowns in the posterior teeth and veneer or full-coverage crowns in the anterior teeth. In the primary dentition, the goal should be reduction of sensitivity and caries risk in the posterior teeth through the use of stainless steel crowns and improvement of esthetics in the anterior teeth with preveneered crowns or prefabricated zirconia crowns. In the permanent dentition, stainless steel crowns on molars may serve as a temporary restoration, but for older adolescents and young adults, permanent crowns are recommended. If the enamel quality is sufficient to allow bonding of composite restorations, veneers in the anterior teeth are good choices for young adolescents. If the enamel quality is poor, full coverage may be required. These are challenging restorative cases that would benefit from the expertise of a prosthodontist (Millet *et al.*, 2015).

Common complications associated with eruption anomalies

Ectopic eruption and impaction of permanent teeth

Permanent incisors, canines, and molars may exhibit aberrant eruption patterns with distinct etiology. Identification of an accurate cause of the ectopic eruption or impaction is important for the development of an appropriate treatment plan. The goal of early management of the eruption anomaly is to minimize the potential extent of the malocclusion. However, the patient may still need comprehensive orthodontic treatment even after the localized issue is addressed.

Ectopic eruption and impaction of permanent incisors

Permanent maxillary incisors may erupt ectopically or become impacted for several reasons. The presence of a supernumerary tooth may alter the eruption of the permanent successor. Pulpal necrosis of a primary incisor from trauma or caries may also result in the altered eruption of the permanent successor (Figure 8.18). Additionally, one study (Coll and Sadrian, 1996) found that after a primary incisor has been treated with a pulpectomy, there is a 20% probability of its permanent successor erupting palatally or in anterior crossbite.

Prevention

It is pertinent to monitor for the ectopic eruption of a permanent incisor after a primary incisor has experienced trauma and has been treated with a pulpectomy

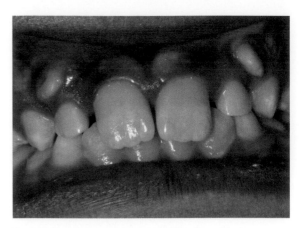

Figure 8.18 Ectopic eruption of maxillary lateral incisors.

or if a supernumerary tooth has been identified. The asymmetric eruption of an incisor relative to its contralateral match may indicate an ectopic eruption pattern and the presence of an impacted tooth and/or a supernumerary tooth.

Treatment

Once ectopic eruption of a maxillary incisor is diagnosed, it is important to minimize the potential impact by addressing the associated etiology. If a supernumerary tooth (unerupted or erupted) has been identified, which is impeding or altering the path of eruption of a permanent incisor, the supernumerary tooth should be removed. If the primary tooth is over-retained, necrotic, or pulpally involved, it should be removed. After the permanent incisor has erupted into the dental arch, either removable or fixed appliance therapy may be used to move the ectopically erupted tooth into a more desirable position.

Ectopic eruption and impaction of permanent canines

Permanent maxillary canines are impacted in 1–2% of the population. 85% of impacted canines occur palatally while 15% occur buccally (Richardson and Russell, 2000). Maxillary canine impaction has a genetic predisposition. A maxillary canine that is impacted buccally is frequently associated with inadequate arch length (dental crowding) and may erupt vertically, buccally, and higher in the alveolus. Palatally impacted maxillary canines are associated with other dental abnormalities such as congenitally missing teeth and small,

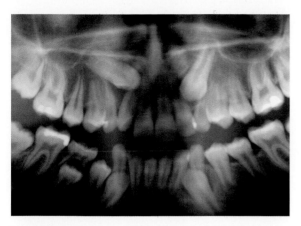

Figure 8.19 Radiograph of palatally impacted canines.

peg-shaped or missing lateral incisors. A palatally impacted maxillary canine may cause root resorption and possibly result in loss of the permanent incisors if left untreated (Figure 8.19).

Prevention

Early detection of an impacted permanent canine can be accomplished by clinical and radiographic evaluation. Clinically, a canine bulge that is not palpable by the age of 9–10 years, asymmetric canine eruption pattern, over-retention of the primary canine, distal tipping of the permanent lateral incisor, and other dental anomalies, such as a peg-shaped or missing lateral incisor, should alert the provider that an aberrant eruption pattern of the canine is possible. Radiographic survey including a panoramic radiograph as well as two periapical views or computed tomography will locate the impacted canine in the alveolus in relation to the other teeth.

Treatment

If a maxillary canine is determined to be erupting buccally or palatally, or has the potential to become impacted, extraction of the primary canine is the interceptive treatment of choice before the age of 11 years (Ericson and Kurol, 1988; Bedoya and Park, 2009). If radiographic signs of root resorption of the maxillary permanent incisors from an ectopically erupting permanent canine are evident, the primary canine should be extracted. Studies have found that extraction of the primary canine results in 68–78% rates of normal permanent canine eruption (Ericson and Kurol, 1986; Power and Short, 1993). However, if there is no improvement in the eruption path

of the permanent canine after 12 months, surgical exposure and orthodontic eruption may be indicated. It may be prudent to consult with an orthodontist at any stage of this process.

Ectopic eruption and impaction of permanent molars

Ectopic eruption of the first permanent molar may occur when the tooth erupts both in vertical and in mesial directions within the alveolus. The erupting permanent molar may resorb the distal root of the second primary molar crown and can become impacted under the distal portion of the primary molar. Ectopically erupted first permanent molars occur in up to 3% of the pediatric population and are more common in pediatric patients with cleft lip and palate (Barberia-Leasche, Suarez-Clus, and Seavedra-Ontiveros, 2005). Usually, no pain or discomfort is associated with the condition unless communication develops between the oral cavity and the pulpal tissue of the primary molar, resulting in an abscess. Sixty-six percent of ectopically erupting first permanent molars will spontaneously self-correct by moving distally and erupting into the correct position by age 7 years. In other instances, the permanent molar gets "stuck" under the primary molar crown and no longer erupts (Yaseen, Naik, and Uloopi, 2011). They are often identified because of an asymmetric eruption pattern or via radiographic evaluation with a bitewing or panoramic radiograph. Ectopically erupting first permanent molars may resorb a significant portion of the second primary molar and cause early exfoliation of that tooth and a potential 6–8 mm of space loss if the condition is not managed upon initial occurrence.

Prevention

Early identification and monitoring are indicated in order to prevent the possible early loss of the second primary molar (Figure 8.20). If self-correction does not occur by age 7 years, treatment is necessary. Additionally, if the second primary molar has a stainless steel crown restoration, the permanent molar can become positioned under the crown itself and may be unable to self-correct.

Treatment

The goal of the treatment is to move the ectopically erupting tooth away from the tooth it is resorbing, allow it to erupt, and retain the second primary molar. The

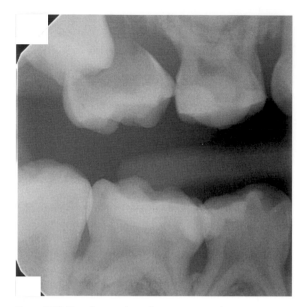

Figure 8.20 Ectopic eruption of permanent molar.

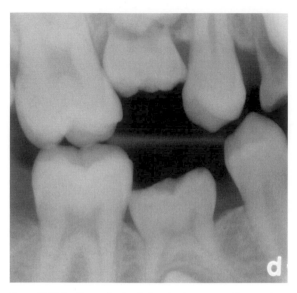

Figure 8.21 Radiograph of ankylosed primary maxillary and mandibular second molars.

extent of resorption of the primary root structure, the amount of movement needed, and the amount of permanent molar visible determine the intervention options available. A minimal impaction may be treated with an orthodontic separator placed interproximally between the second primary molar and the first permanent molar. A more severe impaction may require the use of a brass wire or tipping orthodontic appliance to distally tip the first permanent molar. In the case where the permanent molar is trapped under the stainless steel crown of the second primary molar, removal of the stainless steel crown is indicated. In the most severe presentation of ectopic eruption of the first permanent molar, the second primary molar must be extracted and the first permanent molar distalized once it is erupted.

Ankylosis

Ankylosis is the union of the radicular cementum with the alveolar bone due to a localized lack of periodontal ligament (PDL). An ankylosed tooth is diagnosed clinically by infraocclusion, a high-pitched metallic sound with percussion (as opposed to the cushioned sound of a normal tooth with an intact PDL), and lack of tooth mobility. An area of missing PDL space may also be evident radiographically.

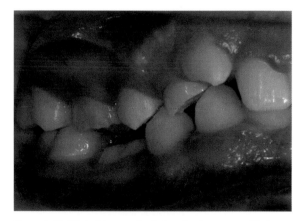

Figure 8.22 Clinical image of ankylosed primary mandibular second molar with significant infraocclusion.

Primary tooth ankylosis

Ankylosis of primary teeth occurs most frequently in mandibular molars followed by the primary maxillary molars. McKibben and Brearlley (1971) reported an incidence of 7–14% in primary teeth. Additionally, 50% of children with an ankylosed tooth will have at least one additional ankylosed tooth. Several sequelae are reported with the presence of an ankylosed primary molar, including arch length loss, alveolar bone defects, and occlusal disturbances; however, these are transient and will resolve once the permanent successor erupts (Figures 8.21 and 8.22).

Treatment

In a recent systematic review (Tieu *et al.*, 2013), the authors concluded that most ankylosed primary teeth tend to resorb and exfoliate on their own and therefore recommended monitoring ankylosed molars for 6–12 months past the expected exfoliation period. If, however, the permanent successor is erupting ectopically or if the adjacent teeth have tipped sufficiently over the infraoccluded tooth as to prevent the eruption of the permanent successor, then extraction of the ankylosed tooth should be considered. Ankylosed teeth without permanent successors may be retained and restored in the absence of dental crowding, unless the ankylosed tooth is associated with a significant vertical step in bone height compared to the adjacent teeth. In that instance, extraction of the ankylosed tooth and an appropriate orthodontic or prosthetic treatment plan should be developed. Extraction of ankylosed primary molars that do not have permanent successors may also be considered to alleviate dental crowding. Additionally, an ankylosed primary anterior tooth should be extracted if it is interfering in the eruption of its permanent successor (Ekim and Hatibovic-Kofman, 2001).

Permanent tooth ankylosis

Ankylosis of a permanent tooth occurs most often following a traumatic luxation injury. The most common location is the anterior region. This type of ankylosis is also termed replacement resorption. In this instance, the root structure is replaced by bone either rapidly or gradually. The remodeling process may be transient or result in an eventual loss of the tooth (Lin *et al.*, 2014). If ankylosis of a permanent tooth occurs during active eruption or during continued growth of the anterior maxilla, the adjacent teeth will continue to erupt while the ankylosed tooth remains in the same position. Eventually, there will be a distinct discrepancy between the positions of the ankylosed tooth and the adjacent teeth (Figure 8.23).

Prevention

Because replacement resorption most often occurs following a luxation injury, timely and appropriate treatment of the injury is necessary to minimize the potential development of replacement resorption (see section "Dental trauma to permanent teeth").

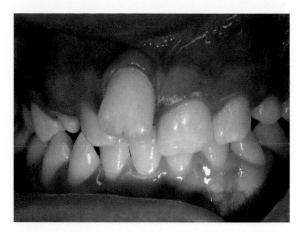

Figure 8.23 Ankylosed permanent maxillary incisor following traumatic dental injury.

Treatment

When a permanent tooth is undergoing replacement resorption, treatment options for the tooth include the following: monitoring, extraction, and decoronation. Decoronation is a procedure that involves laying a gingival flap to expose the crown and alveolar bone. The crown of the tooth is removed along with any root canal filling material placed previously. Irrigation with sterile saline and instrumentation of the canal is performed to bring blood from the apical area of the tooth into the canal space. The gingival flap is then sutured to cover the exposed root. Clinical and radiographic evaluation is done on a regular basis to monitor replacement root resorption (Cohenca and Stabholz, 2007). An appropriate short- and long-term orthodontic and prosthetic plan should be developed.

Common complications associated with dental trauma

The risk for dental trauma in children begins with their first step and continues through adolescence. Eighteen percent of all injuries in children 0–6 years of age involve the mouth and teeth (Malmgren *et al.*, 2012). In school-aged children, 25% have experienced dental trauma (DiAngelis *et al.*, 2012). In the age group between 1 and 3 years, most injuries to the mouth are due to falls (Malmgren *et al.*, 2012), while in the older age groups, sports injuries, automobile accidents, and assaults are frequent causes (Kambalimath *et al.*, 2013).

The timeliness and appropriateness of treatment for traumatic dental injuries are critical for the best long-term prognosis. Guidelines published by the International Association for Dental Traumatology are considered the standard of care for the management of traumatic injuries to both primary and permanent teeth (http://www.iadt-dentaltrauma.org/).

Dental trauma to primary teeth

Oral injuries are the second most common type of injury based on location and account for 18% of all somatic injuries in children aged 0–6 years (Glendor *et al.*, 1996; Petersson *et al.*, 1997; Glendor and Andersson, 2007). Maxillary incisors are the most often injured teeth; the frequency of trauma to these teeth is two to three times more likely in children with a pronounced overjet and protruding incisors. Trauma to the primary dentition and the alveolus may result in one or more of several potential sequelae to the succedaneous teeth including discoloration, hypoplasia, impaction, and eruption abnormalities (Andreasen *et al.*, 1971; Holan and Ram, 1999; do Espirito Santo Jacomo and Campos, 2009). Additionally, following luxation injuries, primary teeth often become discolored yellow, brown, pink, or gray color, either transiently or permanently (Borum and Andreasen, 1998) (Figure 8.24).

Prevention

It is important to provide the family with appropriate age-based anticipatory guidance that includes trauma prevention and management at regular recall visits. Health-care providers who treat children should

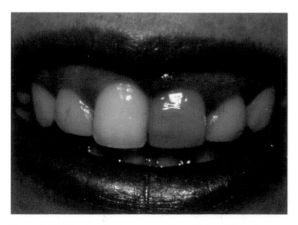

Figure 8.24 Discolored primary maxillary incisor following traumatic dental injury.

provide guidance to families about ways to child-proof their home as infants start learning to walk to prevent tripping over or bumping their mouths onto low tables. Injuries that are unexplained or do not fit the description provided by the parent or caregiver should be investigated to rule out child abuse. Dental providers are mandated reporters of any suspected instances of child abuse and neglect to state child protective services or law enforcement agencies.

Treatment

Treatment of injuries to the primary detention should follow the guidelines set forth by the International Association of Dental Traumatology (IADT) (Table 8.1).

Prior to addressing any hard and soft tissue injuries, it is important to review the patient's medical history, including tetanus immunization status, perform an accurate head and neck examination, and refer to a physician if there are any systemic concerns. Additionally, the patient's ability to cooperate for an examination, taking of radiographs, and treatment should be considered when developing a treatment plan. The IADT treatment recommendations are focused on minimizing any subsequent risks of damage to the permanent successors. Avulsed primary teeth are not reimplanted. Minor luxation injuries to primary teeth that do not result in occlusal interference may be left without an intervention. Severely luxated primary incisors that have resulted in occlusal interference are treated by repositioning (with possible need for splinting) or extraction. Simple crown fractures are either repaired by composite or left to be monitored. Teeth that have complex crown fracture (with resulting pulp exposure) must either receive pulp treatment followed by restorative repair or be extracted.

It is important to stress to the patient and caregiver that the mouth needs to be kept very clean to promote healing of the injured tissues. Chlorhexidine gluconate (0.12%) may be prescribed with the following instructions: 1–2 times daily, apply a small amount to the affected area with cotton applicator. Systemic antibiotics are not recommended unless the child has a compromised health status or if there is a soft tissue wound that appears to be dirty or contaminated.

Injured primary teeth that become discolored may be monitored, as long as they are asymptomatic with no signs of infection.

Table 8.1 Summary of treatment for primary tooth traumatic injuries.

Primary tooth	Description	Treatment	Follow-up
Concussion	Slight mobility, bleeding around gums	Observe, soft foods for 1 week, radiograph to rule out root fracture	1 week, 6–8 weeks
Luxation	Displacement of tooth laterally or incisally, mobility	Reposition tooth or extract, do not splint	1 week, 2–3 weeks, 6–8 weeks[a], 1 year[a]
Intrusion	Displacement of tooth apically, may appear to be missing	Occlusal radiograph, observe and allow to re-erupt, extract if alveolar plate is compromised	1 week, 6–8 weeks[a], 6 months[a], 1 year[a]
Extrusion	Partial displacement of tooth out of its socket	Occlusal radiograph, if minor (<3 mm) reposition or allow to realign, extract with severe extrusion. Soft foods for 1 week	1 week, 6–8 weeks[a], 6 months[a], 1 year[a]
Simple crown fracture	Fracture of tooth leaving either enamel or dentin exposed, may or may not be mobile	Restore tooth, smooth sharp edges, radiograph to rule out root fracture	3–4 weeks
Complicated crown fracture	Fracture of tooth leaving pulp tissue exposed	Pulp treatment, restore or extract tooth, observe for infection	1 week, 6–8 weeks[a], 1 year[a]
Root fracture	Tooth is fractured below the gum line, moderate to severe mobility	Occlusal radiograph, extract if root fracture is in middle or cervical third of root	1 week, 2–3 weeks, 6–8[a] weeks, 1 year[a]
Avulsion	Tooth is out of the socket	Do not replant, make radiograph to rule out intrusion	1 week, 6 months, 1 year, yearly

[a] Clinical and radiographic follow-up. In instances where the treatment was extraction, clinical and radiographic evaluation at 1 year and then every year thereafter until eruption of the permanent successor.

Dental trauma to permanent teeth

Traumatic injuries to permanent teeth may present ranging from mild (concussion) to severe (avulsion) with variations in between including crown fractures that are limited to the enamel and/or dentin, crown fractures with pulp exposure, root fracture, intrusion, extrusion, and luxation. Without proper treatment, the sequelae of traumatic injury to permanent teeth may become severe and include pulp necrosis, abscess, bone resorption, or serious systemic infection. Table 8.2 summarizes the types of permanent tooth trauma and recommended treatment.

Prevention

Although it is not possible to completely prevent accidental traumatic dental injuries, there are steps that can be taken to prevent or minimize harm. Children participating in sports should be encouraged to wear athletic mouthguards and other protective equipment such as helmets or facemasks. Injuries that are unexplained or do not fit the description provided by the parent or caregiver should be investigated to rule out child abuse. Dental providers are mandated reporters of any suspected instances of child abuse and neglect to state child protective services or law enforcement agencies.

Treatment

Most dental trauma is considered a dental emergency and should be addressed as soon as possible. Avulsion of a permanent tooth is the most urgent of all dental traumatic injuries. Reimplantation of an avulsed tooth within 30 min greatly increases the long-term prognosis of the tooth (Andersson *et al.*, 2012). If the

Table 8.2 Summary of treatment for permanent tooth traumatic injuries.

Permanent dentition	Description	Treatment
Concussion	Slight mobility, bleeding around gums	Observe, soft foods for 1 week, X-ray to rule out root fracture
Luxation	Displacement of tooth laterally or incisally, mobility	Radiograph, reposition tooth, splint for 2 weeks
Intrusion	Displacement of tooth apically, may appear to be missing	Occlusal radiograph, observe and allow to re-erupt, surgical or orthodontic repositioning, root canal treatment
Simple crown fracture	Fracture of tooth leaving either enamel or dentin exposed, may or may not be mobile	Restore tooth, smooth sharp edges, radiograph to rule out root fracture
Complicated crown fracture	Fracture of tooth leaving pulp tissue exposed	Pulp treatment, restore tooth, observe for infection, may require root canal treatment
Root fracture	Tooth is fractured below the gum line, moderate to severe mobility	Occlusal radiograph, splint, may require root canal treatment, if in cervical third, may need to extract
Avulsion	Tooth is out of the socket	Replant within 30 min or place in recommended transport medium: Hank's balanced saline, cold milk, saline. Radiograph, replant, and splint ASAP. Systemic antibiotics, soft diet, chlorhexidine, close follow-up, root canal therapy (RCT) within 3–7 days
Alveolar fracture	Teeth are luxated and there is mobility of the entire segment including the teeth	Reposition teeth and alveolar segment; place semirigid splint for 4 weeks; soft diet, chlorhexidine, close follow-up

avulsed permanent tooth cannot be reimplanted immediately, it should be placed in an appropriate storage medium such as Hank's balanced salt solution, cold skim milk, or saliva. Tap water should be avoided. It is important to use a standard protocol to assess traumatic injuries that includes questions about what, where, when, and how the injury occurred; tetanus immunization status; loss of consciousness; extraoral and intraoral findings; and documentation of injuries. Using a standardized trauma form for recording relevant information should be a part of the electronic health record or may be downloaded from the AAPD (http://www.aapd.org/media/Policies_Guidelines/R_AcuteTrauma.pdf) and stored as part of the patient's record. If the patient lost consciousness or if there are other more serious injuries, the patient should be seen in a hospital emergency room or by their primary care physician for a thorough assessment. To determine whether a patient should be seen urgently after sustaining dental trauma, the provider should be guided by the description of the injury; the presence of pain, bleeding, and swelling; and how the injury affects the child's ability to sleep and eat (Figures 8.25 and 8.26). Often, it is recommended to see the child emergently, assess the injury, and then provide either definitive treatment or palliative treatment with a plan for more definitive care at a follow-up visit. Table 8.2 summarizes the treatment recommended for each type of injury, and more details can be found in the guidelines developed by the IADT (Andersson *et al.*, 2012; DiAngelis *et al.*, 2012).

Soft tissue trauma

The oral soft tissues may sustain significant injuries during oral facial trauma. There may be open wounds, abrasions, burns, and puncture wounds. Trauma to gingival tissues may be associated with an injured tooth and varies in presentation from hemorrhage at the time of the injury, torn frenum, large laceration, to penetrating lesion of the lip or cheek.

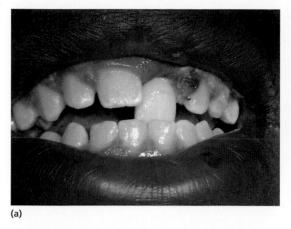

(a)

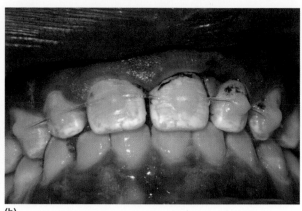

(b)

Figure 8.25 (a and b) Luxated teeth pre- and postsplinting.

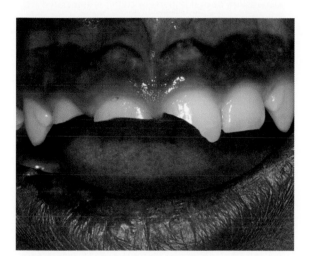

Figure 8.26 Complicated fracture of maxillary incisors requiring an urgent treatment.

Prevention

Appropriate anticipatory guidance that includes injury prevention should be discussed at regular intervals based on the child's age and stage of development. For young children, it is important to discuss the risk for oral burns from chewing on live electrical cords. Parents should be reminded of the importance of using a child safety car seat or a seatbelt. Dentists should also discuss the importance of wearing a mouth guard and/or helmet as appropriate during various sporting activities. And as the child ages, discussing the injuries that may occur due to oral piercings is prudent.

Treatment

Treatment of soft tissue injuries depends on the type and extent of the injury. The wound must be adequately cleaned. Debridement, compression, or suturing should be performed as indicated. It is important to review the patient's tetanus immunization status and to refer the patient to a physician if it is not up to date. It cannot be assumed that a child's immunization status is up to date since a growing number of US parents are declining immunizations for their children. If a foreign body is suspected to be embedded in the soft tissue, a radiograph of the area should be taken. To visualize a foreign body in the lip, the film is placed in the vestibule between the lip and the teeth. The soft tissue film should be taken at 25% of the normal exposure time. Lateral external radiographs may also be taken to better elucidate the position of the foreign body using 50% of the normal exposure time. Depending on the extent and location of the soft tissue injury, conferring with an oral and maxillofacial surgeon or plastic surgeon to participate in the patient's care may be beneficial. Chlorhexidine gluconate (0.12%) may be prescribed with the following instructions: 1–2 times daily, apply a small amount to the affected area with cotton applicator. Systemic antibiotics are not recommended unless the child has a compromised health status or the soft tissue wounds appear to have been contaminated by extrinsic bacteria or if there are other associated injuries, which have an increased risk of infection, such as open fractures or joint injuries.

Alveolar fractures

Fractures of the alveolus may occur when one or more teeth are severely laterally luxated, causing the roots to perforate the buccal or lingual plate. A common finding with this type of injury is movement of an entire segment with multiple teeth affected. Frequently the occlusion is also out of alignment.

Treatment

Alveolar fracture combined with luxation of the teeth requires reposition of the displaced segment and splinting for a minimum of 4 weeks (DiAngelis *et al.*, 2012). Patients should be instructed to eat a soft diet for 2 weeks, avoid contact sports, maintain good oral hygiene, and rinse twice daily with chlorhexidine rinse. One or more teeth may require root canal treatment in the future. Close clinical and radiographic monitoring is indicated.

Common complications associated with patients with special needs or developmental disabilities

G-tube fed

Children who are unable to meet their fluid and nutritional needs orally and who depend on gastrostomy tube feedings are at significantly increased risk of poor oral health, particularly a buildup of calculus and subsequent gingivitis (Jawadi *et al.*, 2004; Thikkurissy and Lal, 2009). Frequently children who are G-tube dependent have other developmental disabilities that make it difficult or impossible for them to perform oral hygiene procedures. Calculus removal by a dental professional is required on a regular basis (Figure 8.27).

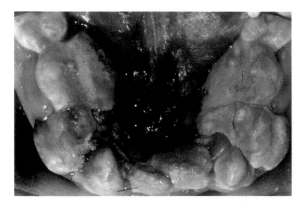

Figure 8.27 Extensive calculus in a G-tube-fed patient.

Treatment

Patients who can tolerate treatment in the traditional dental office setting should have regular scaling of buccal and lingual tooth surfaces to remove calculus at or below the gingiva. It may be necessary to position the patient somewhat upright to minimize the risk for aspiration. Patients who cannot tolerate treatment in the traditional dental setting should be treated under general anesthesia in an environment where the airway is protected from aspiration of bacteria, saliva, and calculus fragments. When children are 100% tube fed, their risk for caries is significantly decreased. However, treatment in the operating room provides an opportunity to obtain intraoral radiographs and provide dental treatment as needed.

Oral aversion

Oral aversion, or oral hypersensitivity, is associated with several different systemic diagnoses. In medically complicated children with a history of gastrostomy tube feeding, oral aversion is thought to arise in response to the child having had minimal opportunities to learn to eat orally and thus having had fewer opportunities for oral stimulation (Dyment and Casas, 1999; Davis, Bruce, and Mangiaracina, 2009). Children with a history of gastrostomy tube feeding may consequently experience physical or psychological discomfort with eating or other oral stimulation, such as tooth brushing. Oral aversion is also a common finding in children with neurodevelopmental disorders such as autism. Perceived invasive contact, such as that experienced with different textures of food or during tooth brushing, may cause a child with a neurodevelopmental disorder physical or psychological trauma.

Management

While prevention of oral aversion may not be possible, it is best to help the family develop a plan early on during which they are working with the child daily in order to decrease hypersensitivity, such as with eating utensils and brushing the teeth. As many of these children will also be seeing an occupational therapist, coordinating an individualized oral care plan may provide the most favorable outcomes for each child (Zangen *et al.*, 2003).

Severe bruxism

Bruxism is grinding of the teeth and is common during sleep. Bruxism can result in trauma to the occlusion, manifesting as abnormal wear patterns and even tooth fractures. It can lead to gingival recession and tooth loss. Bruxism is common in individuals with disabilities such as sleep disorders and malocclusion. One study showed significantly more physical signs of bruxism in children who had autism spectrum disorders (ASDs) (DeMattei, Cuvo, and Maurizio, 2007). Children and adults with cerebral palsy may also have increased incidence of bruxism with resultant extreme wear of permanent teeth. Temporomandibular joint and muscle soreness and pain have been associated with bruxism.

Erosion

Acid erosion is the progressive loss of tooth substance, which may be caused by an acid or chemical dissolution. Most commonly, erosion of enamel is due to gastro-esophageal reflux disease (GERD), bulimia, or frequent consumption of acidic beverages (Figure 8.28a and b).

Prevention

Recognition of the cause of erosion in a specific patient is a prerequisite to prevention. This becomes a challenge if the patient denies all the likely causes. It is important to ask detailed questions about diet, including citrus fruit and carbonated beverages consumed on a regular basis. It is also important to note that young children may have symptoms of GERD without being able to recognize or describe these symptoms. A history of frequent indigestion or having "hot burps" may warrant further evaluation by the child's primary care provider. A history of frequent regurgitation should also warrant medical evaluation. When a dietary cause for erosion cannot be identified, a workup for GERD by the child's primary care physician is recommended.

Treatment

The most important first step in the treatment of erosion is to identify and eliminate the cause, if possible. If the child has GERD, medication prescribed by the physician will often manage the symptoms. For children or adolescents with suspected bulimia, referral to a health-care professional who specializes in the treatment of eating disorders is essential. Where diet is suspected to be the main etiology, eliminating or changing the frequency of acidic beverages and other dietary factors should be strongly encouraged. When acidic challenges to the oral cavity are a regular occurrence, the use of a sodium bicarbonate rinse or chewing antacid tablets to neutralize the pH and use of fluoride toothpaste or fluoride rinse can help to balance the loss of enamel (Barron *et al.*, 2003). In extreme cases of significant tooth structure loss, full-coverage restorations may be necessary.

Cleft lip and palate

Clefts of the lip and/or palate are the most common of the craniofacial anomalies and result from a failure of the embryonic structures to merge or fuse during in utero growth and development. Clefts of the lip and palate can occur simultaneously or separately and bilaterally or unilaterally (Stanier and Moore, 2004). The presence of clefts of the lip and palate may be associated with a genetic predisposition, a teratogenic influence, or an unknown cause. Additionally, cleft lip and palate may present as an isolated condition or as a component of a complex syndrome.

Pediatric patients with clefts of the lip and/or palate may present with several dental anomalies and

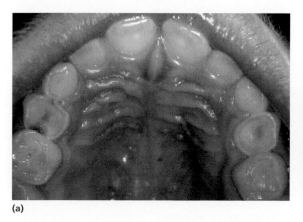
(a)

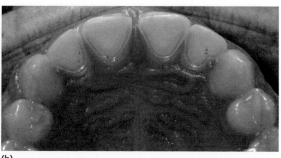
(b)

Figure 8.28 (a and b) Erosion on posterior and anterior teeth.

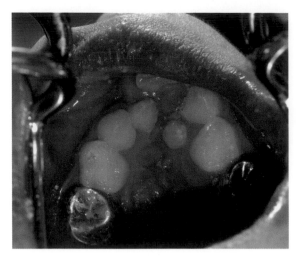

Figure 8.29 Cleft lip palate with extra and malformed teeth.

malocclusions due to the clefting itself or secondary to the surgical corrections of the cleft. There may be supernumerary or missing teeth, most commonly the maxillary lateral incisor as well as premolars (Figure 8.29). The lateral incisors and canines may erupt ectopically and be rotated. Additionally, there may be anomalies in tooth morphology such as enamel hypoplasia, microdontia, macrodontia, fused teeth, and alterations in shape. There is also an increased potential for the ectopic eruption of a maxillary first permanent molar. Given the multiple oral anomalies possible as well as the other stressors associated with managing the cleft, children with cleft lip and/or palate are at an increased risk for the development of dental caries.

Management

From birth until adulthood, children born with lip and palate clefts require assessment and treatment from a diverse team of specialists including pediatric dentistry, audiology, genetics, nursing, oral and maxillofacial surgery, orthodontics, otolaryngology/head and neck surgery, plastic surgery, psychology, social work, and speech–language pathology. They may undergo complex orthodontic treatment and multiple surgical interventions. As the dentist of a child with any craniofacial anomaly, it is imperative to provide preventive counseling and caries control to maintain the child's oral health. The dentist should discuss the possible dental anomalies that may be observed in a child with a cleft lip or palate. It is important to seek input from members of the child's craniofacial team when the dental treatment plan involves the treatment of teeth associated with or adjacent to the cleft. It is preferred to have ectopically erupted or supernumerary teeth associated with the cleft retained in the mouth in order to maintain any bone associated with the teeth.

Autism spectrum disorder

ASD is a chronic neurodevelopmental disorder characterized by impairments in social interaction, language development, behavior, and cognitive function. Twin and family studies suggest a genetic link in the etiology of the disorder (Szatmari *et al.*, 1998). Males are 3–4 times more likely to be affected than females. It is thought that the varied clinical presentations of people with ASD are due to a combination of environmental factors and the wide range of variability of abnormalities of multiple genes existing in different combinations (Johnson, Myers, and American Academy of Pediatrics Council on Children with Disabilities, 2007; Vierck and Silverman, 2015).

A child with ASD may have one or more of the following characteristics:

1 Impaired social interactions, for example, lack of eye contact
2 Impaired verbal and nonverbal communication
3 Restricted, repetitive patterns of behavior
4 Poor body awareness and clumsiness
5 Distorted sensory input, for example, taste or texture sensitivities, oral aversion, and self-injurious behavior

Children with ASD are managed medically with an early diagnosis and intensive education intervention (Myers, Johnson, and American Academy of Pediatrics Council on Children with Disabilities, 2007). They may also be prescribed medication to treat specific behaviors that interfere with the intervention, for example, fluoxetine (Prozac), an antidepressant to decrease compulsive behaviors and self-mutilation.

Dental management

Children with ASD have a caries rate that is similar to that of the neurotypical population. Oral hygiene may be difficult for a child with ASD to accept. The diet may be limited due to their restricted food choices. Children with ASD may have evidence of bruxism or erosion as well as bruising or scarring due to falls because of their decreased coordination or self-injurious behavior (Friedlander *et al.*, 2006).

A child with ASD may do best with consistency in the dentist, staff, and treatment room. Parents are often very helpful in helping to manage a child with ASD. Multiple short visits to the dental office during which the routine is repeated and the child is gradually desensitized may be effective in helping the child to more readily accept the treatment (Luscre and Center, 1987). For a child with whom there is limited cooperation and there are concerns about oral health, dental treatment under general anesthesia may be needed. Long-term considerations for the oral health of a child with ASD include teaching the family about ways to promote optimal oral health and prevent the disease (Klein and Nowak, 1999).

Summary

Dental providers who treat children in their practice should expect to encounter both complications and challenges that are different from those encountered in adult patients. Referral to a specialist such as a pediatric dentist is recommended when the treatment indicated is beyond the comfort level of the general dentist.

Acknowledgments

The authors would like to thank the editor of this text for the opportunity to contribute to this chapter and to the reviewers who provided helpful suggestions that improved the overall content of the chapter.

References

American Academy of Pediatric Dentistry (AAPD) (2014a) Guideline on the use of nitrous oxide for pediatric dental patients. *Pediatr Dent*, **36**, 204–208.

AAPD (2014b) Guideline for monitoring and management of pediatric patients during and after sedation for diagnostic and therapeutic procedures. *Pediatr Dent*, **36**, 209–225.

AAPD (2014c) Guideline on use of anesthesia personnel in the administration of office-based deep sedation/general anesthesia to the pediatric dental patient. *Pediatr Dent*, **36**, 226–229.

AAPD (2014d) Guideline on protective stabilization for pediatric dental patients. *Pediatr Dent*, **36**, 192–196.

AAPD (2014e) Guideline on informed consent. *Pediatr Dent*, **36**, 310–312.

Andersson, L., Andreasen, J.O., Day, P., Heithersay, G., Trope, M., Diangelis, A.J., Kenny, D.J., Sigurdsson, A., Bourguignon, C., Flores, M.T., Hicks, M.L., Lenzi, A.R., Malmgren, B., Moule, A.J., Tsukiboshi, M. and International Association of Dental Traumatology (2012) International Association of Dental Traumatology guidelines for the management of traumatic dental injuries: 2. Avulsion of permanent teeth. *Dent Traumatol*, **28**, 88–96.

Andreasen, J.O., Sundstrom, B. and Ravn, J.J. (1971) The effect of traumatic injuries to primary teeth on their permanent successors. I. A clinical and histologic study of 117 injured permanent teeth. *Scand J Dent Res*, **79**, 219–283.

Barberia-Leache, E., Suarez-Clus, M.C. and Seavedra-Ontiveros, D. (2005) Ectopic eruption of the maxillary first permanent molar: characteristics and occurrence in growing children. *Angle Orthodont*, **75**, 610–615.

Barron, R.P., Carmichael, R.P., Marcon, M.A. and Sandor, G.K. (2003) Dental erosion in gastroesophageal reflux disease. *J Can Dent Assoc*, **69**, 84–89.

Baum, V.C. (2007) When nitrous oxide is no laughing matter: nitrous oxide and pediatric anesthesia. *Paediatr Anaesth*, **17**, 824–830.

Bedoya, M.M. and Park, J.H. (2009) A review of the diagnosis and management of impacted maxillary canines. *J Am Dent Assoc*, **140**, 1485–1493.

Borum, M.K. and Andreasen, J.O. (1998) Sequelae of trauma to primary maxillary incisors. I. Complications in the primary dentition. *Endod Dent Traumatol*, **14**, 31–44.

Brothwell, D.J. (1997) Guidelines on the use of space maintainers following premature loss of primary teeth. *J Can Dent Assoc*, **63** (753), 757–760 764–766.

Cameron, A.C. and Widmer, R.P. (eds) (2003) Dental anomalies, in *Handbook of Pediatric Dentistry*, 2nd edn, Mosby, New York, pp. 184–233.

Chi, D., Kanellis, M., Himadi, E. and Asselin, M.E. (2008) Lip biting in a pediatric dental patient after dental local anesthesia: a case report. *J Pediatr Nurs*, **23**, 490–493.

Cohenca, N., Paranjpe, A. and Berg, J. (2013) Vital pulp therapy. *Dent Clin North Am*, **57**, 59–73.

Cohenca, N. and Stabholz, A. (2007) Decoronation – a conservative method to treat ankylosed teeth for preservation of alveolar ridge prior to permanent prosthetic reconstruction: literature review and case presentation. *Dent Traumatol*, **23**, 87–94.

Coll, J.A. and Sadrian, R. (1996) Predicting pulpectomy success and its relationship to exfoliation and succedaneous dentition. *Pediatr Dent*, **18**, 57–63.

College, C., Feigal, R., Wandera, A. and Strange, M. (2000) Bilateral versus unilateral mandibular block anesthesia in a pediatric population. *Pediatr Dent*, **22**, 453–457.

Croll, T.P. (2000) Restorative options for malformed permanent molars in children. *Compend Contin Educ Dent*, **21**, 676–678 680, 682.

Davis, A.M., Bruce, A.S. and Mangiaracina, C. (2009) Moving from tube to oral feeding in medically fragile nonverbal toddlers. *J Pediatr Gastroenterol Nutr*, **49**, 233–236.

DeMattei, R., Cuvo, A. and Maurizio, S. (2007) Oral assessment of children with an autism spectrum disorder. *J Dent Hyg*, **81**, 65.

DiAngelis, A.J., Andreasen, J.O., Ebeleseder, K.A., Kenny, D.J., Trope, M., Sigurdsson, A., Andersson, L., Bourguignon, C., Flores, M.T., Hicks, M.L., Lenzi, A.R., Malmgren, B., Moule, A.J., Pohl, Y., Tsukiboshi, M. and International Association of Dental Traumatology (2012) International Association of Dental Traumatology guidelines for the management of traumatic dental injuries: 1. Fractures and luxations of permanent teeth. *Dent Traumatol*, **28**, 2–12.

do Espirito Santo Jacomo, D.R. and Campos, V. (2009) Prevalence of sequelae in the permanent anterior teeth after trauma in their predecessors: a longitudinal study of 8 years. *Dent Traumatol*, **25**, 300–304.

Dyment, H.A. and Casas, M.J. (1999) Dental care for children fed by tube: a critical review. *Special Care Dent*, **19**, 220–224.

Ekim, S.L. and Hatibovic-Kofman, S. (2001) A treatment decision-making model for infraoccluded primary molars. *Int J Paediatr Dent*, **11**, 340–346.

Ericson, S. and Kurol, J. (1986) Longitudinal study and analysis of clinical supervision of maxillary canine eruption. *Community Dent Oral Epidemiol*, **14**, 172–176.

Ericson, S. and Kurol, J. (1988) Early treatment of palatally erupting maxillary canines by extraction of the primary canines. *Eur J Orthod*, **10**, 283–295.

Friedlander, A.H., Yagiela, J.A., Paterno, V.I. and Mahler, M.E. (2006) Autism: the neuropathology, medical management and dental implications of autism. *J Am Dent Assoc*, **137**, 1517–1528.

Glendor, U. and Andersson, L. (2007) Public health aspects of oral diseases and disorders: dental trauma, in *Community oral health* (eds C. Pine and R. Harris), Quintessence, London, pp. 203–214.

Glendor, U., Halling, A., Andersson, L. and Eilert-Petersson, E. (1996) Incidence of traumatic tooth injuries in children and adolescents in the county of Vastmanland, Sweden. *Swed Dent J*, **20**, 15–28.

Hargreaves, K.M., Diogenes, A. and Teixeira, F.B. (2013) Treatment options: biological basis of regenerative endodontic procedures. *J Endod*, **39**, S30–S43.

Hersh, E.V., Hermann, D.G., Lamp, C.J., Johnson, P.D. and MacAfee, K.A. (1995) Assessing the duration of mandibular soft tissue anesthesia. *J Am Dent Assoc*, **26**, 1531–1536.

Holan, G. and Ram, D. (1999) Sequelae and prognosis of intruded primary incisors: a retrospective study. *Pediatr Dent*, **21**, 242–247.

Jawadi, A.H., Casamassimo, P.S., Griffen, A., Enrile, B. and Marcone, M. (2004) Comparison of oral findings in special needs children with and without gastrostomy. *Pediatr Dent*, **26**, 283–288.

Johnson, C.P., Myers, S.M. and American Academy of Pediatrics Council on Children with Disabilities (2007) Identification and evaluation of children with autism spectrum disorders. *Pediatrics*, **120**, 1183–1215.

Kambalimath, H.V., Agarwal, S.M., Kambalimath, D.H., Singh, M., Jain, N. and Michael, P. (2013) Maxillofacial injuries in children: a 10 year retrospective study. *J Maxillofac Oral Surg*, **12**, 140–144.

Kerosuo, H., Kullaa, A., Kerosuo, E., Kanerva, L. and Hensten-Pettersen, A. (1996) Nickel allergy in adolescents in relation to orthodontic treatment and piercing of ears. *Am J Orthod Dentofacial Orthop*, **109**, 148–154.

Klein, U. and Nowak, A.J. (1999) Characteristics of patients with autistic disorder (AD) presenting for dental treatment: a survey and chart review. *Special Care Dent*, **19**, 200–207.

Kupietzky, A. and Botzer, E. (2005) Ankyloglossia in the infant and young child: clinical suggestions for diagnosis and management. *Pediatr Dent*, **27**, 40–46.

Kusumi, K., Ayoob, R., Bowden, S.A., Ingraham, S. and Mahan, J.D. (2015) Beneficial effects of intravenous pamidronate treatment in children with osteogenesis imperfecta under 24 months of age. *J Bone Miner Metab*, **33** (5), 560–568.

Laing, E., Ashley, P., Naini, F.B. and Gill, D.S. (2009) Space maintenance. *Int J Paediatr Dent*, **19**, 155–162.

Lang, R., White, P.J., Machalicek, W., Rispoli, M., Kang, S., Aquilar, J., O'Reilly, M., Sigafoos, J., Lancioni, G. and Didden, R. (2009) Treatment of bruxism in individuals with developmental disabilities: a systematic review. *Res Dev Disabil*, **30**, 809–818.

Levitan, M.E. and Himel, V.T. (2006) Dens evaginatus: literature review, pathophysiology, and comprehensive treatment regimen. *J Endod*, **32**, 1–9.

Li, D., Du, X., Zhang, R., Shen, B., Huang, Y., Valenzuela, R.K., Wang, B., Zhao, H., Liu, Z., Li, J., Xu, Z., Gao, L. and Ma, J. (2012) Mutation identification of the DSPP in a Chinese family with DGI-II and an up-to-date bioinformatic analysis. *Genomics*, **99**, 220–226.

Lin, F., Sun, H., Yao, L., Chen, Q. and Ni, Z. (2014) Orthodontic treatment of severe anterior open bite and alveolar bone defect complicated by an ankylosed maxillary central incisor: a case report. *Head Face Med*, **10**, 47.

Luscre, D.M. and Center, D.B. (1987) Procedures for reducing dental fear in children with autism. *J Autism Dev Disord*, **26**, 547–556.

Maines, E., Monti, E., Doro, F., Morandi, G., Cavarzere, P. and Antoniazzi, F. (2012) Children and adolescents treated with neridronate for osteogenesis imperfecta show no evidence of any osteonecrosis of the jaw. *J Bone Miner Metab*, **30**, 434–438.

Malmgren, B., Andreasen, J.O., Flores, M.T., Robertson, A., DiAngelis, A.J., Andersson, L., Cavalleri, G., Cohenca, N., Day, P., Hicks, M.L., Malmgren, O., Moule, A.J., Onetto, J., Tsukiboshi, M. and International Association of Dental Traumatology (2012) International Association of Dental Traumatology guidelines for the management of traumatic dental injuries: 3. Injuries in the primary dentition. *Dent Traumatol*, **28**, 174–182.

Mast, P., Rodrigueztapia, M.T., Daeniker, L. and Krejci, I. (2013) Understanding MIH: definition, epidemiology, differential diagnosis and new treatment guidelines. *Eur J Paediatr Dent*, **14**, 204–248.

McKibben, D.R. and Brearlley, L.J. (1971) Radiographic determination of the prevalence of selected dental anomalies in children. *J Dent Child*, **28**, 390–398.

Millet, C., Duprez, J., Khoury, C., Morgon, L. and Richard, B. (2015) Interdisciplinary care for a patient with amelogenesis imperfecta: a clinical report. *J Prosthodont*, **24** (5), 424–431.

Myers, S.M., Johnson, C.P. and American Academy of Pediatrics Council on Children with Disabilities (2007) Management of children with autism spectrum disorders. *Pediatrics*, **120**, 1162–1182.

Nelson, S., Albert, J.M., Geng, C., Curtan, S., Lang, K., Miadich, S., Heima, M., Malik, A., Ferretti, G., Eggertsson, H., Slayton, R.L. and Milgrom, P. (2013) Increased enamel hypoplasia and very low birthweight infants. *J Dent Res*, **92**, 788–794.

Oehlers, F., Lee, K. and Lee, E. (1967) Dens evaginatus (evaginated odontome): its structure and responses to external stimuli. *Dent Pract Dent Rec*, **17**, 239–244.

Oulis, C., Vadiakas, G. and Vasilopoulou, A. (1996) The effectiveness of mandibular infiltration compared to mandibular block anesthesia in treating primary molars in children. *Pediatr Dent*, **18**, 301–305.

Ovental, A., Maron, R., Botzer, E., Batscha, N. and Dolberg, S. (2014) Using topical benzocaine before lingual frenotomy did not reduce crying and should be discouraged. *Acta Paediatr*, **103**, 780–782.

Patel, R.M., Nagamani, S.C.S., Cuthbertson, D., Campeau, P.M., Krischer, J.P., Shapiro, J.R., Steiner, R.D., Smith, P.A., Bober, M.B., Byers, P.H., Pepin, M., Durigova, M., Glorieux, F.H., Rauch, F., Lee, B.H., Hart, T. and Sutton, V.R. (2015) A cross-sectional multicenter study of osteogenesis imperfecta in North America – results from the linked clinical research centers. *Clin Genet*, **87** (2), 133–140.

Pawlak, R., Lester, S.E. and Babatunde, T. (2014) The prevalence of cobalamin deficiency among vegetarians assessed by serum vitamin B_{12}: a review of literature. *Eur J Clin Nutr*, **68**, 541–548.

Pazzini, C.A., Marques, L.S., Pereira, L.J., Corrêa-Faria, P. and Paiva, S.M. (2011) Allergic reactions and nickel-free braces: a systematic review. *Braz Oral Res*, **25**, 85–90.

Petersson, E.E., Andersson, L. and Sorensen, S. (1997) Traumatic oral vs non-oral injuries. *Swed Dent J*, **21**, 55–68.

Power, R.F. and Murphy, J.F. (2015) Tongue-tie and frenotomy in infants with breastfeeding difficulties: achieving a balance. *Arch Dis Child*, **100** (5), 489–494.

Power, S.M. and Short, M.B. (1993) An investigation into the response of palatally displaced canines to the removal of deciduous canines and an assessment of factors contributing to favourable eruption. *Br J Orthod*, **20**, 215–223.

Rafter, M. (2005) Apexification: a review. *Dent Traumatol*, **21**, 1–8.

Richardson, G. and Russell, K.A. (2000) A review of impacted permanent maxillary cuspids – diagnosis and prevention. *J Can Dent Assoc*, **66**, 497–501.

Sanders, R.D., Weimann, J. and Maze, M. (2008) Biologic effects of nitrous oxide: a mechanistic and toxicologic review. *Anesthesiology*, **109**, 707–722.

Selzer, R.R., Rosenblatt, D.S., Laxova, R. and Hogan, K. (2003) Adverse effect of nitrous oxide in a child with 5,10-methylenetetrahydrofolate reductase deficiency. *N Engl J Med*, **349**, 45–50.

Setcos, J.C., Babaei-Mahani, A., Di Silvio, L., Mjör, I.A. and Wilson, N.H.F. (2006) The safety of nickel containing dental alloys. *Dent Materials*, **22**, 1163–1168.

Slayton, R.L. (2013) Congenital genetic disorders and syndromes, in *Pediatric Dentistry: Infancy through Adolescence*, 5th edn (eds P. Casamassimo, H. Fields, D.J. McTigue and A. Nowak), Elsevier Saunders, St. Louis, MO, pp. 231–246.

Slayton, R.L., Brickhouse, T.H. and Adair, S. (2011) Dental development, morphology, eruption and related pathologies, in *The Handbook*, 4th edn (eds A.J. Nowak and P. Casamassimo), American Academy of Pediatric Dentistry, Chicago, IL.

Stanier, P. and Moore, G.E. (2004) Genetics of cleft lip and palate: syndromic genes contribute to the incidences of non-syndromic clefts. *Hum Mol Genet*, **13**, R73–R81.

Szatmari, P., Jones, M.B., Zwaigenbaum, L. and MacLean, J.E. (1998) Genetics of autism: overview and new directions. *J Autism Dev Disord*, **28**, 351–368.

Thikkurissy, S. and Lal, S. (2009) Oral health burden in children with systemic diseases. *Dent Clin North Am*, **53**, 351–357.

Tieu, L.D., Walker, S.L., Major, M.P. and Flores-Mir, C. (2013) Management of ankylosed primary molars with premolar successors. *J Am Dent Assoc*, **144**, 602–611.

Vierck, E. and Silverman, J.M. (2015) Brief report: phenotypic differences and their relationship to paternal age and gender in autism spectrum disorder. *J Autism Dev Disord*, **45**, 1915–1924.

Webb, A.N., Hao, W. and Hong, P. (2013) The effect of tongue-tie division on breastfeeding and speech articulation: a systematic review. *Int J Pediatr Otorhinolaryngol*, **77**, 635–646.

Willing, M.C., Deschenes, S.P., Slayton, R.L. and Roberts, E.J. (1996) Premature chain termination is a unifying mechanism for COL1A1 null alleles in osteogenesis imperfecta type I cell strains. *Am J Hum Genet*, **59**, 799–809.

Winek, C.L., Wahba, W.W. and Rozin, L. (1995) Accidental death by nitrous oxide inhalation. *Forensic Sci Int*, **22**, 139–141.

Wright, J.T., Carrion, I.A. and Morris, C. (2015) The molecular basis of hereditary enamel defects in humans. *J Dent Res*, **94**, 52–61.

Yaseen, S.M., Naik, S. and Uloopi, K.S. (2011) Ectopic eruption – a review and case report. *Contemp Clin Dent*, **2**, 3–7.

Zangen, T., Ciarla, C., Zangen, S., Di Lorenzo, C., Flores, A.F., Cocjin, J., Reddy, S.N., Rowhani, A., Schwankovsky, L. and Hyman, P.E. (2003) Gastrointestinal motility and sensory abnormalities may contribute to food refusal in medically fragile toddlers. *J Pediatr Gastroenterol Nutr*, **37**, 287093.

CHAPTER 9

Orthodontic complications and the periodontal aspects related to clinical orthodontics

Hung V. Vu[1,2,3,4] and Philip R. Melnick[5]

[1] Section of Orthodontics, UCLA School of Dentistry, Los Angeles, CA, USA
[2] US Department of Veterans Affairs Greater Los Angeles Healthcare System, Los Angeles, CA, USA
[3] Vu Orthodontics, Fountain Valley, CA, USA
[4] Department of Mechanical & Aerospace Engineering, California State University Long Beach, Long Beach, CA, USA
[5] Section of Periodontics, Clinical Dental Sciences, UCLA School of Dentistry, Los Angeles, CA, USA

Part I: Orthodontics

Introduction

In practicing orthodontics, one of the major concerns is complications. It would behoove the clinician to recognize the possible complications, so they can be avoided or treated.

Fundamentals and principles should be learned, and then solutions to the orthodontic problems could come naturally. There is no such thing as "cookbook recipes" or "by-the-book" in practicing orthodontics.

Many complications can occur in practicing orthodontics, and any possible problem can occur. In some way, Murphy's law holds true: "What possibly might happen will happen." Some problems cannot be avoided totally, and the clinician may have to accept certain compromises.

Topics are selected based on common occurrence and presented in an alphabetical order.

The goal of this chapter is to present complications in clinical orthodontics and the major periodontal complications associated with it.

Archwire materials

In contemporary orthodontics, the most common materials for archwires are stainless steel (SS), nickel–titanium (NT) alloy, heat-activated NT, and beta-titanium alloy which is also called titanium molybdenum alloy (TMA). These materials have their own unique properties, so they are best used depending on the applications. Cost is also an economic factor that would affect the clinician's decision as well. The archwire materials are listed in the order of increasing cost: SS, NT, heat-activated NT, TMA, and reverse-curve-of-Spee NT archwires. For the same material, archwire with round cross section is less expensive than that of square or rectangular.

SS archwire is typically used for its low cost, stiffness, and formability. Stiffness is the inverse of flexibility (also called springiness). NT archwire is used for its flexibility and shape memory, and it is a little more expensive than the SS (about two to three times as much). Heat-activated NT archwire, which is a little more expensive than the NT archwire, is dead soft when chilled for ease of engagement to the bracket slot, but it regains its normal stiffness when activated by the body temperature in the mouth. TMA archwire is unique in the sense that it has both useful properties: formability (similar to SS) and flexibility (similar to NT). TMA and the reverse-curve-of-Spee NT archwires are among the most expensive. The reverse-curve-of-Spee NT archwire can be 10–30 times more expensive than the SS.

With SS or TMA archwire, it can be placed into plastic deformation with a simple bend. But NT archwire requires special treatment.

Archwire complications

Archwire complications can occur for any patients. Typical complications include pain, broken archwire, archwire bending, archwire slipping/sliding, and the archwire poking the patient's cheek or gingiva.

How to avoid and treat the complications

Pain or discomfort is a major complication or complaint with an orthodontic treatment. To minimize the pain to the patient, the beginning archwire for the initial stage of leveling and aligning should be as flexible as practical. The reason is that most patients would be extremely sensitive at the beginning when the archwires start to exert their forces compressing the periodontal ligament (PDL). The width of the PDL ranges from 0.15 to 0.38 mm, which decreases with age, and its thinnest part is located around the middle third of the root (Nanci, 2003).

The most flexible and practical NT archwire is SPEED 0.016″ Supercable (a stranded wire, even more flexible than 0.010″ NT). Even with this archwire as the initial one, some patients, with moderate crowding, reported significant levels of pain. The Supercable comprises seven small-gauge wires wrapped together to form a larger wire. In this fashion, a stranded archwire is *much* more flexible than a solid archwire of the same total cross-sectional area. But a serious complication is that the small-gauge wires of the Supercable, after being cut to the proper length, would splay (spread out) at the end (tip) and cause irritation.

The next most flexible NT archwire is a round 0.010″ in diameter, followed by 0.012″ NT. It must be emphasized that different orthodontists use different wire sequencings, depending on their own understanding and belief of biomechanics.

In clinical orthodontics, clinicians may write 10 NT to indicate a round NT archwire whose cross section is 0.010″ in diameter. Similarly, a 16 × 16 SS archwire is a square SS archwire with 0.016″ × 0.016″ in cross section. And 16 × 22 SS archwire is a rectangular SS archwire with 0.016″ × 0.022″ in cross section, where 0.022″ is the base and 0.016″ is the height (in the occlusogingival direction).

When the teeth are malaligned, a smaller (cross-sectional) NT archwire, which is used for more flexibility, would exert less force on the dentition, thus less pain to the patient.

Compared to SS, NT has poor toughness, and its archwire is more susceptible to fracture due to fatigue. And this complication often leads to emergency visits.

Archwire sliding

The high flexibility of the NT archwire can be a blessing or a curse. It is a blessing because a small NT archwire can be completely engaged and stayed in the slot of the brackets when the teeth are moderately malaligned, which is a typical condition in the initial stage of leveling and aligning. The smaller the archwire cross section, the higher the archwire flexibility. But the high flexibility can also be a curse because if the archwire is too flexible, it can easily slip (or slide) out of the molar tube and poke the cheek or the gingiva of the patient. This type of complication will indeed result in an emergency call or visit.

How to avoid and treat the complication

For the NT archwire to prevent the slipping complication, the clinician should bend the tip of the archwire distal to the terminal brackets (or molar tubes). Suppose the archwire is from the lower right second premolar (LR5 or #29) to the lower left second premolar (LL5 or #20), then the bends would be distal to LR5 and LL5.

Some may suggest adding a flowable composite onto the archwire to prevent sliding, but this practice is neither effective nor efficient.

For SS archwire, one of the simplest and most effective ways of preventing this sliding complication is shown in Figure 9.1. The middle bends are introduced into the upper and lower archwires. These bends can simply be done by using special orthodontic pliers: the step-bend pliers for the upper and the V-bend pliers for the lower. The middle bend can point either up or down,

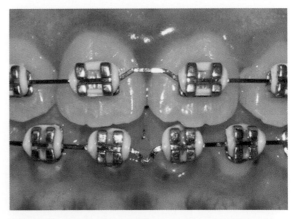

Figure 9.1 Middle bends for the upper and lower archwires to prevent sliding (Reproduced with permission from Dr. Hung Vu).

but for esthetics and consistency reasons, the author prefers that the middle bend points up for the upper and points down for the lower. Note that the reason for using different types of middle bend for the upper and the lower is because of the interbracket distances of the central incisors. The interbracket distance of the upper central incisors is wide, so two (2) step bends are needed, whereas that of the lower central incisors is narrow—thus one single V-bend is used.

Bonding versus banding the molars

A practical question that a clinician would contemplate when providing comprehensive orthodontic treatment to a patient is, should the molars be bonded or banded? What are the advantages (pros) and disadvantages (cons)? What are the possible complications and how to manage them? For patients who have only first molars (erupted in the oral cavity), it is customary to include the first molars in comprehensive orthodontic treatment. But for those who have both first and second molars, the question is, should the second molars be included as well?

The primary advantage of banding the molar is that the band is likely to stay on the molar after the band is cemented onto the molar even when the patient chews or bites on some food that is relatively hard. But to the patient, the major disadvantage of using bands is that when the braces are removed, there will be annoying gaps. Banding also includes other disadvantages as follows:

1 When braces are removed at the end of the orthodontic treatment with a banded molar, a gap that is at least as large as the thickness of the band will exist between the molar and its adjacent tooth/teeth. If two bands are placed on two adjacent teeth, then the gap between these two teeth is double.

2 The band may be pushed under the patient's gingiva and may cause gingival irritation or bleeding or both.

3 The band may abrade the patient's tongue.

4 Due to its limitation, the band may not be positioned in an ideal position and orientation, resulting in non-ideal treatment outcomes: poor occlusion, uneven marginal ridges of posterior teeth, poor root angulation (roots are not parallel), etc.

5 Over a long period of time in orthodontic treatment, caries may develop on the side of the tooth that is inside the band if part of the necessary cement is missing and is difficult to be detected.

The primary disadvantage of bonding is that the bracket may come off if the patient is not careful while eating or if the opposing tooth hits the bracket. When this kind of accident occurs, an emergency call to the office will certainly ensue. A bracket with a molar tube is typically used for the molar, and the advantage of bonding is obvious: it does not have all the disadvantages associated with banding.

In summary, the main advantage of banding for the molars is that it is more secure than bonding so there would be less emergency visits, but in the author's opinion, the risks associated with using bands outweigh the benefits for the patients. Banding may be more convenient for the doctor, but bonding may be better for the patient.

It should be noted that banding the molars is still popular among many clinicians, but the choice is mainly based on personal or professional preferences.

Banding and bonding complications

As an example, Figure 9.2 shows the contrast of banding versus bonding for molars. The case was started with a clinician who banded the molars, and then the patient switched to a new clinician (the author) who bonded the molars.

For the aforementioned reasons, the author would always bond the molars and never band the molars except in some special circumstances. One of the exceptions is with the rapid maxillary expander (RPE): the upper first molars must be banded.

Hereinafter, unless stated otherwise, only bonding is preferred for molars. The next question is when to bond the second molars.

Bonding the second molars

Some clinicians do not want to bond the second molars, but some patients or the parents of the minor patients may request that the second molars to be included in the treatment if they are malaligned.

In addition, one of the requirements for the board cases considered by the American Board of Orthodontics (ABO) is that the malalignment of the second molars must be corrected. And it must be corrected in such a way that their mesial marginal ridge must be even with the distal marginal ridge of the first molars. Of course, the occlusion of the first and second molars with the opposing teeth must also be excellent. To satisfy this requirement, the second molars must be bonded in many cases.

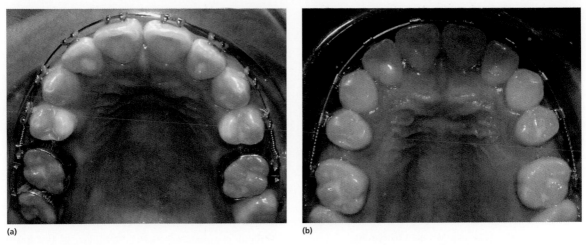

(a)   (b)

Figure 9.2 Molars banding vs. bonding: (a) banding and (b) bonding (Reproduced with permission from Dr. Hung Vu).

Management and treatment

Bonding the second molars may come with certain complications. It is relatively difficult for some clinician to bond brackets on the second molars because these molars are far in the back—if not all the way in the back—for many patients. In addition, second molars erupt only partially for most early teens.

Preadolescent is synonymous to preteen, whereas adolescent comprises early, mid, and late teens. The ages for teenagers can be broken down conveniently, in years, as follows: preteens (10–12), early teens (13–14), mid teens (15–16), and late teens (17–19).

For a typical teenager, the second molars begin to erupt into the oral cavity at around 12 years of age. As a rule of three in dentistry, it takes approximately 3 years for the second molars to fully erupt.

Some patients may experience discomfort or pain when bonding (or banding) the second molars due to the distal end of the bracket (or of the band) abrading the cheek. If the archwire is a bit long—even just a tiny bit—the end of the archwire would stick out of the distal end of the molar tube and cause pain or ulceration.

In typical cases, bracket (or band) with molar tube is used for molars because the end of the archwire would stay inside the molar tube, without any need for ligation. But in some applications of mechanics, if the second molar is bonded (or banded) with molar tube, it may be more advantageous to bond the first molar with a regular bracket without molar tube, for example, when we need to place an open coil spring between the first and second molars.

For some preadolescents or adolescents, the clinician can postpone the bonding (or banding) of the second molars until near the end stage of orthodontic treatment. Doing this would minimize the discomfort/pain to the patients, but the treatment time may be prolonged.

For extraction or partially edentulous cases, the second molars should be bonded in the early stage of orthodontic treatment so the case can be completed in timely manner. If that is the case, care must be taken to ensure that the archwires are cut flush to the distal end of the last molar tubes. It is also important to ensure that the archwire will not slide to one side or another.

One simple way to achieve this goal is to place the middle bend in the archwires so that they would not slide. But the middle bend must be created in such a way that the modified archwire will not create any unwanted tooth movement. The second method is tying the archwire to the bracket such that the wire would less likely slide. The clinician could use color-tie (elastics) with Figure-8 pattern or use the SS ligature. Using elastics is more efficient (faster), and there would be no complication from the elastics itself. On the other hand, using the SS ligature is potentially more hazardous because its tip can turn and cause irritation. Thus, it can be a complication.

Clear aligners versus conventional braces: Quick orthodontic treatment

The correct terminology for the plastic type of *less visible* orthodontic treatment is clear aligner (generic name) which can be Invisalign or ClearCorrect (trade names).

Some general dentists (GDs) (also called general practitioners (GPs)) have expressed that using clear aligners is *easier* than conventional braces. The reason is that, to many if not most GPs, conventional braces are much more difficult, whereas clear aligners may appear easy and more profitable. Some GPs may be led to believe that one needs to only take *polyvinyl siloxane* (PVS) impression and the lab technician will do the rest, and then the GPs just give the aligners to the patients without the need to know anything about orthodontics. But that is not the case for obtaining *ideal* treatment outcomes.

Some programs may advertise an easy way to give quick orthodontic treatment. But the problem is that after about a year of treatment, the case does not progress and the GPs would get into trouble of false promise to the patient by assuring short-term treatment.

Enamel tubercle on premolars

As the name indicates, *enamel tubercle* is a tubercle or protrusion of enamel on the occlusal surface of the crown of a tooth. It is called by various names, such as *Leong tubercle of the premolar*, *dens evaginatus* (Yip, 1974), central cusp, etc.

According to a study, the occurrence of enamel tubercle is at least 2% in the Asian and Native Indian populations (McCulloch *et al.*, 1998). And another study reported that the frequency of occurrence is 0.5–4.3%, in different populations of East Asian countries (Kocsis *et al.*, 2002).

The enamel tubercle has relatively thin enamel and dentin. Due to its nature of formation and location, the enamel tubercle can easily wear out or fracture, and the ultimate consequence is pulpal exposure. When this complication occurs, the tooth will lose its vitality, and a root canal therapy (RCT) will be needed to save the tooth. Thus, the tooth must be protected from being broken by preventive treatment.

In orthodontic cases with premolar extraction, the clinician should be aware of this anomaly and make a wise decision on selecting the appropriate teeth. The principle of keeping the good teeth and extracting the compromised ones should supersede other considerations, in most cases.

How to avoid and treat the complication

The enamel tubercles on the premolars of the lower arch are shown in Figure 9.3a. At the time the initial records were taken, the patient still has the lower left deciduous second molar (Figure 9.3a). Soon after, the deciduous molar exfoliated, and the lower left second premolar erupted into the oral cavity. And it also has the enamel tubercle (not shown).

As a preventive measure, some suggest selective grinding and restoration with either composite or amalgam. But this is a poor choice because an enamel tubercle has thin enamel and dentin; thus grinding—even selective—will inevitably cause pulpal exposure. To prevent fracture, one efficient and effective method is to build around the base of the enamel tubercle with composite to make the structure thicker, but not too thick that it would interfere with the occlusion (Figure 9.3b).

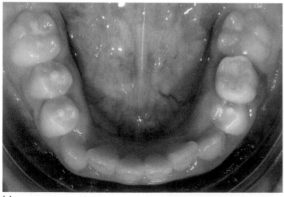
(a)

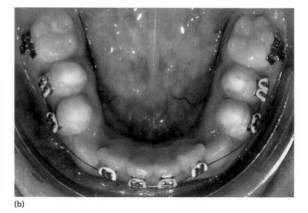
(b)

Figure 9.3 Enamel tubercles on lower premolars: (a) initial and (b) composite buildup, protecting them from being broken (Reproduced with permission from Dr. Hung Vu).

Extraction

Naturally, the majority of orthodontic cases are done by orthodontists. And some GDs and other non-orthodontist dental specialists also treat orthodontic cases as well. For these clinicians, with comprehensive orthodontic treatment, the decision to extract or not to extract, for orthodontic purposes only, may be one of the greatest challenges. Both extraction and non-extraction cases are accompanied with their own complications, and the clinicians must be aware of these complications so they can avoid them or treat them when they occur.

The following case was done by a GD who decided to extract the lower first molars. The teeth had neither decay nor filling/restoration or defect whatsoever, according to the patient and his mother. The *screening* records (photos and panoramic radiograph) are shown in Figure 9.4. This is an example of an extremely poor choice of extraction.

How to avoid and treat the complications

In general, the anterior teeth (canines, lateral incisors, and central incisors) are for both esthetics and function, whereas the posterior teeth (molars and premolars) are mainly for function. Assuming all the teeth are healthy, the premolars are the least important. Thus, if some teeth must be sacrificed, the premolars would be the ones highest in the list.

When the decision of extraction for orthodontic purposes has been made, the next question is, which tooth/teeth? If the premolar is the candidate, then is it the first or second premolar? The answer to this extraction question is relatively complicated, because it depends on multiple factors, but certain guidelines can be given as follows:

1 For severe crowding, extraction is almost always a must. The reason is that if the clinicians try to align all the crowded teeth into the arches, it will inevitably push the anterior teeth and the corresponding alveolar ridges forward. If both the upper and lower arches are involved, then the consequence is bimaxillary alveolar protrusion.

2 With the extraction case of four premolars (two upper and two lower), the bite (occlusion) has a tendency to become deeper. Of course, for certain deep-bite cases, the extraction of the four premolars is still necessary, but the clinician should be aware of the complication that the bite will get deeper.

3 Extraction of impacted canines must be avoided if possible. Although some impacted canines are challenging, they can almost always be saved and brought into the arch (Vu, 2014).

4 Extraction of one lower incisor should be avoided, except for special circumstances. Consider a case in which both canines are in class I, lowers incisors are moderately crowded but normal in size and shape, whereas the upper incisors are significantly smaller than the ideal size. This is an example of tooth-size discrepancy (or Bolton discrepancy) of the anteriors where extracting a lower incisor may be an acceptable compromise. If all the teeth are normal in size and shape, extracting one lower incisor will never yield good occlusion. Optimal occlusion requires the following: all canines and posterior teeth (premolars and molars) in class I, ideal overjet (OJ) and overbite (OB), and anterior teeth with proper inclination.

5 To avoid extraction, some prefer interproximal reduction (IPR) which is also called stripping or slenderizing. But, with this procedure, it is almost impossible to obtain the ideal convex anatomy of the crown in the interproximal area. The evidence of nonideal result can readily be seen from a bitewing (BW) radiograph (Figure 9.5).

Impacted canines

The mandibular (lower) wisdom teeth (third molars) are the most common impacted teeth, and the maxillary (upper) canines are the second common impacted teeth, whereas the upper canine can be considered the most important tooth for both appearance and function.

Canines are the corners of the mouth, so impacted canines must be saved if possible. If an impacted canine cannot be brought in to its arch, then it may be considered for either extraction (only in extremely rare situation) or leaving it alone (if it does no harm).

The best tools for evaluating the status of an impacted canine are the cone beam computed tomography (CBCT) and an appropriate software. With these tools, the clinician would be able to see the exact status of the impacted canine in question. With the information provided by the CBCT scan, the surgical exposure of the impacted canine can be planned and executed accurately. The exposure can be performed with the shortest amount of time, with minimal bleeding and discomfort.

Since CBCT provides the clinician with details of the bone surrounding the impacted canine, most surgical

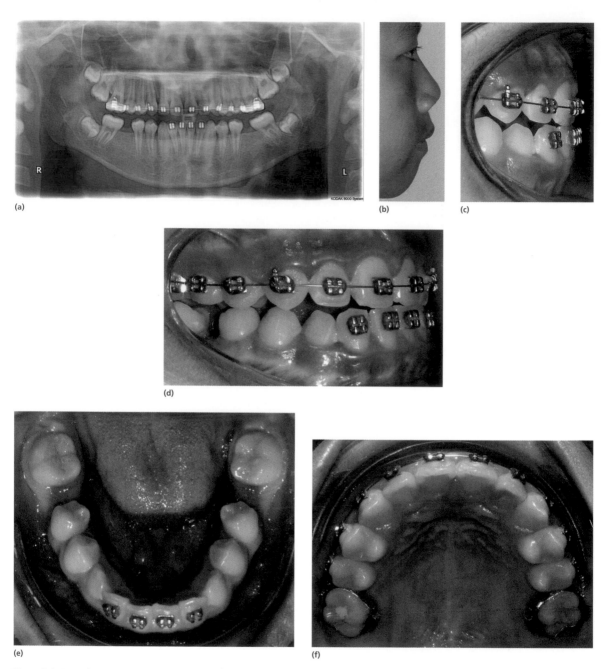

Figure 9.4 Records at *screening*: (a) panoramic radiograph, (b) profile, (c) overjet, (d) right buccal, (e) lower occlusal, and (f) upper occlusal (Reproduced with permission from Dr. Hung Vu).

exposures of impacted canines require only local anesthesia. Thus, this procedure can be done by an able orthodontist, without the help from a periodontist or an oral surgeon.

When an impacted canine is poorly diagnosed and improperly treated, possible complications are devitalization, reexposure (again and again), ankylosis, root resorption (RR) (the impacted tooth itself and/or its

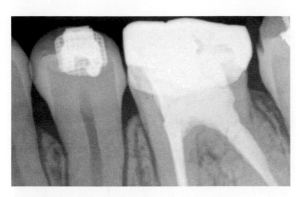

Figure 9.5 IPR. Almost impossible to obtain ideal convexity of crown anatomy (Reproduced with permission from Dr. Hung Vu).

adjacent teeth), periodontal defects (bone loss, gingival recession), tooth loss, etc.

Diagnosis and treatment

In the diagnosis and treatment of impacted canines, the three important considerations are surgical exposure, periodontal issues, and orthodontic traction. There are differences in the surgical management of the labially and palatally impacted canines. In addition, there are different methods of attachment to the canine (right after the surgical exposure) for orthodontic traction.

Depending on the location of the impacted teeth, the traditional techniques that have been established for surgical exposure are given as:

1 Open eruption if the crown of the impacted tooth is near the mucogingival junction:
   (a) Excision if the gingiva is sufficient (Kokich, 2004)
   (b) Apically positioned flap (APF) if the gingiva is insufficient (Vanarsdall and Corn, 1977; Levin and D'Amico, 1974)
2 Closed eruption if the crown of the impacted tooth is far away from the mucogingival junction (Kokich and Mathews, 1993).

For palatal impacted canines, the question is, which technique is superior between closed eruption and open eruption? According to Burden, Mullally, and Robinson (1999), one is *not* better than the other.

Recently, the author has developed a new technique that is classified neither "open" nor "closed" eruption as defined earlier. In this technique, a window is opened on the impacted teeth, almost regardless where and how the teeth are impacted. After studying the details of the impaction with the use of CBCT, including 3D volume rendering, a diode laser is used to remove the soft tissue.

If the crown of the impacted teeth is covered by a bone, then a round bur is used to remove the overlying bone—in low speed. One of the advantages of using a diode laser for this kind of surgery is that a dry field of operation can be obtained readily so that an attachment can be easily bonded on the crown of the impacted teeth. Other advantages include less pain, less complications, and no sutures. Since the surgery is minimally invasive, the wound and its healing are localized to a small area.

A case of challenging impacted upper left canine (UL3 or #11) is shown in Figure 9.6a. The tooth was horizontally impacted and located high up, near the base of the nose. CBCT images clearly revealed the location and orientation of the impacted tooth (Figure 9.6b and c). Many dental specialists thought it would be impossible to save it and recommended extraction. But with proper treatment plan and execution, the tooth has been surgically exposed and brought into the arch using orthodontic traction—though not yet completely done (work-in-progress), without causing any damage to the impacted tooth itself and the roots of the adjacent teeth (Figure 9.6d, radiograph not shown).

Lower lingual arch

Mesial movement of molars will likely occur relatively rapidly with the early loss of deciduous second molars, causing arch length deficiency. It will, in turn, result in crowding or impaction or both to the permanent teeth. For the lower arch, lower lingual arch (LLA) can be used to maintain or minimize the loss of arch length by preventing the molars from moving mesially.

How to avoid and treat the complication

The LLA is constructed in such a way that it has an archwire adapted to the lingual side of the lower teeth, touching the lower incisors. But the use of the LLA is at the expense of lower incisor proclination.

The following is an example of an incorrect use of the LLA (by a GD). After extracting the perfectly good lower first molars—for the wrong reason—he proceeded with placing the LLA. But for what? The usual purpose of LLA is to prevent the mesial movement of the molars. If that is the case, the loop of the LLA should touch the lingual side of the lower incisors, but Figure 9.7 shows otherwise.

Midlines

To some people, one of the most important treatment goals in orthodontics is to obtain coincident midlines. Thus, noncoincident midline can be considered a critical

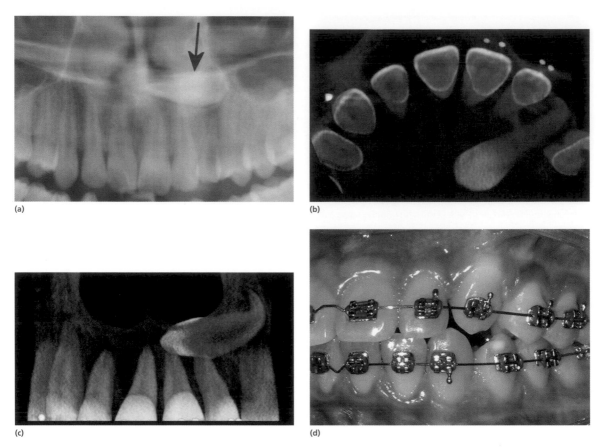

(a)   (b)   (c)   (d)

Figure 9.6 Challenging impacted canine, tooth #11. (a) Initial panoramic, showing horizontally impacted canine, high up, near the base of the nose. (b) CBCT image, just before surgical exposure: front view. (c) CBCT image, just before surgical exposure: occlusal view. (d) Progress photo (Reproduced with permission from Dr. Hung Vu).

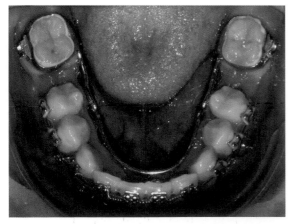

Figure 9.7 LHA. The loop is supposed to touch the lingual side of the lower anteriors (Reproduced with permission from Dr. Hung Vu).

complication. Essentially, there are three midlines: facial, upper, and lower midlines. Facial midline is the line that divides the face into two mirror image halves. Upper midline is the one that is in the middle of the two upper central incisors. Similarly, lower midline is the middle line between the two lower central incisors. Ideally, all these three midlines should be coincident. An example of a perfect alignment of all three midlines is shown in Figure 9.8a and b. Only a few people would naturally have perfect midlines (perfect alignment of the three midlines). For example, a patient has coincident facial and upper midlines, but her nose tip is tilted to her left—a bit (Figure 9.8c), and her lower midline is also shifted to her left—about 1 mm (Figure 9.8d).

Some may argue that there are subjective variations in the level of acceptance or recognition of the midline

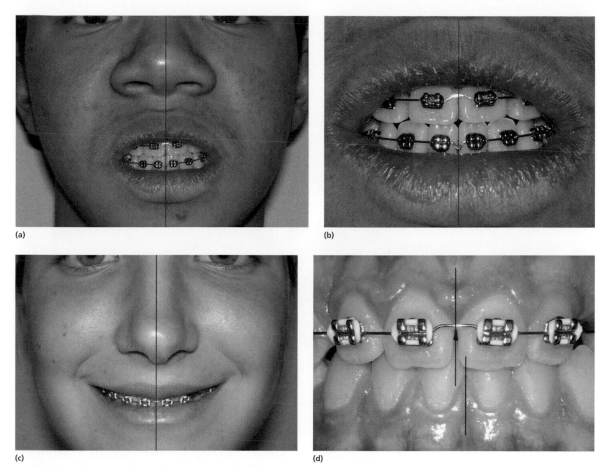

Figure 9.8 Midlines. (a) Perfectly line up of all three midlines: facial, upper, and lower midlines. (b) Closeup view of (a) for upper and lower midlines. (c) Slightly imperfectly line up of all three midlines: facial, upper, and lower midlines. (d) Closeup view of (c) for upper and lower midlines (Reproduced with permission from Dr. Hung Vu).

discrepancy among laypeople, GDs, and dental specialists. But, objectively, when the midlines are not absolutely matching, it is undeniably imperfect.

It is important to recognize that the occlusion of the molars has a significant role in midline discrepancy. In some cases, when the molars are in occlusion, the deflected bite can cause the midline shift. The second molars are often the cause of this complication. Thus, correcting the malalignment of the second molars may correct the midline discrepancy in some individuals. But the complication is compounded with some teenagers whose second molars have not yet fully erupted even near the end of their orthodontic treatment.

For midline consideration, complications typically arise when closing spaces. In the premolar-extraction case, obtaining coincident midlines for all three midlines is achievable when there are spaces (gaps) in the intraarch. If the clinician does not pay attention to the midlines and closes all the spaces, the window of opportunity will be lost. It is difficult or almost impossible to obtain all three midlines (facial, upper, and lower) coincident when all the spaces are closed. When it happens, the game is practically over.

How to avoid and treat the complication

Consider the following example shown in Figure 9.9. The upper and lower midlines are coincident, and the upper arch has some spaces (see arrows). It may be natural for some clinicians to jump immediately into the action of closing the space, and it may be equally natural

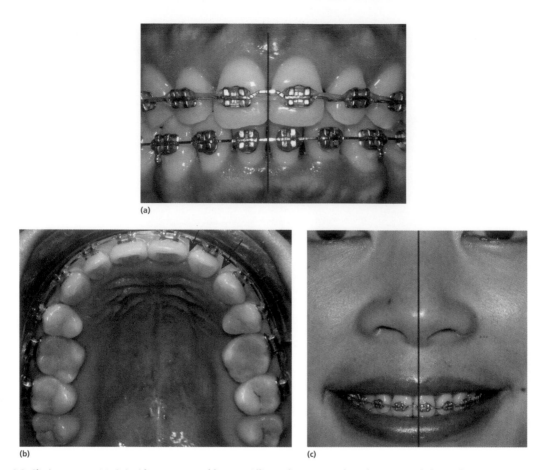

Figure 9.9 Closing spaces. (a) Coincident upper and lower midlines. (b) Upper arch with spaces and elastic chain. (c) Upper and lower midlines are not coincident with the facial midline (Reproduced with permission from Dr. Hung Vu).

for them to forget about the facial midline. Since the upper and lower midlines are coincident, one method of closing the space is using elastic chain from molar to molar, one side to the other. But an analysis of all three midlines (facial, upper, and lower) reveals the hidden truth (Figure 9.9): the upper midline is shifted to the patient's right (with respect to the facial midline).

To some people, the correct course of action would be moving the upper midline to her left to match the facial midline. For this patient, the spaces in the upper left work in our favor. But one may ask, what about the lower midline? What if the lower midline cannot be moved? If that is the case, some compromise may have to be accepted. Esthetically, the decision would have to be made based on the patient's preference. Functionally, the clinician must consider important factors of occlusion, including canine relationship.

In this case, the task of moving the upper midline can be accomplished by using either pulling action on the patient's left or pushing action on the patient's right. Pulling action can be done by using either an elastic chain or a closing coil spring, whereas pushing action can be accomplished by using an open coil spring.

Closing coil is the term that describes the desired outcome: closing the space. It is also called the coil in tension, in which its physical state of being in tension is described. Similarly, open coil or coil in compression is for creating the space, and its physical state is in compression. It should be noted that elastic chain can only support tension—not compression.

In closing spaces, the use of elastic chain is efficient but may not be effective, whereas the use of closing coil is effective but may have some limitations. When attaching the closing coil to a bracket that does not have a hook, the clinician would have to either replace the bracket with the one that has a hook or to add a sliding hook. Kobayashi ligature could be used, but only as a temporary solution because its hook is too flimsy.

Open bite

There are three classification for facial types: hyperdivergent (long face), hypodivergent (short face), and normodivergent (normal face). An open bite can be associated with long face. Other causes of open bite include the following habits: tongue thrusting, thumb sucking, nail biting, mouth breathing, pacifier, etc.

Complications and how to treat them

Open bite is one of the most challenging problems. If the open bite is due to patient's oral habit, then the bad habit must be stopped. If the case is treated successfully with orthodontic treatment, but the patient does not stop the habit, then the inevitable relapse will certainly ensue.

There are different techniques in orthodontic treatment for open bites. For mild anterior open bite, one of the simplest methods is using the reverse-curve-of-Spee NT and the accentuated-curve-of-Spee NT archwires. These two are the same archwire, but the actions are opposite.

Let us assume that the patient does not have a gummy smile and the anterior open bite is only mild. To close the bite, the reverse-curve-of-Spee and accentuated-curve-of-Spee NT archwires are used on the upper arch and lower arch, respectively, to extrude the anterior teeth.

For severe open bite, orthognathic surgery may be indicated. It should be emphasized that the proposed treatment here is oversimplified. Since all patients are different, a careful diagnosis must be done first for every single case before a definitive treatment plan is provided with certain biomechanics utilized.

Orthodontic records: Danger of not reviewing radiograph

Collecting a complete set of orthodontic records must be done before coming up with a correct diagnosis and a primary treatment plan with alternative(s), and it is dangerous if the clinician does not review the radiograph when seeing orthodontic patients in routine visits.

For comprehensive orthodontics, with standard of care, the following records must be obtained:

1 Dental and medical history, informed consent, and financial agreement
2 Panoramic radiograph

3 Dental casts (also called Study Model)
4 Photos (dentofacial, extra-oral, and intraoral), at least eight images must be taken as follows:
  (a) Three extra-oral images for face and head: front without smile, front with smile, profile
  (b) Five intraoral images for dentition: center, buccal right, buccal left, upper occlusal, lower occlusal
5 Lateral cephalometric radiograph and its cephalometric tracing
6 Diagnosis and treatment plan with alternative(s)

For adult patients, in addition to the above items, the records should also include BW and periapical (PA) radiographs.

In modern orthodontics, with the advent of CBCT, orthodontic records regarding radiographs are modified. For comprehensive orthodontic treatment, a CBCT scan should be taken, but the decision is up to the clinician and the patient. Of course, the patient's parent or his/her legal guardian must decide if the patient is a minor (not having reached the legal age for full civil rights). Some people may claim that CBCT would always expose patients to a much higher dose of radiation. But this is not true. It is true that a CBCT scan of a full head, with a large field of view (FoV), has much higher radiation dose than that of a focus scan, with a smaller FoV. For a CBCT with short scan time (in seconds or s) and with reduced values of voltage (in kV) and current (in mA), the radiation dose can be much less than a set of full-mouth "X-rays" (FMX), but the decision of taking a certain type of radiograph (BW, PA, panoramic, lateral cephalometric, CBCT) depends on the need of obtaining the accurate diagnosis for a particular problem.

One may ask, with a full-head CBCT scan, should we also take a 2D lateral cephalometric radiograph for orthodontic records? The answer is yes for two reasons. First, 2D cephalometric is needed for traditional 2D tracing and analysis. A lateral cephalometric image can be obtained from a full-head CBCT scan, but it does not include the calibration marks for 2D cephalometric tracing and analysis. The radiation dose is very small for 2D lateral cephalometric radiograph. Second, in order to obtain a high-quality image of CBCT scan, it is inevitable that the soft tissue of the chin is distorted. To get a clear CBCT image, the head of the patient must be strapped tightly to the stationary part of the CBCT machine, resulting in severe distortion of the soft tissue of the chin.

When adjusting braces in every visit, the clinician should quickly review the patient's orthodontic records.

In some cases, it is simply dangerous not reviewing the records in routine orthodontic visits.

How to avoid and treat the complication

The following example shows a severe complication that results in an irreversible damage due to failure of not reviewing the records when actively treating orthodontic patient. Specifically, the cause was an apparent lack of reviewing the radiograph to see what lies beneath.

This case involves an orthodontic patient that has been treated by a well-known clinician for a few years. The patient had small gaps between the upper first premolars and first molars. Seeing the small gaps, the clinician tried to close them by using elastic chains (not shown)—pulling action. Apparently, he was not aware or did not remember that the patient had impacted upper second premolars. The patient did report painful experience during some period. A review of the patient's panoramic radiograph (at that time, not shown) showed that the patient indeed had impacted upper second premolars. Only after the author recommended the remedy to the patient's parents, the clinician then placed the open coils between the upper first premolars and first molars to create the spaces (Figure 9.2a)—pushing action. Without a radiograph for cases like this, it would be natural for some clinicians to jump to the action of closing the gaps. After the transfer, the patient's orthodontic records were taken, and the panoramic radiograph and photo (upper arch) are shown in Figure 9.10a and b (after the existing braces were removed) and Figure 9.10a does *show* the impacted upper second premolars. Subsequently, in the initial stage of retreatment, photos were taken, and the upper arch is shown in Figure 9.2b. Notice that it is much cleaner with the bonding compared to banding for the molars (cf. Figure 9.2a). A few years later, at the conclusion of the orthodontic retreatment, the upper left second premolar (tooth #13) was brought into the upper arch, and Figure 9.10c shows irreversible damage near the cementoenamel junction (CEJ) on the mesial side of the upper left first molar (tooth #14). This damage is consistent with the panoramic image taken at the beginning of the retreatment (Figure 9.10a), though the panoramic radiograph is only 2D. A CBCT scan would have shown the extent of the damage in 3D.

This case would have been classified as idiopathic external RR if one did not know the history of the patient's orthodontic treatment. But the truth of the matter is that

the cause of this external RR is not idiopathic. The evidence shows that the resorption is caused simply because the previous clinician did not pay attention to the radiograph. The clinician forgot the existence of impacted second premolars and tried to close the gaps.

Overcorrection

In clinical orthodontics, it is challenging to have both efficiency and effectiveness. With this goal in mind, the clinician should use the best possible mechanics to obtain the treatment outcome in the shortest amount of treatment time, with doing no harm. As an example, in certain applications, the clinician can reposition the bracket with a bit of overcorrection so the intended outcome can be obtained in a shorter amount of time.

Overbite and overjet

OB and OJ are best illustrated in the midsagittal plane. OB is the *vertical* overlap of the incisal edge of the upper (maxillary) central incisors over that of the lower (mandibular) central incisors. On the other hand, OJ is the *horizontal* overlap of the incisal edge of the upper central incisors over that of the lower central incisors. The ideal OB should be about a quarter (1/4) of the height of the crown of the lower incisors. The ideal OJ is about 1–2 mm—depending on the inclination of the upper and lower incisors—and the lingual side of the incisal third of the upper central incisor just barely touches the labial side of the incisal third of the lower incisor in intercuspal position (ICP).

When patients have severe OJ, they would often have deep bite (or deep OB) as well. This situation is typical with malocclusioned patients of class II division 1 where the inclination of the upper central incisors is either normal or excessive.

For malocclusioned patients of class II division 2 where the upper central incisors are retroclined, the OJ may be normal.

Complications and how to avoid and treat them

When the patient has deep bite, the orthodontic treatment is expected to be much longer than the typical case. This would be a major complication in terms of estimating the treatment time if the clinician did not realize that. For deep-bite cases, extraction of four premolars would make the orthodontic treatment more challenging because the bite would become even deeper in the process of closing the spaces of missing

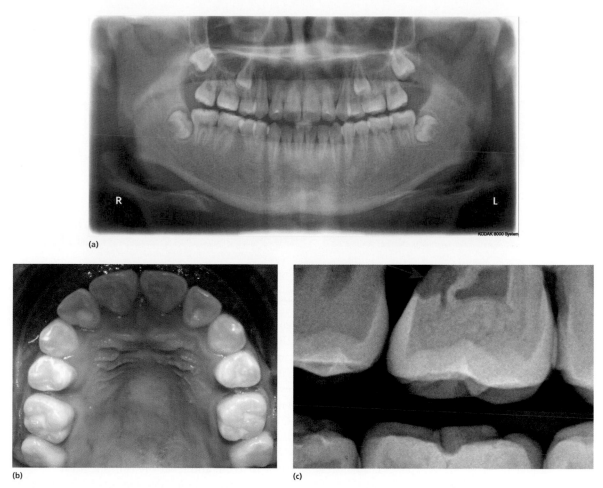

Figure 9.10 After removing existing braces. (a) Panoramic. (b) Upper arch. After orthodontic retreatment: (c) irreversible damage near the CEJ on the mesial side of tooth #14 (Reproduced with permission from Dr. Hung Vu).

premolars—unless some special mechanics are to be employed to control the bite. One of the simplest methods of opening the bite (or controlling the bite) is the use of the RCOS NT archwire for the lower and the ACOS NT archwire for the upper.

When the patient has severe OJ, one of the proposed treatments would be extracting only the two upper first premolars—provided that the upper second premolars are healthy and worth keeping. Another method is extracting four premolars: two upper first premolars and two lower second premolars, assuming the rest of the teeth are healthy and worth keeping. It should be noted that these extraction recommendations are oversimplified because the decision of which teeth to be extracted should be based on multiple factors, including the possibility of orthognathic surgery if the case required.

Push and pull

In the applied mechanics of clinical orthodontics, one of the most important considerations is push or pull. Pushing action is accomplished by using an NT open coil spring (Figure 9.11a). On the other hand, pulling action can be done by using either an NT closed coil spring or an elastic chain (Figures 9.11b and 9.3d). Typical orthodontists use the terms closed coil spring and open coil spring for the intended goal of closing and opening the space, respectively. But others may prefer the terms coil-spring-in-tension and coil-spring-in-compression, respectively. If only material cost per one use is

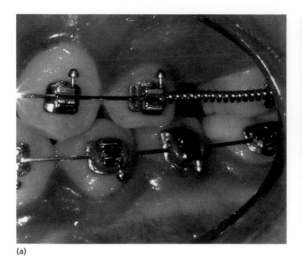
(a)

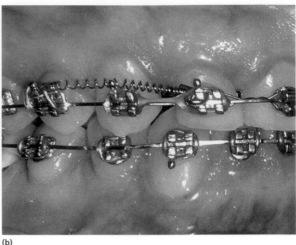
(b)

Figure 9.11 NT coil springs and elastic chain. (a) Open coil spring—push. (b) Closed coil spring and elastic chain—pull (Reproduced with permission from Dr. Hung Vu).

considered, elastic chain is much less expensive than an NT coil spring. But an NT coil spring is much more effective. The reason is that elastic chain provides pulling action fully only at the beginning, but it loses its elasticity soon after being stretched—especially when it is overstretched, which is often the case. A NT coil spring performs consistently over a long period of time as long as it is not permanently deformed by being overstretched beyond limit.

Some orthodontists use the term power chain instead of elastic chain. But it is a misnomer because the word power normally referred to a device that can be powered with an external energy source, for example, from a battery or an electrical outlet. Elastic chain neither uses any battery nor connects to any electrical outlet.

Elastic chain usually comes in three different types: continuous, short, and long. The clinician should select the proper type for each particular application in closing the space, in such a way that the elastic chain is stretched properly and moderately—not too much and not too little.

NT closed coil springs are typically available in different lengths: 9, 12, 14, 16, and 18 mm. Each chain may be classified as L (light) or M (medium) regarding force.

The clinician should not overstretch the elastic chain. Some orthodontists use the term "overpower" to refer to overstretching the elastic chain.

Elastic chain can only support tension, but coil springs can support either tension (with closed coil spring) or compression (with open coil spring). When the elastic chain or the closed coil spring is understretched, it does not provide the necessary tension for tooth movement. On the other hand, if they are overstretched, it could exert excessive pulling force that may either weaken the bond of the bracket or cause pain to the patient. So how much stretching is the proper amount? The answer to this question is given in the following section.

How to avoid and treat the complication
Of course, for curiosity, one can use a force gauge to measure the pulling force. For elastic chain, it is much simpler and more practical for the clinician just to observe the deformation of the circle of the elastic chain and estimate the level of the pulling force.

For example, Figure 9.12a shows closing the gap between the upper central incisors (upper diastema) using an elastic chain. Since the upper central incisors are highly susceptible to RR, it is important to pull these teeth together using a light force. For this particular situation, it is typical to use an elastic chain of the continuous type with an extra link in between. A three-link continuous piece is a bit longer than a two-link long one. It can be seen that the circle of the extra link has deformed into a quasiellipse, and this is about right. Two extremes can occur: (a) no pulling force if the circle remains the same or (b) excessive force if the quasiellipse is flattened out like a slit. Another example is given in Figure 9.12b: closing the gap between the lower central incisors (lower

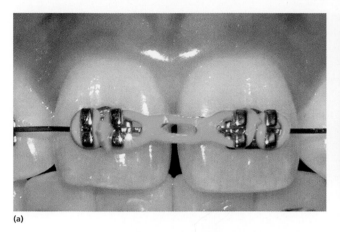
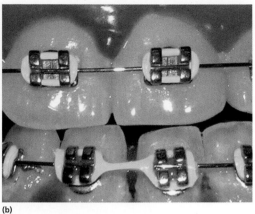

(a)   (b)

Figure 9.12 An example of proper amount of elastic chain stretching. (a) Closing upper diastema. (b) Closing lower diastema (Reproduced with permission from Dr. Hung Vu).

diastema) using an elastic chain. For this application, it is typical to use an elastic chain of the long type. It can be seen that the stretching of the elastic chain is about right by comparing the piece at the deformed and undeformed states. Although it is contraindicated to forcefully move the teeth when they are unclean, this case is used to also illustrate another complication in orthodontics with some children: poor oral hygiene (OH). The recommendation for people with relatively clean teeth and without braces is dental cleaning every 6 months and with braces every 3–4 months. For some individuals, they need to visit a dental office even more frequently. It is critical that the periodontium be healthy when the teeth are actively being moved, with braces.

Root parallelism

Even with the best intention, during the process of orthodontic treatment, the dental condition can become worse—as opposed to be better. One of the common complications is root-parallelism. It is critical that the clinician check for root parallelism before debonding. In some practices, some orthodontists do not own a panoramic machine, so they rely on a third-party lab to take the initial and final records. Due to inconvenience, they are more likely not to have a panoramic radiograph taken for the purpose of checking root parallelism before debonding.

Ideally, the roots of all the teeth must be parallel to those of the adjacent teeth and are perpendicular to the occlusal planes. An example of ideal root parallelism is shown in Figure 9.13a. On the other hand, the case that root parallelism has not been perfectly achieved is shown in Figure 9.13b: upper right canine (tooth #6), and perhaps upper left canine (tooth #11). But the ABO does not even require the roots of the canines to be parallel with the adjacent teeth for the board case (at the time of this writing). This lack of requirement is based on the claim that panoramic radiograph suffers from distortion in the canine region. But with a CBCT scan, one can verify easily if the roots of the canines are parallel with the roots of the adjacent teeth.

Some people use the term *root angulation* to discuss root parallelism. This term may be applicable only for 2D panoramic radiograph, but it is a poor term for 3D imaging. With panoramic radiograph, angulation means mesial–distal tipping, but angulation, in a strict sense, in 3D could also mean buccal–lingual tipping.

It should be emphasized that a panoramic image can be either a conventional 2D panoramic radiograph or one that is reconstructed from the CBCT 3D data that is taken with a sufficiently large FOV scan.

How to avoid and treat the complication

To check for root parallelism, the BW and PA can be utilized if they are available, and the clinician can extrapolate from these radiographs. But these radiographs may not give accurate results because the angles where they are taken may be off.

It would be better to take a panoramic radiograph. But one may ask, what about radiation dose? For the

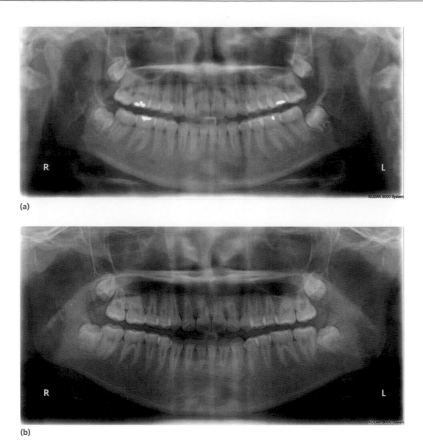

(a)

(b)

Figure 9.13 Root parallelism. (a) Parallel roots—except for the third molars. (b) The root of the upper right canine (tooth #6) is not parallel with those of adjacent teeth (Reproduced with permission from Dr. Hung Vu).

purpose of checking root parallelism, there is no need to see the panoramic image with high degree of clarity using standard settings. All we need to see is the shadow of the roots; thus the parameters kV and mA should be reduced to minimum. In this fashion, the radiation dose may be even less than that of a normal BW or PA.

Root resorption

The cause of RR is multifactorial, and the major risk factor is genetic predisposition or individual susceptibility. RR is unpredictable, but unfortunately it is a common occurrence in orthodontic treatment.

Weltman *et al.* (2010) stated that "Many general dentists and other dental specialists believe that RR is avoidable and hold the orthodontist responsible when it occurs during orthodontic treatment." But this is a wrong belief. Although many studies reported risk factors of RR, the exact etiology is still unknown, hence idiopathic.

The RR associated with orthodontic treatment is typically localized at the root apex; thus, it is called apical root resorption (ARR) or external apical root resorption (EARR). ARR can occur on both deciduous and adult roots, but the resorption of deciduous teeth is a normal physiologic phenomenon, whereas that of adult teeth is not. An example of ARR is given in Figure 9.14. The patient had previous orthodontic treatment elsewhere.

RR can be characterized as internal or external. Inflammation of the pulp is responsible for internal root resorption (IRR), which causes the loss of dentin in the root canal of a tooth. Additional characterization involves two types of internal resorption: replacement and inflammatory resorption. External root resorption (ERR) can be classified into four types: surface resorption, *inflammatory* resorption, replacement resorption, and ankylosis. ERR may occur after injuries, for example, luxation, tooth avulsion, and reimplantation.

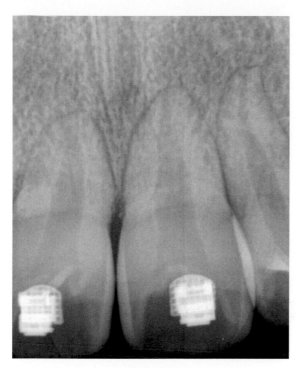

Figure 9.14 Periapical radiograph of upper incisors (Reproduced with permission from Dr. Hung Vu).

External *inflammatory* RR is further categorized into external cervical root resorption (ECRR) and EARR.

Orthodontically induced inflammatory root resorption (OIIRR) is of special concern to clinicians who practice orthodontics. Brezniak and Wasserstein (2002) stated that "orthodontics is the only dental profession that uses the inflammation process to solve esthetic and functional problems."

According to Massler and Malone (1954), RR of adult teeth due to traumatization of the periodontal membrane was first mentioned by Bates in 1856. Reitan (1974) stated that ARR on extracted teeth was first detected by Schwarzkopf in 1887. Schwarz (1931) wrote that orthodontic forces were first experimented on animals by Carl Sandstedt in 1904, and Meikle (2006) reported the same, but the years were 1904–1905 (Sandstedt, 1904, 1905). When Ketcham (1927, 1929) reported ARR associated with orthodontic treatment, it became a major concern for orthodontists. For simplicity, the terms ARR and OIIRR are used interchangeably in this chapter.

For some less fortunate orthodontic patients, ARR is an inevitable outcome.

Biology

Odontoclasts are clastic cells that remove dental tissues, that is, cementum, dentin, and enamel, and they are similar histologically to osteoclasts which are responsible for bone removal. Odontoclasts are derived from monocytes and migrate from the blood vessels to the resorption site, where they fuse to form the multinucleated cells (Nanci, 2003). Odontoclasts are also seen in the cemental and osseous surfaces of the PDL (Newman *et al.*, 2002). The odontoclasts that specifically resorb cementum and dentin can be called cementoclasts and dentinoclasts, respectively. There is no such thing as enamoclast.

According to Newman *et al.* (2002), adult teeth do not undergo physiologic resorption as do deciduous teeth. The cementum of both erupted and unerupted teeth can be resorbed. And the resorption may be microscopic or macroscopic, but the latter can be seen radiographically. Cementum resorption is common, and it could happen to anybody. In one microscopic study reported by Henry and Weinmann (1951) that involves 261 teeth with 922 areas, the resorption occurrence is 91% (236 teeth), and the majority is at the apical third of the root: 77% (708 areas). In this study, 70% of all resorption areas were confined to the cementum, and the dentin was unaffected. The causes of cementum resorption may be local or systemic or by an unknown etiology. Cementum resorption appears microscopically as concavities in the root surface. Multinucleated giant cells and large mononuclear macrophages are generally found adjacent to the cementum that is undergoing active resorption. The resorption may extend into the dentin and even into the pulp. On the root surface, the cementum alternates between resorption and apposition (deposition). Embedded fibers of the PDL reestablish a functional relationship in the new cementum, and the repair of the cementum requires the presence of a connective tissue. Cementum repair can occur in devitalized as well as in vital teeth, but the repair cannot materialize if the epithelium migrates into the resorption area.

Ankylosis is defined as the fusion of the cementum and alveolar bone with disappearance of the PDL. Ankylosis occurs in teeth with cemental resorption, so it appears as an abnormal repair. The root is resorbed and is then replaced by bone. Ankylosis may also develop after chronic periapical inflammation, tooth replantation, and occlusal trauma (Newman *et al.*, 2002). Reimplanted teeth will typically ankylose and subsequently lose their roots.

Osteoclasts and odontoclasts are necessary cells for tooth eruption, but they cause complications when associated with internal or external resorption of adult teeth.

Risk factors of apical root resorption

Pause in orthodontic treatment

A pause in orthodontic treatment seemed useful in minimizing RR since the resorbed cementum has a chance to heal and repair, preventing resorption (Reitan, 1964; Dougherty, 1968). But the jiggling force, associated with an intermittent force, is certainly damaging (Hall, 1978). The practical question regarding this complication is how to apply the concept of pausing in clinical orthodontics, such as how long (duration) and how frequent (frequency) should the *optimal* pause be?

Clear aligners versus braces

The force exerted on a tooth can be considered intermittent with clear aligners but continuous with braces. Roscoe, Meira, and Cattaneo (2015) examined the evidence of association of orthodontic force system and RR with clear aligners and braces. They reported that there was a positive correlation between force magnitude and RR and also between treatment time and RR. In another study comparing clear aligners (ClearSmile, Australia, and Invisalign, United States) and braces (with light and heavy forces), the authors concluded that clear aligners have similar resorption as with light-force braces (Barbagallo *et al.*, 2008). The study of Invisalign aligner by Boyd (2007) showed no measurable RR. But Brezniak and Wasserstein (2008) contradict these studies by showing the case of a patient with severe RR of four upper incisors after 14 months of orthodontic treatment using Invisalign aligner via a case report.

Biologic and mechanical factors

Biologic factors include individual susceptibility, genetics, systemic factors, nutrition, age (chronologic and dental), dilacerations, gender, prior RR, habits, tooth structure, previous trauma, endodontically treated teeth, alveolar bone density, and classification of malocclusion. Mechanical factors include appliances (fixed vs. removable or clear aligners; Begg vs. edgewise), interarch elastics (rubber bands), intraarch elastics (elastic chain), open coil spring, closed coil spring, extraction versus nonextraction, RPE, orthodontic force (continuous vs. intermittent forces), jiggling, and occlusal trauma.

Orthodontic treatment timing

According to Brezniak and Wasserstein (1993a and 1993b), orthodontic treatment should begin as early as possible since there is less RR in developing roots and younger patients show better adaptation to occlusal changes.

Types of tooth movement

Any type of tooth movement can cause RR, and it appeared that intrusion is the most damaging (Reitan, 1985). High incidence of RR is associated with impacted canines (Linge and Linge, 1991). Suppose the surgical exposure of an impacted canine has been performed optimally and the eruption of the canine is not in the colliding path to its adjacent teeth. Then, the extrusive force of orthodontic traction that is applied on the impacted canine will create an intrusive force on its adjacent incisor. This is a direct consequence of action–reaction principle of mechanics, namely, Newton's third law. Thus, according to these references, this intrusive force may cause a high risk for RR.

Predictability

RR is unpredictable, and it could happen to any susceptible orthodontic patient under the care of any orthodontic specialist.

Age

Resorption of the roots of primary teeth is a normal physiologic phenomenon, but that of adult teeth is not (Brezniak and Wasserstein, 1993a and 1993b).

Chronologic age A majority of studies reported that RR is more prevalent in adults since both the periodontal membrane and alveolar bone become less vascular and aplastic (having no tendency to develop into new tissue), causing higher susceptibility to RR (Reitan, 1985). The PDL may adapt to occlusal changes more favorable in young patients. But a few other studies showed no relationship between ARR and patient age, with orthodontic treatment.

Dental age Rosenberg (1972) reported that incompletely formed roots appeared to have less RR than those with completely formed roots, with orthodontic treatment. In other words, RR is more prevalent in late teens and adults. According to Massler and Malone (1954), root resorption incidence increases with age—with or without orthodontic treatment.

Magnitude of applied force

According to Schwarz (1931), RR ceases when pressure from orthodontic force is less than 20–26g_f/cm², but Miura (1975) claimed that the threshold pressure must be higher. Nevertheless, even without orthodontic treatment, ARR occurred in individuals with predisposition (Massler and Malone, 1954). Although properly light force should be used in clinical orthodontics, it would be wrong or over-simplistic if some dental specialist advises another dentist as "in order to *avoid* RR, just use light force!" The reason is that even if the clinician applies the lightest possible force in the mechanics of moving teeth, RR still can occur for unlucky patients who have genetic predisposition or individual susceptibility. Moreover, the high pressure on some root surface may be the consequence of heavy occlusal forces exerting on the tooth, by the patients themselves—regardless how light of the force the clinician applies. The high level of pressure may have nothing to do with the orthodontic treatment, unless the clinician inadvertently creates occlusal trauma in the process of moving teeth.

Postorthodontic treatment

Some people believe that resorption associated with orthodontic treatment should cease once the active treatment is ended. Postorthodontic RR may be related to causes other than the treatment itself, for example, occlusal trauma. A few studies report that some RR occurred even in retention phase.

Treatment duration

Many studies reported that RR is directly related to active orthodontic treatment, but a few other studies disagreed.

Some other factors affecting RR are given as follows:

- Amount of tooth movement (Mirabella and Artun, 1995)
- Ethnicity (Sameshima and Sinclair, 2001).
- Nutrition (Marshall, 1929; Becks, 1936) and previous trauma (Linge and Linge, 1983)
- Biological sex (McNab *et al.*, 1999; Marshall, 1929)
- Systemic factors (McNab *et al.*, 1999)

Tooth-size discrepancy: Upper peg lateral

As stated in the section on extraction, one of the fundamental requirements of a finished orthodontic case is that all the (intraarch) spaces must be closed. But it is impossible to satisfy this requirement by orthodontic means alone in some cases.

For ideal treatment outcomes, especially occlusion, the teeth in the upper arch must match the opposing teeth in the lower arch. The relationship is analogous to that of a lock and its key or a lid and its pot. Unlike plastic teeth, natural teeth sometimes do not come with ideal sizes and shapes. If the tooth-size discrepancy is significant, the treating orthodontist would need to team up with a GD to offer the patient the options of changing the abnormal tooth/teeth to the proper size and shape.

How to avoid and treat the complication

Some patients present with small upper lateral incisors, also called peg lateral. Consider the following case of a female patient with small upper lateral incisors (Figure 9.15a and b).

Recognizing the tooth-size discrepancy complication, the orthodontist explained to the patient and her mother that she would need a GD helping her near the conclusion of orthodontic treatment. The patient then proceeded with conventional twin metal brackets for braces (not shown).

Near the end of orthodontic treatment, the patient was ready for her GD. It must be emphasized that before the patient is seen by the GD, the lateral and central incisors must be in proper position and orientation, with their roots parallel to the adjacent roots.

In this case, for the upper peg lateral incisors, a composite bonding procedure was performed by a skilled GD (Dr. Mindy Nguyen) to yield the proper size and shape (Figure 9.15c). The patient was also considering tooth whitening at a later time.

Underbite

Underbite is the term that a layperson would typically use, but dentists would use the correct term: anterior crossbite or negative OJ. This condition is often associated—but not always—with class III malocclusion.

Complications and how to avoid and treat them

There are many different techniques that can be used to treat this kind of problems. A thorough discussion of these techniques is beyond the scope of this chapter.

For some patients with mild anterior crossbite and class III malocclusion, class III mechanics with rubber bands could be used successfully if the patient is highly motivated.

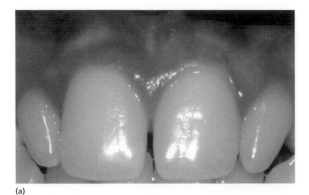

(a)

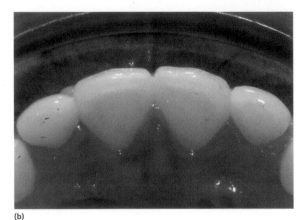

(b)

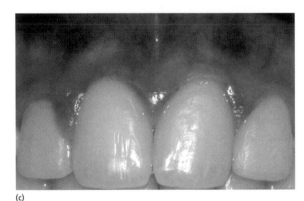

(c)

Figure 9.15 Small upper lateral incisors: (a) front, (b) occlusal, and (c) cosmetic bonding toward the end of orthodontic treatment (Reproduced with permission from Dr. Hung Vu).

When the patient has moderate negative OJ, one of the proposed treatments would be extracting the lower first premolars and upper second premolars—provided that the rest of the teeth are healthy and worth keeping. For class III malocclusion, extracting only the lower first premolars often leads to poor occlusion at the end of orthodontic treatment. Again, it should be emphasized that these extraction recommendations are oversimplified because the decision of which teeth to be extracted is based on multiple factors, including the possibility of orthognathic surgery especially for young adults with severe skeletal Class III.

White spot lesion

White spot lesion (WSL) on teeth is typically a manifestation of either mild fluorosis (slightly excessive intake of fluoride) or demineralization/decalcification (loss of minerals or mineral salts). Although these two have a similar appearance on the enamel of the teeth, namely, a white spot, they have distinct physical characteristics.

Fluorosis is a defect of the enamel (hypomineralization or hypoplasia) due to excessive intake of fluoride during enamel formation. For young children, this problem is typically from the ingestion of fluoridated toothpaste. Mild fluorosis results in white flecks or white lines or opaque patches in the enamel, whereas moderate and severe fluorosis would display chalky and opaque or mottling enamel (Cameron, 2003). Enamel with mild fluorosis would be smooth, shiny, and noncarious. Lesion is derived from the Latin word *laesio*, meaning *injury*, so mild fluorosis should not be considered as a lesion.

On the other hand, demineralization is defined as "… subsurface enamel porosities from carious" with "a milky white opacity…" (Summitt *et al.*, 2006; Maxfield *et al.*, 2012).

Dental plaque and dental caries

Dental plaque comprises mainly microorganisms and their extracellular products, and one of the damaging products is acid. Most of the microorganisms are bacteria; some microorganisms in the plaque are still not yet identified; nonbacterial microorganisms include *Mycoplasma* species, yeasts, protozoa, and viruses (Contreras and Slots, 2000); the plaque also contains some host cells, that is, epithelial cells, macrophages, and leukocytes (Newman *et al.*, 2002).

Dental caries or carious lesion is an infectious disease, and the Gram-positive bacteria group mutans streptococci of which the species *Streptococcus mutans* and *Streptococcus sobrinus* are primarily responsible for causing decay (Balakrishnan *et al.*, 2000). These bacteria can survive in an acidic environment (low pH).

The saliva's mean pH is between 6.75 and 7.25, which supports the growth of many bacteria, and its ionic composition promotes buffering properties as well as remineralization of the enamel (Marsh, 2000). When the pH in the plaque is below the critical level of 5.5, the produced acid begins to demineralize the enamel (Cameron, 2003). If the acid demineralization predominates, it results in carious lesion which is opaque, rough, and chalky (porous). And this lesion is known as WSL.

In a healthy oral condition, the plaque microflora is composed of certain microorganism species that are maintained in a healthy equilibrium, but in disease the composition shifts away from that.

With braces (fixed orthodontic appliance), it may be difficult or time consuming for a orthodontic patients to keep the brackets and teeth always free of plaque. Thus, for those patients who do not maintain good OH, unfortunately, one of the permanent outcomes is WSL, and its common place is around the edge of the bracket that is bonded to the enamel. It can also be at the gingival line.

In the oral environment, there exist dynamic and competing processes between demineralization and remineralization of the enamel, and WSL occurs when the former predominates. WSL begins as demineralization followed by a cavitated lesion and then finally becomes cavitated lesion (Fejerskov and Kidd, 2003; Guzmán-Armstrong *et al.*, 2010).

WSL detracts from otherwise successful orthodontic treatments. Although the responsibility of keeping the teeth clean rests solely on the patient, WSL can be prevented if there is good communication among the cooperating/complying patient (and patient's parent if patient is minor), the orthodontist, and the GD.

An example of a patient with WSL is given in Figure 9.16. Certain spots can also have yellow stains.

This individual had orthodontic treatment elsewhere and came to the author's office for replacing his retainers that he had lost. The demineralization is extensive, but the irreversible damage could have (or should have) been prevented. In this case, it is unknown if the patient did not comply with the given oral hygiene instruction (OHI) or refused to visit his GD for cleaning or the orthodontist did not enforce good OH practice during regular orthodontic visits.

Another instance of poor OH is given in Figure 9.17. This individual had orthodontic treatment elsewhere and came to the author's office for an evaluation/consult. She had severe gingivitis and heavy plaque buildup. This condition, could have certainly lead to WSL.

Prevention and treatment

The best way to prevent WSL is by having good OH. It is a well-known fact that patients with poorly controlled diabetes are more susceptible to dental caries (Falk,

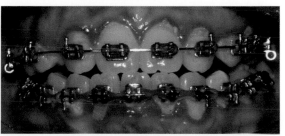

(a)

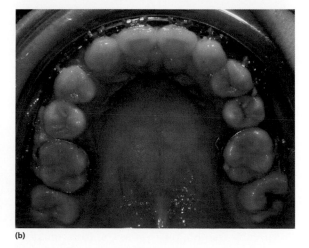

(b)

Figure 9.17 Poor OH: (a) center and (b) upper (Reproduced with permission of Dr. Hung Vu).

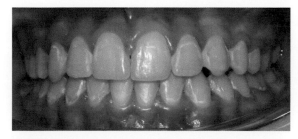

Figure 9.16 Postorthodontic treatment with WSL and some yellow spots (Reproduced with permission from Dr. Hung Vu).

Hugoson, and Thorstensson, 1989; Galea, Aganovic, and Anganovic, 1986). But for patients with poor OH or poor compliance what could be done?

For prevention, McDonald, Avery, and Dean (2004) recommended that dental plaque should be controlled with two specific goals: (i) removal of supragingival plaque for the prevention of caries, which is directly reducing the numbers of mutans streptococci (Gram positive), and (ii) removal of subgingival plaque for the prevention of gingivitis, which is directly reducing Gram-negative bacteria since the plaque associated with gingival inflammation is predominantly occupied by Gram-negative bacteria (or indirectly promoting the microflora that is associated with gingival health, i.e., Gram-positive bacteria). Note that *Aggregatibacter actinomycetemcomitans* and *Porphyromonas gingivalis* (both Gram negative) are periodontal pathogens (Newman *et al.*, 2002).

For prevention and treatment of WSL, Guzmán-Armstrong *et al.* (2010) recommended the following (depending upon patient condition): "fluoride toothpastes, gels, varnishes, and mouth rinses; antimicrobials; xylitol gum…."

Fluoride toothpastes and gels

The use of high-concentration fluoride toothpastes and gels (1500–5000 ppm) twice daily (during orthodontic treatment) has shown a tendency to inhibit demineralization (Derks *et al.*, 2004; Baysan *et al.*, 2001).

Fluoride varnish

It is recommended that moderate-risk and high-risk orthodontic patients should have an in-office fluoride varnish application every 6 months or even every 3 months if necessary (Am. Dent. Assoc. Council of Scientific Affairs, 2006a and 2006b).

Fluoride varnish, which typically has 5% sodium fluoride (NaF) or 22 600 ppm fluoride, is not a permanent varnish, but it provides a highly concentrated fluoride to the tooth surface. The varnish, which is a suspension of sodium fluoride in alcohol- and resin-based solution, sets quickly upon contacting saliva. When applied, the varnish is recommended to remain on the teeth for at least 4–6 h, approximately. Fluoride varnish must be delivered by a dental professional in most states (ASTDD, 2007).

Examples of fluoride varnishes are Colgate® PreviDent® Varnish, MI Varnish™ (GC America), Clinpro™ White Varnish (3M ESPE), and Premier® Enamel Pro® Varnish. Different manufacturers make different fluoride varnishes, and these products release varying amounts of fluoride, calcium, and phosphate ions. MI Varnish is a topical fluoride varnish with calcium and phosphate, but it releases the most amounts of fluoride and calcium ions, whereas Premier® Enamel Pro® Varnish releases the most amount of phosphate ions (Cochrane *et al.*, 2014).

Note that the contraindication of fluoride varnish is *necrotizing ulcerative gingivostomatitis* which is also called *acute necrotizing ulcerative gingivitis* (ANUG) or *trench mouth*.

According to ASTDD (2007), fluoride varnish has been found effective in preventing caries on both primary and permanent teeth. But the US Food and Drug Administration (FDA) approved fluoride varnish only for dentin hypersensitivity treatment or for cavity varnish—not for caries prevention or protection.

Fluoride mouth rinse

It is thought that fluoride mouth rinse may reduce the severity of WSL during orthodontic treatment, but there is little evidence supporting this idea.

Antimicrobials: Chlorhexidine gluconate

As an antimicrobial agent, chlorhexidine mouth rinse may be beneficial in preventing WSL when patients are having orthodontic braces, based on the idea of shifting the ecology from an unfavorable to favorable microflora in the oral cavity. But chlorhexidine mouth rinse causes staining quickly, so it would be unacceptable.

Xylitol gum

Guzmán-Armstrong *et al.* (2010) stated that xylitol chewing gum is noncariogenic and seems to be antimicrobial. From a 40-month cohort study in 1989–1993, Makinen *et al.* (1995) concluded that xylitol is the most effective agent in reducing caries compared to other chewing gums.

Part II: Periodontal complications associated with orthodontic therapy

Introduction

The importance of understanding the relationship between periodontal health and orthodontic tooth movement cannot be overstated. Clinicians providing orthodontic services should be familiar with the reciprocal relationship between common periodontal conditions and orthodontic therapy. This would include a basic understanding of the development, prevention, and treatment of the periodontal inflammatory diseases—gingivitis and periodontitis, gingival hyperplasia, mucogingival deformities, and periodontal abscess.

Treatment that did not have a coordinated plan

Avoiding complications: periodontal treatment planning for an orthodontic patient (Mathews and Kokich, 1997; Vanarsdall, 1981; AAP, 2003; Diedrich, Fritz, and Kinzinger, 2004, adapted from Milano and Milano, 2012).

Combined orthodontic and periodontal treatment requires a coordinated plan, a "roadmap," from the inception to the conclusion of the treatment.

Preceding orthodontic therapy
- Comprehensive periodontal examination
- Diagnosis
- Prognosis
- Treatment planning and coordination with orthodontic therapy
- OHIs
- Nonsurgical therapies (scaling, root planing, correction of plaque-retaining sites, e.g., faulty restorations, caries)
- Reevaluation
- Periodontal surgery of sites not responding to scaling and root planing and not amenable to control by routing preventive maintenance
- Gingival augmentation (e.g., gingival recession, thin tissue, root exposure)
- Frenulectomy
- Canine exposure surgery

During orthodontic therapy
- Preventive maintenance
  - OH reinforcement
  - Control plaque-associated gingival inflammation
  - Monitoring of at-risk sites
  - Coordination of visits between the orthodontist and providers of preventive/general care
- Canine exposure surgery
- Emergency care

During and after orthodontic therapy
- Definitive corrective surgery: pocket reduction by osseous surgery and regenerative therapy.

Definitive corrective surgery for periodontitis and soft-tissue grafting may be elected at any time before, during, or after orthodontic therapy. The timing of these treatments is based on clinical findings. Efforts to arrest active periodontal diseases are made before orthodontic tooth movement. The most common treatment for plaque-associated inflammatory periodontal diseases is nonsurgical, for example, OHIs and periodontal scaling (Sanders, 1999). However, if the treatment response is found to be inadequate or there is disease recurrence during orthodontic tooth movement, an additional treatment should be undertaken to control periodontal inflammation and disease progression. If the inflammation can be controlled via repeated nonsurgical treatment or limited periodontal surgery, definitive osseous or regenerative surgery may be delayed until after the completion of orthodontic therapy. This takes into consideration the morphological bone changes that can occur during orthodontic movement, which may reduce the extent of surgery required. Postponement of orthodontic tooth movement is recommended during the healing period of any surgical intervention (Brown, 1973; Diedrich, Fritz, and Kinzinger, 2004).
- Periodontal soft-tissue grafting, including possible root coverage surgery

Progression of gingival recession during orthodontic treatment is an indication for soft-tissue grafting (AAP Parameters of Care, 2000a–2000d; Zachrisson, Lang, and Lindhe, 2008). However, teeth with narrow zones of keratinized attached tissue can be successfully maintained with good OH (Wennström, 2014). However, teeth with thin periodontal tissues, when moved beyond the envelope of the alveolar housing, are at risk for gingival recession (Wennström, 1996). If such tooth movement is planned, preemptive soft-tissue grafting intended to stabilize the tissue attachment by increasing tissue volume (thickness) may be considered. If there is a decision to monitor these sites and changes in tissue levels are noted, orthodontic treatment may be temporarily suspended in favor of soft-tissue augmentation. After a healing period of approximately 6 weeks, active orthodontic tooth movement can be continued (Wennström et al., 2008).

- Crown lengthening

  Crown lengthening surgery may be accomplished during and after orthodontic therapy to assist with necessary restorative dentistry (Camargo et al., 2007).

- Gingival reshaping (e.g., hyperplastic gingiva)

  Gingival reshaping may be accomplished during orthodontic therapy to remove overgrown tissues that interfere with the placement of orthodontic appliances and with OH procedures. After the completion of orthodontic therapy, gingival reshaping is done to improve gingival health, OH access, and esthetics.

- Emergency care

  During orthodontic treatment, emergency care should be considered in the event of periodontal or endodontic infections, dental pain due to caries, and orofacial trauma (Polson et al., 1984).

After orthodontic therapy

- Preventive (supportive) maintenance
- Monitoring for changes (e.g., gingivitis, periodontitis, gingival recession)

Prevention

Avoiding complications—comprehensive periodontal examination (AAP Parameters of Care, 2000a–2000d).

Orthodontic patients are also periodontal patients. Orthodontic treatment should be preceded by a comprehensive periodontal examination, irrespective of the patient's age (AAP, 2011; Milano and Milano, 2012):

- **Up-to-date medical and dental history**. The patient's medical and dental history can have a significant impact on the course and success of orthodontic treatment. As with many types of dental treatment, common medical conditions to be considered may include diabetes mellitus, bleeding disorders, active viral illness, and conditions requiring antibiotic prophylaxis. Patients with a high caries experience, current or treated, and periodontal disease require additional attention (Zachrisson, Land, and Lindhe, 2008).
- **Chief complaint**. The chief complaint is the primary reason for the patient seeking treatment.
- **Extra- and intraoral examination**. Extra-and intraoral examination for pathological conditions should be completed before treatment is rendered (AAP, 2003).
- **Current PA and BW radiographs of diagnostic quality**. Current radiographs are required to provide for assessment of periodontal bone levels and the presence of mineralized dental deposits.
- **Presence and distribution of plaque, calculus, and OH adequacy**. A key element in the periodontal management of orthodontic patients with a history of susceptibility to periodontitis is the control of dental plaque-associated inflammation. It is important to establish a baseline of patient personal OH and preventive care before and during orthodontic treatment (Zachrisson, Lang, and Lindhe, 2008).
- **Degree and distribution of gingival inflammatory changes**. Severity of gingival inflammation is often described as slight, moderate, or severe. These may all be found within a single dentition. The distribution is expressed as localized (<30% of teeth) or generalized (>30% of teeth) (Armitage, 2004; Fiorellini et al., 2012; Hujoel, 2015).
- **Periodontal soft tissues**. Periodontal soft tissues are often described by their color, size contour, shape, consistency, surface texture, and gingival margin position (Fioriellini and Stathopoulou, 2015).
- **Periodontal probing depths**. The measurement of the gingival sulcus or periodontal pocket, extending from the gingival margin to where the probe tip stops within the gingival sulcus, at a consistent probing force (Gabathuler and Hassell, 1971).
- **Clinical attachment levels**. Clinical attachment levels are the point at which the periodontal tissues attach to the tooth. This is measured from a fixed point, such as the CEJ to the point where the periodontal probe tip stops within the gingival sulcus (AAP Glossary of Periodontal Terms, 2001).
- **Periodontal bone loss**. Radiographic evidence of bone loss is the clinical reflection of a history of periodontitis. Past periodontitis is considered a risk factor for possible future periodontal breakdown (Dommisch and Kebschull, 2015).
- **Bleeding on probing**. Bleeding on probing is an important indicator of subgingival inflammation. Sites that consistently lack bleeding on probing are considered to be less likely to suffer from future periodontitis. Consequently, clinicians should strive to achieve this treatment endpoint (Lang et al., 1986).
- **Furcation invasions**. Periodontitis lesions often extend between the roots of multirooted teeth. These defects are the most challenging to treat successfully

and require special monitoring during orthodontic treatment. Rapid increases in severity should be addressed without delay (Hirshfeld and Wasserman, 1978).

- **Dental mobility and fremitus**. Significantly increased dental mobility and fremitus could be signs of lost periodontal attachment (bone loss) and/or excessive occlusal forces (Lindhe and Ericsson, 1976).
- **Mucogingival relationships**. The extension of a periodontal pocket beyond the mucogingival junction should be considered for treatment. These sites are difficult to maintain and are at risk for continuing progression (Maynard and Wilson, 1980).
- **Gingival recession**. Baseline measurements will assist in specific treatment planning: the direction of proposed tooth movement relative to an area of recession, pretreatment gingival grafting, monitoring, and posttreatment needs (Maynard and Wilson, 1980; Zachrisson, Lang, and Lindhe, 2008).
- **Width of keratinized tissue**. Narrow bands of keratinized gingiva are at no greater risk of recession, as long as inflammation is controlled (Wennström et al., 1987).
- **Thickness of gingival marginal tissue**. Thin marginal tissues are at greater risk of recession due to inflammation and orthodontic tooth movement in the direction of a thin cortical plate and out of the normal contour of the alveolus (Maynard and Ochsenbein, 1975; Maynard and Wilson, 1980; Zachrisson, Lang, and Lindhe, 2008)
- **Abnormal frenulum insertions**. The participation of the maxillary anterior frenum in the formation of a midline diastema is controversial (Zachrisson, Lang, and Lindhe, 2008). When reaching the gingival margin, they can contribute to tissue retractability, compromising OH and promoting gingival inflammation and hyperplasia. Fan-shaped, hyperplastic midline frenum attachment can interfere with space closure and is an indication for removal (Zachrisson, Lang, and Lindhe, 2008). With the frenotomy procedure, care should be taken not to damage interproximal papilla (Zachrisson, Lang, and Lindhe, 2008).
- **Vestibular depth**. A shallow vestibule can reduce access for OH, and the soft tissues of the cheek may be subject to trauma from the orthodontic appliances.
- **Tooth/root prominence**. Root prominence may indicate thin gingival tissues and thin or absence of underlying bone. Tooth movement in the direction of tooth prominence, beyond the envelope of the genetically determined bone profile, is a risk for gingival recession (Wennström et al., 1987, 2008).
- **Root proximity**. Roots in close proximity are more difficult to clean and are therefore at a greater risk of periodontal inflammation and bone loss (Vermylen et al., 2005).
- **Periodontal biotype**. The relative anatomical morphology of the periodontium has been described as thin (scalloped), average, and thick (flat) (Zweers et al., 2014). It has been suggested that a thin (scalloped) biotype, suggesting a reduced periodontal tissue volume, has a greater tendency for gingival recession. This could present a risk in orthodontic tooth movement, as previously noted (Krishnan et al., 2007).

Orthodontic treatment in conjunction with inflammatory periodontal diseases: Gingivitis and periodontitis

Periodontal disease is a chronic inflammatory disease that affects the gingival tissues (gingivitis) and can extend to the alveolar bone supporting the teeth (periodontitis) (AAP, 2014b). If left untreated, periodontitis can lead to tooth loss (Martin et al., 2009). Consequently, it is essential for the treating clinicians to identify and treat patients with active periodontal disease (or those at risk), prior to orthodontic therapy. If more than one clinician is involved in the patient's care, interdisciplinary collaboration is essential to avoid the sequelae of untreated disease. The team approach is critical to the diagnosis, treatment, and monitoring of the periodontium during the course of orthodontic therapy.

Periodontal diseases as infections

Gingivitis and periodontitis, the two major forms of periodontal diseases, have been described as infections, initiated by microorganisms that colonize and grow at or apical to the gingival margin (Socransky and Haffagee, 2008). While the relationship between these microorganisms and their host is usually benign, specific bacteria may overgrow, change, or be newly introduced, upsetting the homeostatic equilibrium. This can result in the clinical manifestations of the disease process, including periodontal bone loss. Periodontal disease progression was previously thought to be slow and continuous. However, it is now also believed to progress episodically, with "bursts" of activity, followed by periods of quiescence (Socransky *et al.*, 1984). Reestablishment of the equilibrium can occur either spontaneously or as the result of treatment (Socransky and Haffagee, 2008). Unfortunately, these episodes of attachment loss are not predictable, and continuous efforts should be made at preventing their occurrence and progression.

While periodontal microorganisms are required to initiate the disease process, other factors can influence susceptibility, rate of progression, and the potential success of treatment (Kornman, 2008). Risk factors often associated with periodontitis have been categorized as behavioral, host-genetic, environmental, bacterial, modifiable, and nonmodifiable (Ronderos and Ryder, 2004; Kornman, 2008; Van Dyke and Sheilesh, 2005).

Plaque-induced gingivitis in patients undergoing orthodontics

Definition and prevalence

Plaque-induced gingivitis is defined as an inflammation of the gingiva in the absence of clinical attachment or bone loss (AAP Parameters of Care, 2000a–2000d). Gingivitis is the most common form of periodontal disease, with prevalence estimates approaching 100% in children and adolescents (Koch and Lindhe, 1967; Vanarsdall, 1981) and 50–90% of adults (Albandar and Rams, 2000, Albandar and Tinoco, 2002).

Due to the ubiquitous presence of gingivitis, especially in children, there may be a tendency to accept that the periodontium can resist the "stresses" of orthodontic treatment without negative consequences. However, that is not necessarily the case (Vanarsdall, 1981; Polson and Reed, 1984; Joss-Vassalli *et al.*, 2010). While gingivitis does not result in bone or tooth loss, it is considered a precursor of periodontitis, beginning as early as childhood. As such, treatment and control of gingivitis are an essential instrument in the prevention of periodontitis (Quirynen, Dekeyser, and van Steenberghe, 1991).

Clinical signs and symptoms

Gingivitis is commonly identified by its clinical signs including redness, edema, and bleeding on probing. Local factors such as dental plaque and calculus are often present. However, there is no radiographic evidence of bone loss (AAP Parameters of Care, 2000a–2000d).

Prevention

Plaque-associated gingivitis is a reversible condition. Therapy aimed at the reduction of etiologic factors (plaque and calculus) includes initial anti-infective treatment, followed by supportive/preventive care. The goal is to reduce subgingival bacteria below the threshold required to produce the inflammatory response (AAP Position Paper, 2003; Robinson, 1995).

Periodontal disease in patients undergoing orthodontics

Common risk factors for periodontitis (Van Dyke and Sheilesh, 2005)

Modifiable risk factors

- Smoking
- Diabetes mellitus
- Microorganisms
- Psychological factors (stress)

Nonmodifiable risk factors

- Genetics
- Host response
- Aging

The goal of periodontal treatment is to reestablish a "nonactive," healthy state by addressing the modifiable risk factors. This would include reducing the subgingival microorganisms to a level below which they can be controlled by the host's defense mechanisms (Zachcriasson, 1996).

Management

Successful orthodontic therapy and the health of periodontium are inseparably intertwined. Orthodontic tooth movement results from periodontal osteoclastic and osteoblastic activity when controlled forces are applied to the teeth (Ong, Wang, and Smith, 1998). Compression of the PDL during tooth movement reduces its blood supply, resulting in an avascular "cell-free" zone ("hyalinization"), temporarily halting the tooth movement. This effect is reversed by resorption of the contiguous alveolar bone ("undermining resorption"), paving the way for the reorganization of the PDL and the continuation of the tooth movement. Regeneration of the PDL does not proceed normally when the periodontal tissues are inflamed (Ericsson *et al.*, 1977). Therefore, the periodontal remodeling required for orthodontic tooth movement is one that should be undertaken under periodontally healthy conditions. This is particularly true in patients with a history of periodontitis susceptibility or other factors predisposing patients to periodontal complications:

1 OHIs. The short- and long-term value has been clearly demonstrated (Löe et al., 1965; Theilade et al., 1966). As orthodontic appliances can be obstacles to OH effectiveness, professional reinforcement of plaque control activities is important in maintaining a consistent result (Suomi et al., 1971).

2 Correction of plaque-retentive elements, such as active caries, defective restorations, and overhanging margins, should be considered part of the OH continuum (AAP Report, 2001).

3 Use of a power toothbrush with a 2 min timer and an oral irrigator with or without medicaments can be useful adjuncts to prevention (AAP Position Paper, 2003, 2005; Gugerli et al., 2007; Nanning et al., 2008).

4 Scaling, and root planing, as needed, in sites of previous attachment loss, aimed at removing plaque, calculus, and tooth surface accretions (AAP Report, 2001).

5 Continuing supportive periodontal maintenance. To maximize a successful outcome, effective personal OH and professional preventive care on a regular 3–4-month interval, during orthodontic treatment, should be considered.

6 Close monitoring for OH efficacy, gingival inflammation, and increased probing depths associated with attachment loss (AAP Parameters of Care, 2001).

7 In cases of extremely poor OH, discontinuance of orthodontic tooth movement should be considered until OH and periodontal health status improves sufficiently to reinstitute an active treatment.

Complication: Undetected periodontal disease for patients undergoing orthodontic treatment

Definition and prevalence

Chronic periodontitis is defined as an inflammation of the gingiva extending into the adjacent attachment apparatus (AAP Parameters of Care, 2000a–2000d).

Adult patients are and will be seeking orthodontic care (AAO, 2013). Patients, including children and adolescents, with an undiagnosed and untreated periodontal disease can worsen during orthodontic treatment. Clinicians must be prepared to manage these potentially complicating conditions. With an early diagnosis and treatment, even patients with periodontally compromised dentitions can be successfully treated (Kokich, 2013).

Prevalence (United States)

47.2% 30 years and older (64.7 million adults) (Dye et al., 2012)

70.1% 65 years and older (Dye et al., 2012)

0.2–2.75% children and adolescents (Albandar, 2002, Albandar, Brown, and Löe, 1997)

0.2–0.5% children and adolescents with severe attachment loss (Loe and Brown, 1991).

The disease is characterized by the loss of clinical attachment due to destruction of the PDL and loss of the adjacent supporting bone. Tooth loss can result as the ultimate complication (AAP Parameters of Care, 2000a–2000d).

Clinical signs and symptoms

Periodontitis is commonly identified by the clinical signs of gingival redness, edema, bleeding on probing, periodontal pockets, and radiographic evidence of bone loss. Local factors such as dental plaque and calculus are often present. Periodontal pockets associated with bone loss are the major distinguishing factors for gingivitis (AAP Parameters of Care, 2000a–2000d).

Prevention

The key to preventing periodontitis is to control plaque-associated gingivitis (Loe and Brown, 1991; Socransky and Haffagee, 2008). Sites free of gingivitis are much less likely to progress to periodontitis (Lang et al., 1986). Therapy is aimed at reducing the factors etiologic to gingivitis (e.g., plaque and calculus). This includes anti-infective treatment, followed by supportive/preventive care. The technical goal of treatment is to reduce the potency of the subgingival biofilm below the threshold required to produce the inflammatory response (AAP Position Paper, 2003). The treatment of gingivitis can be found in the previous section.

Treatment (Carranza and Takei, 2012)

1 OHIs

2 Scaling and root planing

3 Reevaluation

4 Periodontal surgery of sites not responding to nonsurgical treatment to remove residual deposits, reduce periodontal pocket depth, and correct the bony defects caused by the disease process

5 Preventive (supportive) periodontal maintenance

Complication: Gingival hyperplasia (enlargement, overgrowth)

Gingival hyperplasia is an enlargement of the gingival tissues, resulting from the proliferation of gingival epithelium and connective tissue elements (fibroblasts). It is most often an inflammatory response to plaque accumulation (Hong, 2007) (see Chapter 2). Mouth breathing and delayed eruption may serve as cofactors. Gingival hyperplasia can interfere with proper plaque control, complicate orthodontic treatment, and be esthetically displeasing. It can mask disease progression, gingivitis to periodontitis. Consequently, proper diagnosis and treatment is an essential part of overall therapeutic success (Sanders, 1999; Weinberg and Eskow, 2000; Doufexi, Mina, and Ioannidou, 2005) (Figure 9.18: gingival hyperplasia).

Diagnosis

The diagnosis is made primarily through clinical presentation and medical history (Seymour, Thomason, and Ellis, 1996; Marshall and Bartold, 1998; Seymour, Ellis, and Thomason, 2000). The gingival tissues are often enlarged and may be fibrotic or edematous.

Prevention

1 Provide OHIs and remove dental deposits before initiating orthodontic treatment.
2 Maintain high levels of plaque control during orthodontic treatment, understanding that orthodontic appliances may complicate OH measures.

Treatment

1 Gingival hyperplasia may resolve after removal of the orthodontic appliances.
2 Nonresolving gingival hyperplasia, especially that which is associated with delayed eruption, may require surgical treatment before, during, or after orthodontic treatment (Camargo *et al.*, 2001) (Figure 9.18).

Mucogingival deformities and orthodontic care
Definition and prevalence

Mucogingival deformities are deviations from the normal anatomic relationship between the gingival margin and the mucogingival junction (AAP Parameters of Care, 2000a–2000d). The two most common mucogingival deformities that may complicate orthodontic care are gingival recession and aberrant frenal attachments.

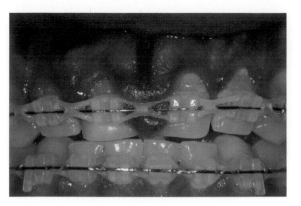

Figure 9.18 Gingival hyperplasia during orthodontics.

Gingival recession has been defined as "the migration of the marginal soft tissue to a point apical to the cemento-enamel junction of a tooth or the platform of a dental implant" (AAP, 2014a). This condition can be localized or generalized. It has been found to affect a significant percentage of the population, the prevalence increasing with age (Kassab and Cohen, 2003). In children and adolescents, the prevalence of gingival recession was 5% at 7 years, 39% at 12 years, and 74% at 17 years of age (Ainamo *et al.*, 1986). It has been reported that more than 50% of 18–50-year-olds and 88% of people 65 years and older have one or more sites of gingival recession. A multifactorial etiology has been proposed (Löe *et al.*, 1992). Inflammation due to trauma from OH procedures, plaque-induced periodontal infections, and dental treatment, superimposed on underlying alveolar bone deficiencies, have been identified as the most likely causes (Geiger, 1980; Watson, 1984).

Clinical signs and symptoms

The migration of the gingival margin to a position apical to the CEJ or the progression of previous recession.

Complications

1 **Progressive gingival recession related to orthodontic tooth movement**. Gingival recession during orthodontics most often occurs when the tooth is moved through the cortical plate and outside the envelope of the alveolus. This may indicate the need for soft-tissue grafting as a preventive measure (Ong, Wang, and Smith, 1998; Sanders, 1999; Zachrisson, Lang, and Lindhe, 2008).

2 Clinical attachment loss. Clinical attachment loss indicates a reduced connection between a tooth and its surrounding periodontium. This could be the result of inflammatory periodontal disease or a mucogingival deformity (gingival recession). These findings could indicate the need for immediate or future treatment for active periodontitis or soft-tissue grafting (AAP Position Paper, 2003).

3 Root exposure to the oral environment. Root exposure to the oral environment increases the possibility of root damage related to cervical abrasion and acid erosion. Both reduce the structural integrity of the tooth and increase the risk of dentinal sensitivity and caries (Ravald and Hamp, 1981; West *et al.*, 2013; Bignozzi *et al.*, 2014).

4 Esthetics. Gingival recession involving the teeth located in the esthetic zone can be a concern for patients who display their gingiva on smiling (Needleman *et al.*, 2004).

5 Dentinal sensitivity. Discomfort due to dentinal exposure can result in alterations in lifestyle, for example, eating, smiling, oral cleanliness, and periodontal health (Gillam *et al.*, 2013).

6 Compromised OH. Gingival recession can result in reduced OH efficacy by exposing sensitive dentin (Addy, 2005).

Prevention

It had been suggested that 2 mm of keratinized gingiva, with 1 mm attached, is an adequate dimension for maintaining gingival health and stability (Lang and Loe, 1972). However, it was subsequently determined that even narrow zones of keratinized tissue would remain stable if good OH practices were instituted (Dorfman, Kennedy, and Bird, 1982; Kennedy *et al.*, 1985). Wennström and Lindhe (1983) proposed that insufficient buccolingual gingival thickness, rather than apicocoronal height of keratinized tissue, is a predisposing factor for gingival recession. If the tooth is moved within the envelope of the alveolus, there is little risk of recession (Steiner *et al.*, 1981; Wennström *et al.*, 1987). Gingival inflammation, inadequate OH, thin gingival tissues, and tooth movement beyond the natural genetically determined envelope (often to the buccal) can represent a risk for gingival recession, and sites showing these characteristics should be approached with caution when orthodontic treatment is considered.

Treatment

1 Periodontal examination for sites showing gingival recession, thin gingival tissues, and inadequate OH.
2 OHIs.
3 Consultation with the dentist performing orthodontic treatment regarding the direction and extent of tooth movement.
4 If the tooth is to be moved in the direction of reduced gingival thickness, the site should be considered for gingival enhancement by periodontal soft-tissue grafting.
  Evidence indicates that reduced tissue volume (often on the buccal side) offers reduced resistance to gingival recession. Risk for the development of recession defects in conjunction with tooth movement is present if the tooth is moved out of the alveolar bone housing, creating an alveolar bone dehiscence (Wennström, 1996).
5 Any borderline sites should remain under close observation for progressive gingival recession.
6 In the event that progressive recession is observed, the orthodontic treatment should be temporarily suspended, gingival augmentation procedure completed, and orthodontic treatment reinstituted after a suitable healing period.
7 Aberrant frenal attachments that reduce OH efficacy or prevent the closure of a diastema may be surgically revised or removed.

Periodontal abscess during orthodontic treatment

A periodontal abscess is a localized, frequently purulent inflammatory reaction, often as an exacerbation of preexisting chronic periodontitis (Carranza and Camargo, 2012). It may be chronic or acute. The latter is more frequently symptomatic. This condition can result in rapid, irreversible bone loss and should be treated immediately upon discovery (Sanz, Herrera, and van Winkelhoff, 2008). As previously noted, the inflammatory periodontal lesion can interfere with successful orthodontic tooth movement by preventing the regeneration of PDL and bone on the diseased root surface. Detailed treatment of the periodontal abscess is discussed in Chapter 2.

Prevention

1 Complete periodontal examination, diagnosis, and treatment to remedy active periodontal disease.

2 Preventive periodontal therapy, adjusted to the patient's particular risk profile and susceptibility. The value of good OH cannot be overstated.

Orthodontic specific treatment recommendations

1 Establish a definitive periodontal diagnosis (see Chapter 2).

2 Once the acute lesion has been diagnosed, halt active tooth movement.

3 Treat the abscess as described in Chapter 2 with a combination of establishing drainage, removing plaque and calculus, and implementing antibiotic therapy, as needed.

4 Reinitiate tooth active movement once the inflammation has resolved.

5 Periodontal surgery may be required to attain a satisfactory result.

6 Continue preventive periodontal maintenance, with close observation for recurrence.

References

AAP. (2003) Guidelines for Periodontal Therapy. AAP, Chicago, IL.

AAP. (2011) AAP Comprehensive Periodontal Therapy: A Statement by the American Academy of Periodontology. AAP, Chicago, IL.

AAP. (2014a) Glossary of Terms. AAP, Chicago, IL.

AAP. (2014b) Periodontal Disease Fact Sheet. AAP, Chicago, IL.

AAP Parameters of Care (2000a) Parameter on comprehensive periodontal examination. *J Periodontol*, **71** (5 Suppl.), 847–848.

AAP Parameters of Care (2000b) Parameter on periodontal maintenance. *J Periodontol*, **71** (5 Suppl.), 849–850.

AAP Parameters of Care. (2000c) Parameter on plaque-induced gingivitis. *J Periodontol*, **71** (5 Suppl.), i–ii, 851–852.

AAP Parameters of Care. (2000d) Chronic periodontitis with slight to moderate loss of periodontal support. *J Periodontol*, **71** (5 Suppl.), 853–855.

AAP, Position Paper. (2003) Periodontal Diseases of Children and Adolescents. AAP, Chicago, IL.

AAP, Position Paper (2005) The role of supra- and subgingival irrigation in the treatment of periodontal diseases. *J Periodontol*, **76**, 2015–2027.

Academy Report. (2001) Treatment of plaque-induced gingivitis, chronic periodontitis, and other clinical conditions. AAP, Position Paper, Vol. **72**, No. 12, 1790–1800.

Addy, M. (2005) Tooth brushing, tooth wear and dentine hypersensitivity—are they associated? *Int Dent J*, **55** (4 Suppl. 1), 261–267.

Ainamo, J., Paloheimo, L., Norblad, A. and Murtomaa, H. (1986) Gingival recession in schoolchildren at 7, 12 and 17 years of age in Espoo, Finland. *Community Dent Oral Epidemiol*, **14** (5), 283–286.

Albandar, J.M. (2002) Periodontal disease in North America. *Periodontology*, **29**, 31–69.

Albandar, J. and Rams, T. (2002) Global epidemiology of periodontal diseases. *Periodontology*, **29**, 7–10.

Albandar, J.M. and Tinoco, E.M.B. (2002) Global epidemiology of periodontal diseases in children and young persons. *Periodontology*, **29** (1), 153–176.

Albandar, J.M., Brown, L.J. and Löe, H. (1997) Clinical features of early-onset periodontitis. *J Am Dental Assoc*, **128** (10), 1393–1399.

American Academy of Periodontology (AAP). (2001) AAP Glossary of Terms. AAP, Chicago, IL.

American Association of Orthodontists (AAO) (2013) *Survey on the Number of Adult Patients Seeking Orthodontic Treatment during 2010–2012*, Economics of Orthodontics, AAO Press Release, St. Louis, MO.

American Dental Association Council of Scientific Affairs (2006) Caries risk assessment. *J Am Dent Assoc*, **137**, 1151–1159.

American Dental Association Council on Scientific Affairs (2006) Professionally applied topical fluoride: evidence-based clinical recommendations. *J Am Dent Assoc*, **137**, 1151–1159.

Armitage, G. (2004) Periodontal diagnosis and classification of periodontal diseases. *Periodontology*, **34**, 9–21.

Association of State and Territorial Dental Directors Fluorides Committee (ASTDD). (2007) *Fluoride Varnish: An Evidence-Based Approach*. Research Brief. ASTDD, Reno, NV.

Balakrishnan, M., Simmonds, R.S. and Tagg, J.R. (2000) Dental caries is a preventable infectious disease. *Aust Dent J*, **45** (4), 235–245.

Barbagallo, L.J., Jones, A.S., Petocz, P. and Darendelilerd, M.A. (2008) Physical properties of root cementum: Part 10. Comparison of the effects of invisible removable thermoplastic appliances with light and heavy orthodontic forces on premolar cementum. A microcomputed-tomography study. *Am J Orthod Dentofacial Orthop*, **133**, 218–227.

Bates, S. (1856) Absorption. *Brit J Dent Sci*, **1**, 256.

Baysan, A., Lynch, E., Ellwood, R., Davies, R., Petersson, L. and Borsboom, P. (2001) Reversal of primary root caries using dentifrices containing 5000 and 1100 ppm fluoride. *Caries Res*, **35**, 41–46.

Becks, H. (1936) Root resorptions and their relation to pathologic bone formation. *Int J Orthod Oral Surg*, **22**, 445–482.

Bignozzi, I1., Crea, A., Capri, D., Littarru, C., Lajolo, C. and Tatakis, D.N. (2014) Root caries: a periodontal perspective. *J Periodontal Res*, **49** (2), 143–163.

Boyd, R.L. (2007) Complex orthodontic treatment using a new protocol for the invisalign appliance. *J Clin Orthod*, **41** (9), 525–547.

Brezniak, N. and Wasserstein, A. (1993a) Root resorption after orthodontic treatment: Part 1. Literature review. *Am J Orthod Dentofacial Orthop*, **103**, 62–66.

Brezniak, N. and Wasserstein, A. (1993b) Root resorption after orthodontic treatment: Part 2. Literature review. *Am J Orthod Dentofacial Orthop*, **103**, 138–146.

Brezniak, N. and Wasserstein, A. (2002) Orthodontically induced inflammatory root resorption. Part II: The clinical aspects. *Angle Orthod*, **72**, 180–184.

Brezniak, N. and Wasserstein, A. (2008) Root resorption following treatment with aligners. *Angle Orthodontist*, **78** (6), 1119–1124.

Brown, I.S. (1973) The effect of orthodontic therapy on certain types of periodontal defects. I. Clinical findings. *J Periodontol*, **44**, 742–756.

Burden, D.J., Mullally, B.H. and Robinson, S.N. (1999) Palatally ectopic canines: Closed eruption versus open eruption. *Am J Orthod Dentofacial Orthop*, **115**, 634–639.

Camargo, P.M., Melnick, P.R., Pirih, F.Q.M., Lagos, R. and Takei, H.H. (2001) Treatment of drug-induced gingival enlargement: aesthetic and functional considerations. *Periodontology*, **27**, 131–138.

Camargo, P.M., Melnick, P.R. and Camargo, L.M. (2007) Clinical crown lengthening in the esthetic zone. *J Calif Dental Assoc*, **35**, 487–498.

Cameron, A.C. (2003) *Handbook of Pediatric Dentistry*, 2nd edn, Mosby Elsevier Health Science, London.

Carranza, F.A. and Camargo, P.M. (2012) in *The Periodontal Pocket. Carranza's Clinical Periodontology*, 11th edn (eds M.G. Newman, H.H. Takei, P.R. Klokkevold and F.A. Carranza), Elsevier/W.B. Saunders, St. Louis, MO, pp. 127–139.

Carranza, F.A. and Takei, H.H. (2012) The treatment plan, in *Carranza's Clinical Periodontology*, 11th edn (eds M.G. Newman, H. Takei, P.R. Klokkevold and F.A. Carranza), Elsevier /Saunders, St. Louis, MO, pp. 384–386.

Cochrane, N.J., Shen, P., Yuan, Y. and Reynolds, E.C. (2014) Ion release from calcium and fluoride containing dental varnishes. *Aust Dent J*, **59** (1), 100–105.

Contreras, A. and Slots, J. (2000) Herpesviruses in human periodontal disease. *J Periodontal Res*, **35**, 3.

Derks, A., Katsaros, C., Frencken, J.E., Van't Hof, M.A. and Kuijpers-Jagtman, A.M. (2004) Caries-inhibiting effect on preventive measures during orthodontic treatment with fixed appliances: a systematic review. *Caries Res*, **38**, 413–420.

Diedrich, P., Fritz U. and Kinzinger G. (2004) Interrelationships Between Periodontics and Adult Orthodontics: Clinical and Research Report, pp. 1–16 *Perio*, **1** (3).

Dommisch, H. and Kebschull, M. (2015) Chronic periodontitis, in *Carranza's Clinical Periodontology*, 12th edn (eds M.G. Newman, H. Takei, P. Klokkevold and F.A. Carranza), Elsevier Saunders, St. Louis, MO, pp. 309–319.

Dorfman, H.S., Kennedy, J.E. and Bird, W.C. (1982) Longitudinal evaluation of free gingival grafts. A four-year report. *J Periodontol*, **53**, 349–352.

Doufexi, A., Mina, M. and Ioannidou, E. (2005) Gingival overgrowth in children: Epidemiology, pathogenesis, and complications: a literature review. *J Periodontol*, **76** (1), 3–10.

Dougherty, H.L. (1968) The effects of mechanical forces upon the mandibular buccal segments during orthodontic treatment. Part II. *Am J Orthod*, **54**, 83–103.

Dye, B.A., Wei, L., Thorton-Evans, G.O. and Genco, R.J. (2012) Prevalence of periodontitis in adults in the United States: 2009 and 2010. *J Dent Res*, **91**, 914–920.

Ericsson, I., Thilander, B., Lindhe, J. and Okamoto, H. (1977) The effect of orthodontic tilting movements on the periodontal tissues of infected and non-infected dentitions in dogs. *J Clin Periodontol*, **4**, 278–293.

Falk, H., Hugoson, A. and Thorstensson, H. (1989) Number of teeth, prevalence of caries and periapical lesions in insulin-dependent diabetics. *Scand J Dent Res*, **97**, 198.

Fejerskov, O. and Kidd, E. (2003) *Dental Caries: The Disease and its Clinical Management*, Blackwell Munksgaard, Copenhagen, p. 101.

Fiorellini, J.P., Kim, D.M. and Uzel, N.G. (2012) Clinical features of gingivitis, in *Carranza's Periodontology*, 11th edn (eds T. Newman and C. Klokkevold), Elsevier Saunders, St. Louis, MO, pp. 76–83.

Fioriellini, J. and Stathopoulou, P. (2015) Anatomy of the periodontium, in *Carranza's Clinical Periodontology*, 12th edn (eds M.G. Newman, H. Takei, P. Klokkevold and F.A. Carranza), Elsevier Saunders, St. Louis, MO, pp. 9–39.

Gabathuler, H. and Hassell, T. (1971) A pressure sensitive probe. *Helv Odontol Acta*, **15** (2), 114–117.

Galea, H., Aganovic, I. and Anganovic, M. (1986) The dental caries and periodontal disease experience of patients with early-onset insulin-dependent diabetes. *Int Dent J*, **36**, 219.

Geiger, A.M. (1980) Mucogingival problems and the movement of mandibular incisors: a clinical review. *Am J Orthod*, **78**, 511–527.

Gillam, D., Chesters, R., Attrill, D., Brunton, P., Slater, M., Strand, P., Whelton, H. and Bartlett, D. (2013) XX. *Dent Update*, **40** (7514–516, 518–520, 523–524).

Gugerli, P., Secci, G. and Mombelli, A. (2007) Evaluation of the benefits of using a power toothbrush during the initial phase of periodontal therapy. *J Periodontol*, **78** (4), 654–660.

Guzmán-Armstrong, S., Chalmers, J. and Warren, J.J. (2010) White spot lesions: prevention and treatment. *Am J Orthod Dentofacial Orthop*, **138** (6), 690–696.

Hall, A. (1978) Upper incisor root resorption during stage II of the begg technique. *Br J Orthod*, **5**, 47–50.

Henry, J.L. and Weinmann, J.P. (1951) The pattern of resorption and repair of human cementum. *J Am Dent Assoc*, **42**, 271.

Hirshfeld, L. and Wasserman, B. (1978) A long-term survey of tooth loss in 600 treated periodontal patients. *J Periodontol*, **49** (5), 225–237.

Hong, C. and the American Academy of Oral Medicine Web Writing Group (2007) Gingival Enlargement. Available at website for the American Academy of Oral Medicine, under the title "Gingival Enlargement" Updated on January 22, 2015).

Hujoel, P. (2015) Fundamentals in the methods of periodontal disease epidemiology, in *Carranza's Clinical Periodontology*, 12th edn (eds M.G. Newman, H. Takei, P. Klokkevold and F.A. Carranza), Elsevier Saunders, St. Louis, MO, pp. 68–75.

Joss-Vassalli, I., Gebenstein, C., Topouzelis, N., Sculean, A. and Katsaros, C. (2010) Orthodontic therapy and gingival recession: a systematic review. *Orthod Craniofac Res*, **13** (3), 127–141.

Kassab, M. and Cohen, R.E. (2003) The etiology and prevalence of gingival recession. *J Am Dental Assoc*, **134** (2), 220–225.

Kennedy, J.E., Bird, W.C., Palcanis, K.G. and Dorfman, H.S. (1985) A longitudinal evaluation of varying widths of attached gingiva. *J Clin Periodontol*, **12**, 667–675.

Ketcham, A.H. (1927) A preliminary report of an investigation of apical root resorption of vital permanent teeth. *Int J Orthod*, **13**, 97–127.

Ketcham, A.H. (1929) A progress report of an investigation of apical root resorption of vital permanent teeth. *Int J Orthod*, **15**, 310–328.

Koch, J. and Lindhe, J. (1967) The effect of supervised oral hygiene on the gingiva of children. *J Periodontal Res*, **2** (1), 64–69.

Kocsis, G.S., Marcsik, A., Kókai, E.L. and Kocsis, K.S. (2002) Supernumerary occlusal cusps on permanent human teeth. *Acta Biologica Szegediensis*, **46** (1–2), 71–82.

Kokich, V.G. (2004) Surgical and orthodontic management of impacted maxillary canines. *Am J Orthod Dentofacial Orthop*, **126**, 278–283.

Kokich, V.G. (2013) It's worse than we thought. *Am J Orthod Dentofacial Orthop*, **143** (2), 155.

Kokich, V.G. and Mathews, D.P. (1993) Surgical and orthodontic management of impacted teeth. *Dent Clin North Am*, **37**, 181–204.

Kornman, K.S. (2008) Mapping the pathogenesis of periodontitis: a new look. *J Periodontol*, **79**, 1560–1568.

Krishnan, V., Ambili, R., Davidovitch, Z. and Murphy, N.C. (2007) Gingiva and orthodontic treatment. *Semin Orthod*, **13**, 257–271.

Lang, N.P. and Loe, H. (1972) The relationship between the width of keratinized gingiva and gingival health. *J Periodontol*, **43**, 623–627.

Lang, N.P., Joss, A., Orsanic, T., Gusberti, F.A. and Siegrist, B.E. (1986) Bleeding on probing. A predictor for the progression of periodontal disease? *J Clin Periodontol*, **13** (6), 590–596.

Levin, M.P. and D'Amico, R.A. (1974) Flap design in exposing unerupted teeth. *Am J Orthod Dentofacial Orthop*, **65** (4), 419–422.

Lindhe, J. and Ericsson, I. (1976) The influence of trauma from occlusion on reduced but healthy periodontal tissues in dogs. *J Clin Periodontol*, **3** (2), 110–122.

Linge, B.O. and Linge, L. (1983) Apical root resorption in upper anterior teeth. *Eur J Orthod*, **5**, 173–183.

Linge, L. and Linge, B.O. (1991) Patient characteristics and treatment variables associated with apical root resorption during orthodontic treatment. *Am J Orthod Dentofacial Orthop*, **99**, 35–43.

Loe, H. and Brown, L.J. (1991) Early on-set periodontitis in the United States of America. *J Periodontol*, **62** (10), 608–616.

Löe, H., Theilade, E. and Jensen, S.B. (1965) Experimental gingivitis in man. *J Periodontol*, **36**, 177–187.

Löe, H., Anerud, A. and Boysen, H. (1992) The natural history of periodontal disease. In man: prevalence, severity, and extent of gingival recession. *J Periodontol*, **63**, 489–495.

Makinen, K.K., Bennett, C.A., Hujoel, P.P., Isokangas, P.J., Isotupa, K.P., Pape, H.R., Jr and Makinen, P.L. (1995) Xylitol chewing gums and caries rates: a 40-month cohort study. *J Dent Res*, **74** (12), 1904–1913.

Marsh, P.D. (2000) Role of the oral microflora in health. *Microb Ecol Health Disease*, **12**, 130–137.

Marsh, P.D. (2003) Are dental diseases examples of ecological catastrophes? *Microbiology*, **149**, 279–294.

Marshall, J. (1929) A comparison of resorption of roots of deciduous teeth with the absorption of roots of the permanent teeth occurring as a result of infection. *Int J Orthod*, **15**, 417.

Marshall, R.I. and Bartold, P.M. (1998) Medication induced gingival overgrowth. *Oral Diseases*, **4**, 130–151.

Martin, J.A., Page, R.C., Kaye, E.K., Hamed, M.T. and Loeb, C.F. (2009) Periodontitis severity plus risk as a tooth loss predictor. *J Periodontol*, **80** (2), 202–209.

Massler, M. and Malone, A.J. (1954) Root resorption in human permanent teeth. *Am J Orthod*, **40**, 619–633.

Mathews, D. and Kokich, V. (1997) Managing treatment for the orthodontic patient with periodontal problems. *Semin Orthod*, **3**, 31–38.

Maxfield, B.J., Hamdan, A.M., Tufekci, E., Shroff, B., Best, A.M. and Lindauer, S.J. (2012) Development of white spot lesions during orthodontic treatment: perceptions of patients, parents, orthodontists, and general dentists. *Am J Orthod Dentofacial Orthop*, **141**, 337–344.

Maynard, J.G. and Ochsenbein, C. (1975) Mucogingival problems, prevalence and therapy in children. *J Periodontol*, **46** (9), 543–552.

Maynard, J.G., Jr and Wilson, R.D. (1980) Diagnosis and management of mucogingival problems in children. *Dent Clin North Am*, **24** (4), 683–703.

McCulloch, K.J., Mills, C.M., Greenfeld, R.S. and Coil, J.M. (1998) Dens evaginatus: review of the literature and report of several clinical cases. *J Can Dent Assoc*, **64** (2), 104–6, 110–113.

McDonald, R.E., Avery, D.R. and Dean, J.A. (2004) *Dentistry for the Child and Adolescent*, 8th edn, Mosby, St. Louis, MO.

McNab, S., Battistutta, D., Taverne, A. and Symons, A.L. (1999) External apical root resorption of posterior teeth in asthmatics after orthodontic treatment. *Am J Orthod Dentofacial Orthop*, **116**, 545–551.

Meikle, M.C. (2006) The tissue, cellular, and molecular regulation of orthodontic tooth movement: 100 years after Carl Sandstedt. *Eur J Orthodont*, **28**, 221–240.

Milano, F. and Milano, L.G. (2012) Interdisciplinary collaboration between orthodontics and periodontics, in *Adult Orthodontics*, 1st edn (ed B. Melsen), Wiley-Blackwell Publishing, Hoboken, NJ, pp. 261–290.

Mirabella, A.D. and Artun, J. (1995) Risk factors for apical root resorption of maxillary anterior teeth in adult orthodontic patients. *Am J Orthod Dentofacial Orthop*, **108**, 48–55.

Miura, F. (1975) Effect of orthodontic force on blood circulation in periodontal membrane, in *Transactions of the Third Orthodontic Congress* (ed J.T. Cook), St. Louis, MO, CV Mosby, pp. 35–41.

Nanci, A. (2003) *Ten Cate's Oral Histology: Development, Structure, and Function*, 6th edn, Mosby, St. Louis, MO.

Nanning, A.M. *et al.* (2008) Comparison of the use of different modes of mechanical oral hygiene in prevention of plaque and gingivitis. *J Periodontol*, **79**, 1386–1394.

Needleman, I., McGrath, C., Floyd, P. and Biddle, A.J. (2004) Clinical impact of oral health on the life quality of periodontal patients. *J Clin Periodontol*, **31** (6), 454–457.

Newman, M.G., Takei, H.H. and Carranza, F.A. (2002) *Carranza's Clinical Periodontology*, 9th edn, W.B. Saunders Company, Philadelphia, PA.

Ong, M.A., Wang, H.L. and Smith, F.N. (1998) Interrelationship between periodontics and adult orthodontics. *J Clin Periodontol*, **25**, 271–277.

Polson, A. and Reed, B. (1984) Long-term effect of orthodontic treatment on crestal alveolar bone levels. *J Periodontol*, **55** (1), 28–34.

Polson, A., Caton, J., Polson, A.P., Nyman, S., Novak, J. and Reed, B. (1984) Periodontal response after tooth movement into intrabony defects. *J Periodontol*, **55** (4), 197–202.

Quirynen, M.L., Dekeyser, C. and van Steenberghe, D. (1991) The influence of gingival inflammation, tooth type, and timing on the rate of plaque formation. *J Periodontol*, **62**, 219–222.

Ravald, N. and Hamp, S.-E. (1981) Prediction of root surface caries in patients treated for advanced periodontal disease. *J Clin Periodont*, **8** (5), 400–414.

Reitan, K. (1964) Effects of force magnitude and direction of tooth movement on different alveolar bone types. *Angle Orthod*, **34**, 244–255.

Reitan, K. (1974) Initial tissue behavior during apical root resorption. *Angle Orthod*, **44**, 68–82.

Reitan, K. (1985) Biomechanical principles and reactions, in *Orthodontics: Current Principles and Techniques* (eds T.M. Graber and B.F. Swain), C.V. Mosby, St. Louis, MO, pp. 101–192.

Robinson, P.J. (1995) Gingivitis: a prelude to periodontitis? *J Clin Dent*, **6**, 41–45.

Ronderos, M. and Ryder, M.I. (2004) Risk assessment in clinical practice. *Periodontology*, **2000** (34), 120–135.

Roscoe, M.G., Meira, J.B.C. and Cattaneo, P.M. (2015) Association of orthodontic force system and root resorption: a systematic review. *Am J Orthod Dentofacial Orthop*, **147**, 610–626.

Rosenberg, M.N. (1972) An evaluation of the incidence and amount of apical root resorption and dilaceration occurring in orthodontically treated teeth, having incompletely formed roots at the beginning of Begg treatment. *Am J Orthod*, **61**, 524–525.

Sameshima, G.T. and Sinclair, P.M. (2001) Predicting and preventing root resorption: part II. Treatment factors. *Am J Orthod Dentofacial Orthop*, **119**, 511–515.

Sanders, N.L. (1999) Evidenced-based care in orthodontics and periodontics. *J Am Dental Assoc*, **130** (4), 521–527.

Sandstedt, C. (1904) Einige Beiträge zur Theorie der Zahnregulierung. *Nordisk Tandläkare Tidskrift*, **5**, 236–256.

Sandstedt, C. (1905) Einige Beiträge zur Theorie der Zahnregulierung. *Nordisk Tandläkare Tidskrift* **6**, 1–25, 141–168.

Sanz, M., Herrera, D. and van Winkelhoff, A.J. (2008) The periodontal abscess, in *Clinical Periodontology and Implant Dentistry*, 5th edn (eds J. Lindhe, N.P. Lang and T. Karring), Wiley Blackwell, Hoboken, NJ, pp. 496–503.

Schwarz, A.M. (1931) Tissue Changes Incidental to Orthodontic Tooth Movement. Read at the Second International Orthodontic Congress, London, July.

Schwarzkopf, E. (1887) Resorption der Zahnwurzeln bei Regulierung. *Dtsch. Monatschr. f. Zhk.*, **5**, 180.

Seymour, R.A., Thomason, J.M. and Ellis, J.S. (1996) The pathogenesis of drug-induced gingival overgrowth. *J Clin Periodontol*, **23**, 165–175.

Seymour, R.A., Ellis, J.S. and Thomason, J.M. (2000) Risk factors for drug-induced gingival overgrowth. *J Clin Periodontol*, **27**, 217–223.

Socransky, S. and Haffagee, A. (2008) Periodontal infections, in *Clinical Periodontology and Implant Dentistry* (eds J. Lindhe, N.P. Niklaus and T. Karring), Wiley-Blackwell, Hoboken, NJ, pp. 207–267.

Socransky, S.S., Haffajee, A.D., Goodson, J.M. and Lindhe, J. (1984) New concepts of destructive periodontal diseases. *J Clin Periodontol*, **11** (1), 21–32.

Steiner, G.G., Pearson, J.K. and Ainamo, J. (1981) Changes of the marginal periodontium as a result of labial tooth movement in monkeys. *J Periodontol*, **52**, 314–320.

Summitt, J.B., Robbins, J.W. and Schwartz, R.S. (2006) *Fundamentals of operative dentistry: a contemporary approach*, 3rd edn, Quintessence Publishing, Hanover Park, IL, pp. 2–4.

Suomi, J., Greene, J.C., Vermillion, J.R., Doyle, J., Chang, J.J. and Leatherwood, E.C.D. (1971) The effect of controlled oral hygiene procedures on the progression of periodontal disease in adults: results after third and final year. *J Periodontol*, **42** (3), 152–160.

Theilade, E., Wright, W.H., Jensen, S.B. and Löe, H. (1966) Experimental gingivitis in man. II. A longitudinal clinical and bacteriological investigation. *J Periodont Res*, 1–13.

Van Dyke, T. and Sheilesh, D. (2005) Risk factors for periodontitis. *J Int Acad Periodontol*, **7** (1), 3–7.

Vanarsdall, R. (1981) Periodontal problems associated with orthodontic therapy. *Pediatr Dent*, **3**, 154–157.

Vanarsdall, R.L. and Corn, H. (1977) Soft-tissue management of labially positioned unerupted teeth. *Am J Orthod Dentofacial Orthop*, **125**, 284–293.

Vermylen, K., De Quincey, G.N., Wolffe, G.N., van't Hof, M.A. and Renggli, H.H. (2005) Root proximity as a risk marker for periodontal disease: a case-control study. *J Clin Periodontol*, **32** (3), 260–265.

Vu, H.V. (2014) CBCT, Surgical Exposure and Orthodontic Treatment of Impacted Canines. American Association of Orthodontists 2014 Annual Session—Doctors Scientific Program, New Orleans.

Watson, P.J. (1984) Gingival recession. *J Dent*, **12** (1), 29–35.

Weinberg, M.A. and Eskow, R.N. (2000) An overview of delayed passive eruption. *Compend Contin Educ Dent*, **21** (6), 511–514.

Weltman, B., Vig, K.W.L., Fields, H.W., Shanker, S. and Kaizare, E.E. (2010) Root resorption associated with orthodontic tooth movement: a systematic review. *Am J Orthod Dentofacial Orthop*, **137**, 462–476.

Wennströ, J. and Lindhe, J. (1983) Plaque-induced gingival inflammation in the absence of attached gingiva in dogs. *J Clin Periodontol*, **10**, 266–276.

Wennström, J.L. (1996) Mucogingival considerations in orthodontic treatment. *Semin Orthod*, **2** (1), 46–54.

Wennström, J.L. (2014) Treatment of periodontitis: Effectively managing mucogingival defects. *J Periodont*, **85**, 1639–1641.

Wennström, J.L., Lindhe, J., Sinclair, F. and Thilander, B. (1987) Some periodontal tissue reactions to orthodontic tooth movement in monkeys. *J Clin Periodontol*, **14** (3), 121–129.

Wennström, J.L., Zucchelli, G. and Pini Prato, G.P. (2008) Mucogingival therapy-periodontal plastic surgery, in *Clinical Periodontology and Implant Dentistry*, 5th edn (eds N.P. Lang and J. Lindhe), Blackwell Munksgaard, Oxford, pp. 955–1028.

West, N.X., Lussi, A., Seong, J. and Hellwig, E. (2013) Dentin hypersensitivity: pain mechanisms and aetiology of exposed cervical dentin. *Clin Oral Investig*, **17** (1), S9–S19.

Yip, W.K. (1974) The prevalence of dens evaginatus. *Oral Surg Oral Med Oral Pathol*, **38**, 80–87.

Zachcriasson, B. (1996) Clinical implications of recent orthodontic-periodontic research findings. *Semin Orthod*, **2** (1), 4–12.

Zachrisson, B., Lang, J. and Lindhe, J. (2008) Tooth movements in the periodontally compromised patient, in *Clinical Periodontology and Implant Dentistry*, 5th edn (eds L.P. Lang and J. Lindhe), Blackwell Munksgaard, Oxford, pp. 1241–1279.

Zweers, J., Thomas, R.Z., Slot, D.E., Weisgold, A.S. and Van der Weijden, F.G. (2014) Characteristics of periodontal biotype, its dimensions, associations and prevalence: a systematic review. *J Clin Periodontol*, **41** (10), 958–971.

Index

Page numbers in *italics* refer to illustrations; those in **bold** refer to tables

---

Avoiding and Treating Dental Complications: Best Practices in Dentistry, First Edition. Edited by Deborah A. Termeie.
© 2016 John Wiley & Sons, Inc. Published 2016 by John Wiley & Sons, Inc.